HANDBOOK OF

HARNESSING BIOMATERIALS IN NANOMEDICINE

edited by
DAN PEER

HANDBOOK OF HARNESSING BIOMATERIALS IN NANOMEDICINE

PREPARATION, TOXICITY, AND APPLICATIONS

PAN STANFORD PUBLISHING

Published by

Pan Stanford Publishing Pte. Ltd.
Penthouse Level, Suntec Tower 3
8 Temasek Boulevard
Singapore 038988

Email: editorial@panstanford.com
Web: www.panstanford.com

British Library Cataloguing-in-Publication Data
A catalogue record for this book is available from the British Library.

Handbook of Harnessing Biomaterials in Nanomedicine: Preparation, Toxicity, and Applications

ISBN 978-981-4316-46-0 (Hardcover)
ISBN 978-981-4364-27-0 (eBook)

Contents

Preface

Nanomedicine has emerged as a novel field in medicine integrating nanoscale technologies with materials sciences, chemistry and biology. The medical application of nanotechnology has the potential to revolutionize diagnosis and therapy and bring this new field from a notion into reality while impacting the lives of millions around the world.

Innovative therapeutic and diagnosis modalities are emerging with several products already in clinical use while many more under clinical evaluation. A variety of nanomaterials made from naturally occurring biopolymers (protein-, lipid-, polysaccharides-, and nucleic-acid-based nanocarriers, to name a few), polymeric nanoparticles, carbon nanotubes, fullerenes, capsules, nanoshells, nanocages, microbubbles, dendrimers, engineered viral envelops and various inorganic materials (silicon oxide nanoparticles, gold, magnetic, and quantum dots) are already in different stages of laboratory, pre-clinical and clinical investigations. Yet, the race for improved, bio-inspired, and safer biomaterials for medical applications is still a vibrant field of research.

There are several books focusing on biomaterials for biological applications and other books on nanomedicine, however, there are fewer books that integrate the use of biomaterials in nanomedicine that enlighten the readers with the variety of medical applications and at the same time discuss the potential toxicity with special emphasis on immune toxicity, which led me to commence this book.

The readers are exposed to the state-of-the-art in this active field where biomaterials are used as building blocks to generate assortment of nanostructures for medical applications. This book includes contributions from world experts starting with an overview on biomaterials-based nanocarriers, discussing success stories and failures in the field with examples from polymer therapeutics, liposomes, polysaccharides as building blocks for nanotherapeutics, the promise of RNA interference as a new class of nanomedicines and its potential as a platform for personalized medicine, integrating nanomedicine with stem cells as platform for drug discovery and validation, nanomedicine in the context of diagnosis and disease management, and immuno-nanotoxicity, understanding how the immune system looks at different nanocarriers made of variety of biomaterials.

The arsenal of nanocarriers and new therapeutic molecules (including pathway-targeted small molecules, monoclonal antibodies or their fragments and RNAi (siRNAs, micro (mi)RNA mimic and anti-miRNAs) are opening new avenues for treatment and diagnosis of cancer, inflammation, infection diseases, neurodegenerative, cardiovascular diseases, and metabolic disorders and are providing physicians with the opportunity to tailor the best potential treatment (with its appropriate carrier) to each patient. I hope the reader will find in this book the appropriate mixture of basic and applied knowledge on nanomedicine and their applications as novel therapeutic modality.

I am grateful to all the authors that contributed to this book among them Prof. R. Margalit, from Tel Aviv University, Dr. I. Loinas from CIDETEC, Prof. L. Forrest, from the University of Kansas, Dr. R. Satchi-Fainaro, from Tel Aviv University, Prof. D. Dykxhoorn from the university of Miami, Prof. P. Kumar from Yale School of Medicine, Dr. J. Dearling and Prof. A. Packard from Harvard Medical School, Dr. M. Weil from Tel Aviv University, Prof. T. Vorup-Jensen from Aarhus University, Prof. J. Szebeni from Miskolc University, and Prof. Y. Barenholz from the Hebrew University in Jerusalem.

Special thanks to my wife, Shlomit, and my children Dor, Barak, and Naama for their unrestricted support.

This book is dedicated to the memory of my parents, Itta and Alexander Peer, who educated me to strive for knowledge and excellence.

Dan Peer

Tel Aviv, October 2011.

Chapter 1

Biomaterial-Based Particulate Drug Carriers

Rimona Margalit
Department of Biochemistry and Molecular Biology,
George S. Wise Faculty of Life Sciences, Tel Aviv University, Tel Aviv 69978, Israel
rimona@post.tau.ac.il

This chapter focuses on biomaterial-based particulate carriers, starting with issues that are common to all carriers: the needs that drive carrier-mediated therapy, essential carrier requirements and carrier mediated drug targeting. The advantages of biomaterial-based systems are then discussed in terms of the wide choice of raw materials, of utilizing nature's sites for targeting and of lowered risks for treatment safety. Also brought up are drawbacks for such carriers, in meeting requirements of pharmaceutical products and in potential adverse immune responses. The drawbacks are expected to be resolved in the future and even today the benefits of biomaterial-based carriers outweigh their downside. The concept of pathology-driven selection of carrier specifications, in particular, size and the route of administration, is introduced and discussed for a variety of pathologies. Specific examples are drawn from systemic, oral and local administrations for the treatment of cancer, diabetes and osteoarthritis. In conclusion, future prospects for biomaterial-based particulate drug carriers are deemed quite encouraging.

Handbook of Harnessing Biomaterials in Nanomedicine: Preparation, Toxicity, and Applications
Edited by Dan Peer

ISBN 978-981-4316-46-0 (Hardback), 978-981-4364-27-0 (eBook)
www.panstanford.com

1.1 Introduction

1.1.1 The Needs for Drug Carriers

The majority of approved drug formulations as well as those under development, irrespective of dosage form and route of administration, are formulations of free drug. The meeting between a free drug and a living system is often an unfriendly encounter, arising from deficiencies of treatment with free drug — diminishing efficacy and damaging the biological system, as summarized in Figure 1.1

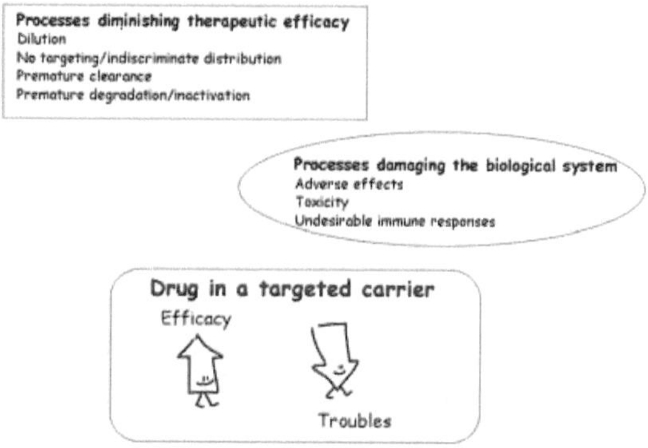

Figure 1.1 Deficiencies of treatment with free drugs.

Four processes, each separately and more so their combinations, reduce treatment efficacy: dilution of the administered dose, irrespective of administration route; lack of self-targeting, hence indiscriminate distribution within the living system; premature (i.e., before reaching the molecular sites of drug action) clearance from the whole system as well as from the target zone; vulnerability to premature enzyme-catalyzed degradation, metabolism, and other processes of inactivation. The end result of all or some of these processes is severely diminished efficacy. A rather small share of the administered dose reaches the target in active form and remains there for a sufficient time span, to generate the desirable therapeutic responses. The other side of the coin is damage to the biological system mostly due to the lack of targeting. Many drugs cause adverse effects, toxicity, and undesirable immune responses. Thus, even if a satisfactory level of efficacy is obtained, the damage severely undermines the therapy. Attempts to increase efficacy by increasing the administered doses, so that the small share reaching the target in active form may be sufficient for therapy, are frequently limited as the increased doses also aggravate the damage to the system.

A major approach to overcoming these deficiencies of treatment with free drug, also illustrated in Figure 1.1, is to formulate the drug in a targeted carrier that would simultaneously increase efficacy and reduced damage [1–10].

1.1.2 Drug Carriers: Essential Requirements

To provide a true solution for the deficiencies of treatment with free drugs, not merely shifting from one set of problems to another, drug carriers should ideally meet two sets of essential requirements, listed in Figure 1.2.

Requirements for task performance
Mutual drug/environment protection
Drug release kinetics matching therapeutic requirements
Drug-targeting
Carrier-retention at target matching therapeutic requirements
Stability

Requirements to avoid new problems
Biodegradability & Bicompatibility
No toxicity
Low to no immunogenicity

Figure 1.2 Drug carriers: essential requirements.

The first set of requirements, designated to address the problems of treatment with free drugs is mostly self-explanatory; yet we find that some additional comments are in place.

Drug release: To minimize losses, drug release rate from the site of administration to the therapeutic targets should obviously be as slow as possible; yet it is not a given that drug release at the target should always be slow. Some treatments may actually need immediate total drug release once the drug-carrier system has reached the target. Accordingly, kinetics of drug release from a designated carrier cannot be generalized nor studied with drug models — they need to be investigated for the specific drug in the selected carrier.

Targeting: Drug targeting and carrier mediated drug targeting are the subject matter of Section 1.1.4.

Retention at the target: The carrier should obviously remain at the target for a sufficient time span to release its drug load. This time span could be short or long depending on the needs of the specific therapy.

Stability: The stability of drug-carrier formulations is required for long-term shelf life as a pharmaceutical product, and also upon administration until the system reaches the target. Stability for a drug-carrier formulation means: chemical stability of the drug and of all carrier materials; retention of drug activity; retention of a carrier's structural integrity; retention of the drug encapsulation-level achieved at the end of production.

The second set of requirements, designated to avoid problems introduced by the carrier itself, is also self-explanatory. As will be discussed later in this chapter, constructing carriers from biomaterials helps toward meeting these requirements.

1.1.3 Major Categories of Drug Carriers

Drug carriers can be divided into two categories (Figure 1.3).

In the first category, the carrier is a macromolecule, from biological or synthetic origins, carrying several drug molecules attached covalently, directly or through spacers [6–10]. The drug-carrier bond should obviously be of a type cleavable at the target. These carriers have been termed soluble or linear, even though the macromolecule is not necessarily linear.

In the second category, the carrier is a particle that can also be made from biological or synthetic components. The drug molecules are encapsulated within the particle with no need for covalent binding [1–5].

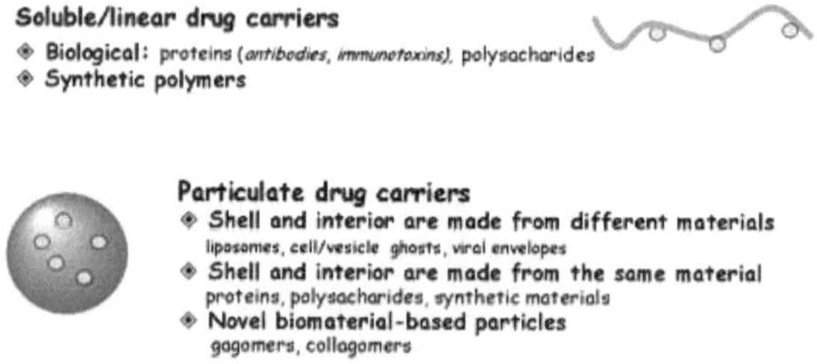

Figure 1.3 The two major categories of drug delivery systems. See also Color Insert.

Particulate carriers can be further divided into several sub-categories (Figure 1.3): particles in which the shell and the interior are made from different components, the interior usually containing an aqueous core; particles in which both the shell and the interior are made from the same material and that may contain water molecules in their interior in nano or microchannels rather than a phase or core; two new types of particulate drug carriers, developed by our group, that do not fall strictly into the previous two sub-categories. These will be introduced and discussed in later sections of this chapter [11–15].

In the remainder of this chapter, we will focus solely on particulate carriers.

1.1.4 Carrier-Mediated Drug Targeting

Even simple searches within scientific databases, using the term "drug targeting" alone or with additional key words, yield many results. It may, therefore, seem that the goal of drug targeting, whether for a free drug for a drug-carrier system, has been achieved long ago and is no longer an issue. The reality is quite different — achieving drug targeting is still an elusive goal and a significant challenge.

The definition of drug targeting is delivery of the drug exclusively to its molecular sites of action. By its very nature, drug targeting is relevant to living systems, not — as will be further discussed — to cell cultures. Striving for drug targeting can be divided into three steps, as illustrated in Figure 1.4:

In the first step, which is relevant to systemic administration, the drug has to reach the anatomic location where the pathological state resides. For example, if the intent is to deliver an antibacterial agent for the treatment of lung bacterial infection and the drug is administered intravenously (IV), the first step means reaching from the systemic port of entry to the lungs.

In the second step the drug has to reach, within that anatomic location, the specific region where its sites of action reside. Continuing with the example of lung bacterial infection, once the drug has reached to lungs, it has to get as close as possible to the bacterial colonies there. In cases of local administration, the drug is delivered directly to the anatomic locations, and one could view it as either achievement or circumvention of step 1. In further continuation of the lungs example, local administration could be by the pulmonary, rather than the IV route. For drugs, small or large, that operate outside the target cell, such as on receptors harbored by the cell membranes — achievement of the second step suffices to provide drug targeting. This is usually sufficient also for small drugs that operate inside the cell.

The third step may be necessary for macromolecules that operate inside the cell. In this respect, it is imperative to differentiate — at the cellular level — between drug targeting and drug internalization. Frequently and especially for carrier-mediated drug targeting, efforts are made to achieve internalization of the complete system. For drugs that operate on the cell membrane, internalization is detrimental and should be avoided, as any drug molecule that has entered the cell is probably lost to its extracellular sites of action.

When it comes to drug targeting, the use of the term "homing" should be avoided as it is erroneous and misleading. Unlike a weapon that can be equipped with homing devices that recognize their target from afar and lock onto it, self-targeting drugs or targeted drug-carrier systems cannot home onto the target immediately upon administration (local or systemic). The forces that drive recognition and binding between the targeting moiety and its counterpart at the target operate at short range, when the administered system is at very close proximity to the target-provided binding counterpart.

Focusing, from here on, on carriers, the question of whether the steps in drug targeting illustrated in Figure 1.4 (obviously mediated by a carrier) have been, and can be, achieved is discussed in Section 1.3.

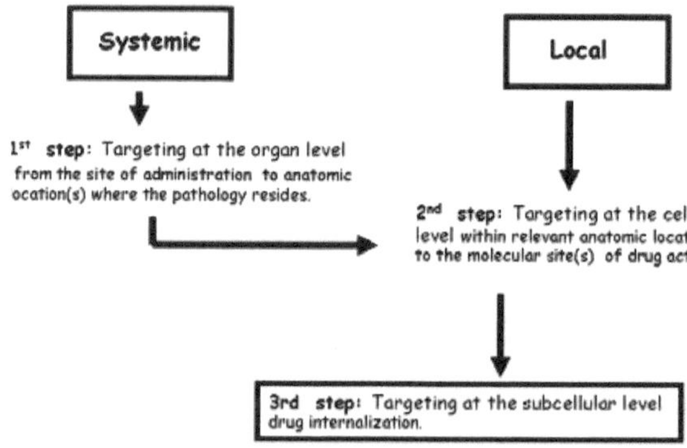

Figure 1.4 Steps in drug targeting.

Finally, we would like to stress that a major share of the experimental work done in the area of drug targeting has been performed *in vitro*, in cell cultures. The extensively investigated case of immunoliposomes — liposomes that are surface modified to carry an antibody against a specific membrane-embedded receptors, in a given cell line — is brought here as an example [16–20]. Incubating immunoliposomes with cells that express the specific receptor usually results in high affinity binding, whereas blocking the receptors prior to binding with free antibody or administering such liposomes to cells that do not express the specific receptor results in negligible binding [16–20]. Such results are important experimental evidence for a key requirement of carrier-mediated drug targeting — the recognition and high affinity binding between the liposome-bound Ab and the specific receptor. Such results may even have higher relevance if local administration is intended. In such cases, the cell monolayer becomes a model system for the designated tissue. *In vitro* binding and recognition are not, however, evidence of drug targeting that should, as already discussed in this section, be pursued in an animal model.

1.2 Biomaterial-Based Particulate Drug Carriers: Advantages and Drawbacks

1.2.1 A Wide Choice of Raw Materials

The continuous ability to make new synthetic raw materials, in addition to those already available, makes the pool of synthetic raw materials available for the construction of drug carriers practically infinite. Against this background, claiming the wide choice of biological raw material for drug carriers may seem odd. Yet, we wish to point out that the existing pool is quite large.

For liposomes and other lipid-based particles, there is a wide choice of lipids for liposomes and other lipid-based carriers. Such carriers can be made from a single lipid: phospholipids such as phosphatidylcholine, phosphatidylserine, phosphatidylinositol, and others (although not from phosphatidylethanolamine alone); sphingomyelin, ceramides [1, 3, 11, 14–21]. Liposomes can also be made from a mixture of lipids, and in that case, cholesterol, fatty acids, and phosphatidylethanolamine can be included in the formulation [1, 3, 11, 14–21]. For a given lipid, there are further choices depending on its source: biological, in which case the hydrocarbon chains can be a mixture of sizes and degrees of saturation; synthetic or semi-synthetic, in which case selections of desired chain length and degree of saturation are possible.

For protein-based microspheres and nanospheres, serum albumin or gelatin seem to be the most-frequent raw material, but other proteins, single or mixtures, can also be selected for the task [21–24].

Alginate and chitosan are prominent polysaccharides used as raw materials for drug carriers [25–27].

Then there are also carriers that contain more than one type of biomaterial: particles derived from living systems (Figure 1.2); new carriers, made from a mixture of several biological components, such as the collagomers (containing collagen and lipid) and gagomers (containing hyaluronan and lipids), developed by our group [11–15].

1.2.2 Utilizing Nature's Sites for Targeting and High-Affinity Binding

In the context of targeting, the ability of a drug-carrier formulation to recognize and bind with high affinity to the target has already been discussed in this chapter (Section 1.1.4). These recognition and binding are key critical requirements to achieve successful therapy.

Using biomaterial-based drug carriers opens the door to utilize the wide repertoire nature provides of sites — membrane-embedded receptors, extracellular matrix components — that offer recognition, specificity, and high-affinity binding. To simplify matters, we will use from here on the term receptor as generic for all types of recognition and binding sites offered by the target, whether they are a biochemically defined receptor or a protein weaved within the ECM, or others. In the context of targeting, the term specificity has dual meaning: specificity of the receptor to a given ligand serving as the targeting agent; specificity of the receptor in terms of its uniqueness to the therapeutic target. To differentiate between the two, we will reserve the term "specificity" for the interaction of a targeting agent with its receptor and apply the term "unique" to the presence of a particular receptor at the therapeutic target compared with the other locations within the living system.

The biological targeting agents can play a single or dual role in biomaterial-based drug carriers. In the single role, which is the prevalent mode, the targeting agent is attached to the carrier in a bond that should be sufficiently stable to avoid separation of carrier and targeter before reaching the target. Monoclonal antibodies (mAbs) including conformational-selective ones, are a wide class of targeting agents, perhaps the most investigated [1–3, 16–20, 28]. Key examples of other extensively investigated targeting agents include LDL, EGF, transferrin, folate, biological haptens, and hyaluronan [2, 29–36]. Additional biologically derived targeting ligands are exemplified by collagen-originating RGD peptides [37–38]. The specificity of bio-originating targeting agents to their respective receptors are clear and well-documented [2, 29–38]. A receptor that nature has developed for a given ligand — serving as a targeting agent — binds that ligand with high affinity and binds other molecules, even if quite similar, with low affinity or none. The dual role biological targets can play in biomaterial-based drug carriers is to serve as both a carrier component and a targeting agent. This dual role is exemplified by two systems developed in our group: gagomers, in which hyaluronan is both the shell of the particulate carrier and a targeting agent [13, 15, 39]; collagomers, in which collagen is both a particle component and a targeting agent [12].

The other side of the coin, receptor target-uniqueness is not as achievable as receptor-targeter specificity. For the most, as exemplified by several following examples, such uniqueness is a quantitative, rather than a qualitative, matter [2, 29–38]. On its face — a membrane-embedded antigen could be considered to also have qualitative target uniqueness. The reality is, however, that mAbs raised against such an antigen may still bind with sufficient affinity to other binding entities, turning the antigen case from qualitative to quantitative, and requiring a case-by-case analysis to evaluate the level of target-uniqueness. As targeters, mAb have other issues that will be discussed in a later chapter. For carrier-mediated cancer therapy, hyaluronan receptors harbored by cell membranes — in particular, the CD44 family and — CD168 are an example of highly quantitative target uniqueness, supported by experimental evidence [2, 13, 15, 30–31, 40 and references within]: In many types of tumor cells, there is overexpression of HA membrane-embedded receptors that are furthermore in an active conformation for high-affinity hyaluronan binding, whereas in most normal cells, these receptors are poorly expressed and in a conformation inactive for HA binding [2, 13, 15, 30–31, 40 and references within]. On the other hand, for carrier-mediated cancer therapy, cell membrane-embedded receptors for RGD peptides and (separately) for LDL, are examples of insufficient quantitative target uniqueness. The differences in receptor expression between cancer and normal cells may not be enough to ensure that carriers endowed by these targeters will be sufficiently selective to the cancer cells over normal cells [29, 33, 37–38]. In summary, target-uniqueness needs to be verified case by case, and drive targeter selection.

1.2.3 Lower Risks of Adverse Effects, Toxicity, and Undesirable Immune Responses

Carrier essential requirements, designed to avoid problems introduced by the carrier itself, have been discussed earlier in this chapter (Section 1.1.2 and Figure 1.2). In these respects, biomaterial-based drug carriers provide significant potential advantages over carriers made of synthetic materials, or a mix of synthetic and biological materials. The biomaterial-based carriers — including targeting moieties of biological origin — are expected to be biocompatible and biodegradable. Carriers composed from, or containing, non-biological matter may have compatibility issues and, if not biodegradable, may require invasive procedures for their removal post drug-load delivery as, for example, in the case of antibiotic-loaded cement particles applied to control/prevent osteomyelitis [41]. Compared with carriers containing synthetic materials, the biomaterial-based carriers have lower potential to be toxic, to generate adverse effects, and to stimulate the immune system in undesirable directions. The boundary between recognition as self and non-self is delicate as can be exemplified by regular vs. cationic liposomes. Regular liposomes made from biological lipids, containing, for example, PC, cholesterol, and PE, are safe in all respects discussed here (see also Figure 1.2) as are also liposomes of the same composition carrying HA as the targeting agent [13, 15, 30, 31, 39]. Cationic liposomes containing these biological lipids, but also a synthetic cationic lipid are toxic and immunogenic [42–44].

1.2.4 Drawbacks of Biomaterial-Based Particulate Drug Carriers

Despite their many advantages, discussed in the previous sections, there are drawbacks to particulate carriers made from biological materials. The shortcomings start from the very fact that the raw materials are of biological origin. These include: material scarcity;

isolation from the biological source and purification to the degree required for therapeutic agents may be difficult to achieve and cause extensive material loss: batch-to-batch reproducibility of each raw material is also a tough call. Quite obviously, not every biomaterial has to be isolated from the biological source, some — for example many types of lipids that constitute a major type of material in biomaterial-based carrier — are commercially available. In such cases, the raw material issues are similar to those of regular synthetic materials, and discussion of such issues is beyond the scope of the present communication. Another aspect of biological raw material that can cause problems in the biological milieu is species specificity, especially for carrier components that are proteins. Conventional phospholipids are usually less restricting in that respect — for example, phosphatidylcholine obtained from soybean can be used without immune limitations for drug carriers administered to mammals. The least restricting in this respect is hyaluronan. It has been approved for clinic use in ocular surgery and osteoarthritis treatment, from both non-mammalian and mammalian sources. As to the biomaterial-based particle itself, drawbacks include: the need to develop the production processes from the inventing lab to industrial levels; sterilization processes; batch-to-batch reproducibility and size uniformity.

A common thread throughout the drawbacks, whether arising from the raw materials or the particle, are high costs, which may significantly exceed those of drug carriers made from synthetic materials.

We would like to stress, however, that not all drawbacks are encountered with each biomaterial-based particulate drug carrier. Weighing the advantages over the drawbacks should be done on a case-by-case basis, and frequently the benefits outweigh the limitations.

1.3 Particle Size, Route of Administration, and Therapeutic Needs

1.3.1 The Conceptual Approach and Definitions of Passive and Active Targeting

The conceptual approach discussed in this section concerns the selection of particle species and dimensions, for carrier-mediated treatment of a particular pathology. We contend that the driving force should be the therapeutic needs and the strongly related choice of administration route. This concept will be discussed below, supported by specific examples.

For particulate carriers, the term "passive targeting"[3] has been coined for cases where the therapeutic targets are cells of the reticuloensothelial system (RES), which tend to internalize particles [45–50]. If, on the other hand, the therapeutic targets are not within the RES, "active targeting" is called for, and requires two types of efforts that may be at odds with each other. One type of effort is to endow the particles with the ability to avoid uptake by the RES and to circulate long. The other type of effort is to endow the carrier with the ability to bind with high affinity to sites unique to the target (as has been discussed in Section 1.1.4). When and how this relates to pathology-driven selection of carrier is discussed below.

1.3.2 Systemic Administration, Passive and Active Targeting

Passive and active carrier-mediated drug targeting are particularly relevant for therapies that require systemic administration. If the pathology to be treated resides within RES cells, then carriers that fit passive targeting are the systems of choice. Veteran and extensive *in vitro* and *in vivo* studies made it clear that RES cells internalize micro-sized particles such as liposomes and microspheres significantly better than nano-sized particles [45–50]. Within microparticles for RES therapy, further selection and caution are required with respect to the loci of drug action. Taking, for example, macrophages as a therapeutic target for a drug that operates inside the cell — for such cases, conventional (regular) multilamellar liposomes (MLV) internalized by these cells are an obvious carrier choice. If, however, the macrophage-intended drug operates on its cell membrane, the conventional MLV are the wrong choice, as they will deliver the drug to the wrong place. For such therapies, even though the therapeutic target is an RES cell, active targeting will be needed — using particles that preferentially bind to the macrophage but are not internalized. As already stated in this chapter, selecting a targeter that can provide the carrier with active targeting is a case-by-case issue; specific examples are given below.

The preference RES cells show for micro- over nanoparticles constitutes an essential, though not sufficient, clue to achieving active targeting to non-RES cells upon systemic administration. It was furthermore shown that when small particles are also coated with agents such as polyethylene glycol (PEG) that delay opsonization, RES avoidance and long circulation are much improved [2, 30, 31, 50–55]. These issues have been extensively reported and reviewed and an interested reader is referred to these sources [2, 30, 31, 50–55]. A prominent example is the well-known clinically approved Doxil, the PEGylated doxorubicin-loaded nano liposomes [51, 54, 56]. PEG, an agent that when coating a nanoparticle confers upon it the ability for long circulation is not, however, a targeting agent. In the area of cancer, efforts are under way to add targeters such as folate or antibodies to Pegylated nanoparticles [35, 57–59]. The success of such approaches will obviously depend on the choice of targeter and whether the opsonization-delay agent and the targeting agent will not interfere with each other. Hyaluronan, when coating particle surfaces, performs a dual role: Rich with hydroxyl residues (much like PEG), hyaluronan coating confers long circulation; it is also, as discussed in section 1.2.2, an effective tumor targeter. We have shown this dual role for nano-sized liposomes encapsulating doxorubicin or mitomycin C, which have hyaluronan as a targeter attached to their surface and for nano-sized gagomers encapsulating paclitaxel, in which hyaluronan is the surface [15, 30, 31].

1.3.3 Administration by Local Injection

For local injections of particulate carriers, restrictions on particle size are less stringent than those discussed above for IV administration. Carrier type and size can be selected to fit the specific treatment modality and drug requirements. Local injection of a carrier encapsulating a macromolecule that operates inside the cell, such as in gene therapy or gene silencing, will require a different type of particle than for the smaller molecules such as antibacterial or chemotherapeutic. As already said, for small drugs operating inside a target cell, internalization may not be necessary. Carrier binding to the cell membrane and retention there to allow sufficient drug diffusion into the cell may well suffice. In such cases, micro-sized particles are also a valid choice.

Local, intra-tumoral injection of biomaterial-based particulate carriers such as liposomes has been applied in cancer therapy [60, 61]. Local injections can be applied for therapeutic indications other than cancer, such as infectious diseases, osteoarthritis, and local anesthesia. The benefits of replacing treatment with free drug, with drug-carrier formulations, with emphasis on biomaterial-based particulate carriers has already been discussed in the previous sections. For treatments of chronic diseases by local injections, drug-carrier formulations may provide an additional benefit by extending the time intervals between injections.

Local injections still require local targeting (Figure 1.4). To that end, the carrier should localize close to the cells in which the drug operates, bind with high affinity, and remain at the site performing as a slow-release drug depot on a time scale of several weeks or more. Needless to say, for carriers expected to remain within the body for prolonged periods, the properties of biomaterial-based carriers (Figure 1.2) are particularly advantageous. As to favored particle size, for these types of treatments, microparticles are probably preferable to nanoparticles. The larger particles usually provide for higher drug loads and do better in avoiding internalization within cells. Such evasion is obviously needed, since internalization of a drug-carrier will lead to relatively fast release of the drug at once, thus losing the slow-release drug-depot performance. Treatment of osteoarthritis (OA) by intra-articular injection to an inflamed rat knee is brought here to illustrate additional potential benefits for carrier-mediated therapy using microparticles. A single injection of an NSAID encapsulated in collagomers (5 μm diameter) or of an NSAID and a corticosteroid co-encapsulated in the same hyaluronan-coated MLV (1–2 μm diameter) reduced inflammation over a 3 week time from two- to fourfold better than untreated controls and free drug [11, 12, 14].

1.3.4 Oral Administration of Drug-Carrier Formulations

The oral route is among the most patient-friendly and the prevailing option (when possible) for drugs that need to reach the circulation either as the final destination or for distribution to their targets. The oral route is not currently feasible for drugs that are biologicals—peptides, proteins, and nucleic acids. Such drugs, when administered in free form, do not survive the hostile gastrointestinal tract (GIT) intact and in active form, suffering acutely from deficiencies of treatment with free drugs as discussed in the introduction (see also Figure 1.1). Formulating biologicals in carriers may conceivably protect them along the GIT but needs careful consideration. The carrier itself has to survive the GIT, which is a tough call for biomaterial-based particulate drug carriers. The encapsulated drug may leak out extensively during exposure of the drug-carrier formulation to the acidic stomach environment. Similar to the inability of particulate carriers — even if nano-sized — to get across walls of intact blood vessels, particles are unable to gain access — intact and with their drug load — from the GIT to the circulation.

Rather, particulate drug carriers administered orally are indicated to act as site-adherent drug depots, allowing the drug itself to gain access into the circulation [62–64].

To perform as drug depots in the GIT, there is no particular advantage to using nano-sized particles. Micro-sized particles may do better in terms of higher drug loads, slower particle degradation, and slower drug loss.

Insulin is a key example, for itself and as a model for other biologicals, for which oral delivery formulated in a particulate carrier — from biological or synthetic materials — has been and is actively pursued. Tested particles include hydrogels, microspheres, nanoparticles, microemulsions, and liposomes, but unfortunately, none has yet merited progression toward approved treatment modalities [39, 62]. Yet, two examples from current ongoing studies are encouraging. We have recently studied oral delivery of insulin in two particulate carrier formulations, both of them micro-sized and encapsulating insulin in a reversible-fibrillar form [39]. Both formulations have hyaluronan on their surface, which turned out to protect both carrier and encapsulated protein along the GIT, and to perform in diabetic mice as a long-acting insulin formulation, reducing blood glucose to satisfactory levels [39]. Another insulin formulation in a particulate carrier, orally administered and peaking at 5 h post administration, has advanced to clinical trials [65].

Thus, despite the difficulties of biomaterial-based drug carriers for oral delivery of biologicals, the needs for such systems and their attraction — for the patient and for improved therapy — are sufficiently strong to drive extensive past and current research efforts. This is a particular area where pros and cons need to be tested anew for each drug-carrier system, but hope should not dwindle, as illustrated by the two examples cited above for insulin.

1.4 Conclusions and Future Prospects

The needs for carrier-mediated drug therapy, in particular for targeted biomaterial-based particulate systems, have been discussed throughout this chapter, as were the advantages and drawbacks.

The road to achieving biomaterial-based targeted particulate drug carriers has been and still is long and difficult. Of the vast amount of investigated systems, only relatively few have reached the clinic to become established treatment modalities. Yet, as discussed throughout this chapter, such systems are acutely needed, and the potential advantages clearly outweigh the drawbacks.

Future prospects of getting more systems to the clinic hinge on several factors that should be addressed from the very beginning. First and foremost, building the carrier-drug system should be driven by the pathology and the drugs for which the carrier formulation is developed. Those, in turn, will drive the selection of administration route, targeting agent, and particle specifications (raw materials, structure, size range). Setting those initial parameters does not guarantee successful development all the way to the clinic. Each drug-carrier formulation will be required to go through all the steps of pre-clinical and clinical studies. We contend, however, that "starting right" as defined above will be a substantial positive contribution toward successful therapy with targeted, biomaterial-based particulate drug carriers.

References

1. Torchilin, V.P. (2006) Multifunctional nanocarriers, *Adv. Drug Deliv. Rev.*, 58, pp. 1532–1555.
2. Peer, D. et al. (2007) Nanocarriers: emerging platforms for cancer therapy, *Nature Nanotechnol.*, 2, pp. 751–760.
3. Puri, A. et al. (2009) Lipid-based nanoparticles as pharmaceutical drug carriers: from concepts to clinic, *Crit. Rev. Ther. Drug. Carrier Syst.*, 26, pp. 523–580.
4. Kurmi, B.D. et al. (2010) Micro- and nanocarrier-mediated lung targeting (2010), *Expert Opin. Drug Deliv.* 7, pp. 781–794.
5. Muzykantov V.R. (2010) Drug delivery by red blood cells: vascular carriers designed by mother nature, *Expert Opin. Drug Deliv.*, 7, pp. 403–427.
6. Senter, P.D. (2009) Potent antibody drug conjugates for cancer therapy, *Curr. Opin. Chem. Biol.*, 13, pp. 235–244.

7. Hetzel, C., et al. (2009) Improved immunotoxins with novel functional elements, *Curr. Pharm. Des.*, 15, pp. 2700–2711.

8. Segal. E., Satchi-Fainaro, R. (2009). Design and development of polymer conjugates as anti-angiogenic agents,. *Adv. Drug Deliv. Rev.*, 61, pp. 1159–1176.

9. Gaspar, R., Duncan, R. (2009) Polymeric carriers: Preclinical safety and the regulatory implications for design and development of polymer therapeutics, *Adv. Drug Deliv. Rev.*, 61, pp. 1220–1231.

10. Astruc, D., Boisselier, E., Ornelas, C. (2010) Dendrimers designed for functions: from physical, photophysical, and supramolecular properties to applications in sensing, catalysis, molecular electronics, photonics, and nanomedicine, *Chem. Rev.*, 110, pp. 1857–1959.

11. Elron-Gross, I., Glucksam,Y., Melikhov, D., Margalit, R. (2008) Cyclooxygenase inhibition by diclofenac formulated in bioadhesive carriers, *Biochim. Biophys. Acta*, 1778, pp. 931–936.

12. Elron-Gross, I., Glucksam, Y., Biton, I.E., Margalit, R. (2009) A novel Diclofenac-carrier for local treatment of Osteoarthritis applying live-animal MRI. *J. Cont. Rel.*, 135, pp. 65–70.

13. Barkay, Z., Rivkin, I., Margalit, R. (2009) Three-dimensional characterization of drug-encapsulating particles using STEM detector in FEG-SEM, *Micron*, 40, pp. 480–485.

14. Elron-Gross, I., Glucksam, Y., Margalit, R. (2009) Liposomal dexamethasone-diclofenac combinations for local osteoarthritis treatment, *Int. J. Pharma.*, 376, pp. 84–91.

15. Rivkin, I. et al. (2010) Paclitaxel-clusters coated with hyaluronan as selective tumor-targeted nanovectors, *Biomaterials*, 31, pp. 7106–7114.

16. Torchilin, V.P. (2006) Recent approaches to intracellular delivery of drugs and DNA and organelle targeting, *Annu. Rev. Biomed. Eng.*, 8, pp. 343–375.

17. Baum, P., Müller, D., Rüger, R., Kontermann, R.E. (2007) Single-chain Fv immunoliposomes for the targeting of fibroblast activation protein-expressing tumor stromal cells, *J. Drug Target.*, 15, pp. 399–406.

18. Rothdiener, M., Beuttler, J., Messerschmidt, S.K., Kontermann, R.E. (2010) Antibody targeting of nanoparticles to tumor-specific receptors: immunoliposomes, *Methods Mol. Biol.*, 624, pp. 295–308.

19. Loomis, K. et al. (2010) Specific targeting to B cells by lipid-based nanoparticles conjugated with a novel CD22-ScFv, *Exp. Mol. Pathol.*, 88, pp. 238–249.

20. Rothdiener, M., et al. (2010) Targeted delivery of SiRNA to CD33-positive tumor cells with liposomal carrier systems, *J. Cont. Rel.*, 144, pp. 251–258.

21. Samad, A., Sultana, Y., Aqil, M. (2007) Liposomal drug delivery systems: an update review, *Curr. Drug Deliv.*, 4, pp. 297–305.
22. Kratz, F. (2008) Albumin as a drug carrier: design of prodrugs, drug conjugates and nanoparticles, *J. Cont. Rel.*, 132, pp. 171–183.
23. Chan, O.C.M., So, K.-F., Chan, B.P. (2008) Fabrication of nano-fibrous collagen microspheres for protein delivery and effects of photochemical crosslinking on release kinetics, *J. Cont. Rel.*, 129, pp. 135–143.
24. Gardner, E.R., Dahut, D., Figg, W.D. (2008) Quantitative determination of total and unbound paclitaxel in human plasma following Abraxane treatment, *J. Chromatogr. B*, 862, pp. 213–218.
25. Yongsheng, M.Y. et al. (2008) Microencapsulation of bacteriophage Felix O1 into chitosan-alginate microspheres for oral delivery, *Appl. Environ. Microbiol.*, 74, pp. 4799–4805.
26. Matricardi, P., Di Meo, C., Coviello, T., Alhaique, F. (2008) Recent advances and perspectives on coated alginate microspheres for modified drug delivery, *Expert Opin. Drug Deliv.*, 5, pp. 417–425.
27. Amidi, M., Mastrobattista, E., Jiskoot, W., Hennink, W.E. (2010) Chitosan-based delivery systems for protein therapeutics and antigens, *Adv. Drug Deliv. Rev.*, 62, pp. 59–82.
28. Peer, D. el al (2008) Systemic leukocyte-directed siRNA delivery revealing cyclin D1 as an anti-inflammatory target, *Science*, 319, pp. 627–630.
29. de Smidt, P.C., van Berkel, T.J. (1990) LDL-mediated drug targeting, *Crit. Rev. Ther. Drug Carrier Syst.*, 7, pp. 99–120.
30. Peer, D., Margalit, R.(2004) Loading Mitomycin C inside long circulating hyaluronan targeted nano-liposomes increases its antitumor activity in three mice tumor models, *Int. J. Cancer* 108, pp. 780–789.
31. Peer, D., Margalit, R. (2004). Tumor-targeted hyaluronan nano-liposomes increase the antitumor activity of liposomal doxorubicin in syngeneic and human xenograft mouse tumor models, *Neoplasia*, 6, pp. 343–353.
32. Nobs, L., Buchegger, F., Gurny, R., Alle'manni, E. (2004) Current methods for attaching targeting ligands to liposomes and nanoparticles, *J. Pharm. Sci.*, 93, pp. 1980–1092.
33. Davis, M.E, Zhuo, G., Chen, Z., Shin, D.M. (2008) Nanoparticle therapeutics: an emerging treatment modality for cancer. *Nature Rev. Drug Discov.*, 7, pp. 771–782.
34. Sega, E.I., Low, P.L. (2008) Tumor detection using folate receptor-targeted imaging agents, *Cancer Metastasis Rev.*, 27, pp. 655–664.
35. Gabizon, A. et al. (2010) Improved therapeutic activity of folate-targeted liposomal doxorubicin in folate receptor-expressing tumor models, *Cancer Chemother. Pharmacol.*, 66, pp. 43–52.

36. Xianjun, Y.X. et al. (2010) Targeted drug delivery in pancreatic cancer. *BBA Rev. Cancer*, 1805, pp. 97–104.

37. Garanger, E., Didier, B. Pascal, D. (2007) Tumor targeting with RGD peptide ligands-design of new molecular conjugates for imaging and therapy of cancers, *Anti-Cancer Agents Med. Chem.*, 7, pp. 552–558.

38. Vivès, E., Schmidt, J., Pèlegrin, A. (2008) Cell-penetrating and cell-targeting peptides in drug delivery, *BBA Rev. Cancer*, 1786, 126–138.

39. Dekel, Y., Glucksam, Y., Margalit, R. (2010) Novel fibrillar insulin formulations for oral administration: formulation and *in vivo* studies in diabetic mice, *J. Cont. Rel.*, 143, pp. 128–135.

40. Platt, V.M., Szoka, F.C. (2008). Anticancer therapeutics: targeting macromolecules and nanocarriers to hyaluronan or CD44, a hyaluronan receptor, *Mol. Pharm.*, 5, pp. 474–486.

41. Kanellakopoulou, K., Giamarellos-Bourboulis, E.J (2000) Carrier systems for the local delivery of antibiotics in bone infections, *Drugs*, 59, pp. 1223–1232.

42. Zhang J-S., Liu, F., Huang, L. (2005) Implications of pharmacokinetic behavior of lipoplex for its inflammatory toxicity, *Adv. Drug Deliv. Rev.*, 57, pp. 689–698.

43. Lv, H. et al. (2006). Toxicity of cationic lipids and cationic polymers in gene delivery, *J. Cont. Rel.*, 114, pp. 100–109.

44. de Ilarduyaa, C.T., Sunb, Y., Duzgunes, N. (2010) Gene delivery by lipoplexes and polyplexes, *Eur. J. Pharm.* Sci., 40, pp. 159–170.

45. Alving, C.R. et al. (1978) Improved therapy of experimental leishmaniasis by use of a liposome-encapsulated antimonail drug, *Life Sci.*, 22, pp. 1021–1026.

46. Raz, A. et al. (1981) Biochemical, morphological, and ultrastructural studies on the uptake of liposomes by murine macrophages, *Cancer Res.*, 41, pp. 487–494.

47. Isaiah, I.J. et al. (1981) The role of plasma membrane receptors and the kinetics of macrophage activation by lymphokines encapsulated in liposomes, *Cancer Res.*, 41, pp. 495–504.

48. Kirsh, R., Bugelski, P.J., Poste, G. (1987) Drug delivery to macrophages for the therapy of cancer and infectious diseases, *Ann. N.Y. Acad. Sci.*, 507, pp. 141–154.

49. Nardin, A. et al. (2006) Liposomal muramyl tripeptide phosphatidylethanolamine: targeting and activating macrophages for adjuvant treatment of osteosarcoma, *Curr. Cancer Drug Targets*, 6, pp. 123–133.

50. Bhowmick, S., Mazumdar, T., Sinha, R.. Ali, N. (2010), Comparison of liposome based antigen delivery systems for protection against *Leishmania donovani*, *J. Control. Release*, 141, pp. 199–207.

51. Gabizon, A., Shmeeda, H., Barenholtz, Y. (2003) Pharmacokinetics of pegylated liposomal Doxorubicin: review of animal and human studies, *Clin. Pharmacokinet.*, 42, pp. 419–436

52. Allen, T.M., Martin, F.J. (2004) Advantages of liposomal delivery systems for anthracyclines, *Semin. Oncol.*, 31, 5–15.

53. Immordino, M.L., Dosio, F., Cattel, L. (2006) Stealth liposomes: review of the basic science, rationale, and clinical applications, existing and potential, *Int. J. Nanomed.*, 1, pp. 297–315.

54. Soloman, R., Gabizon, A.A. (2008) Clinical pharmacology of liposomal anthracyclines: focus on pegylated liposomal doxorubicin. *Clin. Lymphoma Myeloma*, 8, pp. 21–32.

55. Schneider, G.F. et al. (2009) Multifunctional cytotoxic stealth nanoparticles. a model approach with potential for cancer therapy, *Nano Lett.*, 9, pp. 636–642.

56. Grenader, T. el al ((2009) Long-term response to pegylated liposomal doxorubicin in patients with metastatic soft tissue sarcomas, *Anti-Cancer Drugs*, 20, pp. 15–20.

57. Torchilin, V. (2008) Antibody-modified liposomes for cancer chemotherapy, *Exp. Opin. Drug Deliv.*, 5, pp. 1003–1025.

58. Gabizon, A. et al.(2010) Improved therapeutic activity of folate-targeted liposomal doxorubicin in folate receptor-expressing tumor models. *Cancer Chemo. Pharm.*, 66, pp. 43–52.

59. Petros, R.A., DeSimone, J.M. (2010) Strategies in the design of nanoparticles for therapeutic applications, *Nat. Rev. Drug Discov.*, 9, pp. 615–627.

60. Huang Y.-H. et al (2009) Nanoparticle-delivered suicide gene therapy effectively reduces ovarian tumor burden in mice. *Cancer Res.* 69, pp. 6184–6191.

61. Ahmed, M. et al. (2010) Pharmacokinetics of doxorubicin after intratumoral injection using a thermosensitive hydrogel in tumor-bearing mice, *J. Control. Release*, 142, pp. 101–107.

62. Morishita, M., Peppas, N.A. (2006) Is the oral route possible for peptide and protein drug delivery? *Drug Discov. Today*, 11, pp. 905–910.

63. Singh, R., Singh, H., Lillard, J.W. (2008) Past, present, and future technologies for oral delivery of therapeutic proteins, *J. Pharm. Sci.*, 97, pp. 2497–2523.

64. Muller, G. (2010) Oral delivery of protein drugs: driver for personalized medicine? *Curr. Issues Mol. Biol.*, 13, pp. 13–24.

65. Arbit, E., Kidron, M. (2009) Oral insulin: the rationale for this approach and current developments, *J. Diab. Sci. Technol.*, 3, pp. 562–567.

Chapter 2

Single-Chain Polymer Nanoparticles for Application in Nanomedicine

Ibon Odriozola, Miren Karmele Aiertza, Germán Cabañero, Hans-Jürgen Grande, and Iraida Loinaz
New Materials Department, Fundación CIDETEC,
Parque Tecnológico de San Sebastían,
Paseo Miramón 196 Donostia-San Sebastián, 20009, Spain
iloinaz@cidetec.es

The synthesis of polymer nanoparticles with controlled characteristics has become an appealing research topic lately. Nanomedicine and, especially, drug delivery and imaging are fields that require particles with controlled size and tailored arrangement of functional groups. Intramolecular cross-linking or collapse of single polymeric chain has emerged as an alternative to the synthesis of well-defined polymeric nanoparticles. The method allows the synthesis of particles of 1.5–20 nm size with a wide variety of chemical composition and functionalities. This chapter discusses the synthetic strategies described in the literature and groups them into four main methods: homo-functional collapse, hetero-functional collapse, cross-linker-mediated collapse, and one-block collapse of diblock or triblock copolymers. Then, the text describes main characterization techniques and physical properties of single-chain polymeric nanoparticles. Finally, some applications in nanomedicine are discussed and the chapter finishes with future perspectives.

Handbook of Harnessing Biomaterials in Nanomedicine: Preparation, Toxicity, and Applications
Edited by Dan Peer

ISBN 978-981-4316-46-0 (Hardback), 978-981-4364-27-0 (eBook)
www.panstanford.com

2.1 Introduction

The role of nanoparticles in biomedicine has increased in recent years, mainly due to their wide number of applications in the field of nanomedicine. Advances in synthetic techniques have enabled the preparation of particles ranging from a few nanometres up to hundreds of nanometres over a wide range of materials.

Hence, inorganic nanoparticles are being exploited due to their unique physical properties. Silver nanoparticles have demonstrated to be active antibacterial agents. Hydroxyapatite nanoparticles have been investigated due to their osteo-inductive properties. Superparamagnetic properties of ferromagnetic and ferrimagnetic nanoparticles are interesting for their application in MRI, hyperthermia therapy, and biosensors. The optical properties of quantum dots and gold nanoparticles are also a field of interest for their application in imaging. And TiO_2, silica, ZnO, and other nanoparticles are also under development.

However, there is a growing concern over the toxicity of particles of different sizes, shapes, and composition. It is widely known that the size and surface properties of nanomaterials determine their interaction with biological systems, and as such, their potential toxicity [1]. Different types of nanoparticles have been shown to be cytotoxic to human cells [2], induce oxidative stress [3], or induce an immune response [4]. Nanoparticles can accumulate in lung tissue after inhalation and translocate to the bloodstream [5]. Of particular concern is their ability to enter neurons and cross the blood–brain barrier [6].

However, even though there is a concern regarding the toxicity of nanoparticles, and though it may seem contradictory, the use of these nanoparticles could have applications in reducing the toxicity of certain drugs and contrast agents. This could be done with the design of multifunctional biodegradable and biocompatible particles, specifically designed to improve the biodistribution and target site accumulation of systematically applied therapeutics at the pathological site, and so reducing the accumulation in healthy organs and tissues. This would lead to an increase of the efficacy of treatments and a reduction of the toxicity.

For this purpose, nanocarriers based on soft matter have particularly interesting characteristics. The classification of those systems is variable, depending on their nature. Some authors differentiate between polymeric, non-polymeric, and biological nanocarriers [7]. Polymeric nanocarriers include nano-conjugates, polymer nanoparticles, micelles, dendrimers, or polyplexes, for example. Non-polymeric nanocarriers consist on liposomes, ethosomes, solid lipid nanoparticles, lipid nanocapsules, nano-emulsions, and others. Finally, biological nanocarriers include viral and bacterial vectors, erythrocytes, or stem cells.

Soussan and co-workers differentiate matrix systems and vesicles depending on their morphology [8]. They divide them into two categories: those that consist of solid nanoparticles, such as polymer nanoparticles and dendrimers, and those that consist of hollow spheres, such as nanocapsules or polymersomes, liposomes, niosomes, or cationic vesicles.

Irrespective of their nature, size, or morphology, there are interesting developments for a wide number of applications. In particular, polymer nanoparticles are being mostly developed for drug delivery [9], and there are a large number of examples of their applications in many biomedical fields and pathologies. Examples include HIV [7, 10, 11], cancer [12, 13], siRNA delivery [14], malaria [15], Chagas [16], imaging agents [17], image-guided drug delivery [18], and sensors and self-healing systems [19].

We have mentioned many nanoparticulate systems depending on their nature and morphology. Size is also an important parameter. If we focus on solid polymer nanoparticles, most of the examples can be included in three different systems: polymer nanoparticles, micelles, and dendrimers.

Polymer nanoparticles (PNPs) are usually 20–100 nm in size and can be composed of biodegradable or biostable polymers and copolymers. For drug delivery applications, the active agent can be (i) entrapped or encapsulated within the particle, (ii) physically adsorbed on the surface, or (iii) chemically linked to the surface of the particle [20–22]. Polymer nanoparticles can be divided into two main families: nanospheres, which have a homogeneous structure in the whole particle, and nanocapsules, which exhibit a typical core–shell structure [23]. There are two main methods of synthesis: those formed by *in situ* polymerisation in nanoemulsion systems and those synthesised by preformed polymers. Polymer micelles are nanostructures of a mean diameter of 20–50 nm that have been utilized for improving aqueous solubility, intestinal permeability, and disease site targeting of several drug molecules. Compared with the conventional surfactant-based micelles, polymer micelles are composed of block copolymers (having both hydrophobic and hydrophilic parts) or triblock copolymers (with one hydrophobic and two hydrophilic parts or one hydrophilic and two hydrophobic parts). Although the structural "core–shell" arrangement is similar to surfactant-based micelles, polymer micelles self-associate at much lower concentrations (low critical micelle concentration, CMC), typically 10^{-6}–10^{-7} M compared with 10^{-3}–10^{-4} M for surfactant-based micelles.

A dendrimer is a polymeric nanostructure (1–10 nm) built around a core unit. There are several branching units around the core units in a layer-by-layer fashion which defines the growth, size and the microenvironment within the dendrimer. Dendrons are formed after the removal of the core units and can be divided into three areas: the (empty) core, the interior (branching units), and the periphery (end-groups). The empty core of dendrons can be utilized for the entrapment of drug molecules for solubilisation, controlled release, targeting, or protection from surrounding degrading environment. Dendrimers offer unique properties such as uniform particle size (especially for lower generation, i.e. up to G-3), poly-valency of the end groups, which helps in binding to diverse receptors, and an ability to bind a variety of targeting agents to their high density peripheral functional groups.

2.2 Single-Chain Polymer Nanoparticles

Very recently, a new method for producing polymer nanoparticles has emerged as a fascinating alternative to the strategies mentioned earlier in this chapter: the intramolecular cross-linking and collapse of single polymer chains. This elegant method allows the facile preparation of tiny nanoparticles from 1.5 to 20 nm in diameter, with a wide variety of chemical compositions and functionalities. In addition, the sizes of the particles fabricated in such manner can be tuned by (i) controlling the molecular weight of the precursor polymer chain and (ii) the percentage of cross-linking units used to perform the intramolecular chain-collapse. For all these reasons, single-chain polymer nanoparticles (SCPNs) are envisaged as promising candidates for applications in nanomedicine.

In order to control the molecular weight of the precursor polymer chain, these need to be synthesized using polymerisation techniques that permit a high degree of control. The reversible addition-fragmentation chain transfer (RAFT) process, the most recent of the living/controlled free radical polymerisations, is especially convenient for this purpose. The lower the polydispersity of the precursor polymer chains, the narrower will be the size of the final nanoparticles.

2.2.1 Chain-Collapse Strategies

SCPNs can be classified according to the strategy used to effect the intramolecular chain-collapse. Scheme 2.1 illustrates the main approaches for their preparation that have been carried out thus far. The first approach (Scheme 2.1a) involves the functionalisation of the (co)polymer chain with suitable reactive self-complementary "R" groups (i.e. double bonds), and then to promote the intramolecular reaction of such groups under diluted conditions. This can be achieved both by covalent or non-covalent cross-linking. The percentage of reactive groups used is variable, ranging from 10 to 100%.

The second approach consists of inserting two complementary functionalities ("R" and "X") on the same polymer chain (Scheme 2.1b), which are then forced to react intramolecularly, also under diluted conditions.

A third approach uses a polymer chain functionalised with a suitable "R" reactive group and a cross-linker, the latter having two "X" end-groups that react with the "R" groups of the polymer chain (Scheme 2.1c). Usually the reaction is carried out by the slow addition of one component to the other. This method is especially useful, for it simplifies the synthesis of the precursor polymer and permits the insertion of extra functionality through the cross-linking agent.

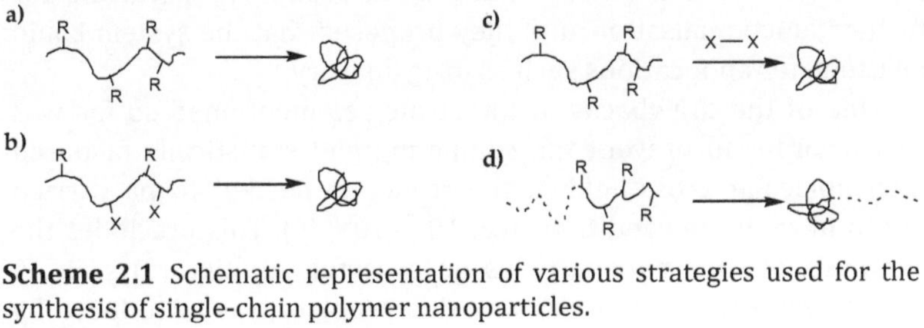

Scheme 2.1 Schematic representation of various strategies used for the synthesis of single-chain polymer nanoparticles.

As a special case, there are also some reports on the use of diblock copolymers for the fabrication of nanoparticle-coil copolymers or molecular "tadpoles". The strategy consists of functionalising just one of the blocks with reactive groups, so that when the intramolecular cross-linking is forced this block collapses into a globule, whereas the other block remains as a coil (Scheme 2.1d). In this case, the intramolecular collapse could be performed using any of the three strategies previously mentioned.

2.2.2 Homo-Functional Chain Collapse

The synthesis of discrete nanoparticles using a strategy that involves the intramolecular coupling of single polymer chains was proposed as early as in the 1980s [24, 25]. Davankov and co-workers published the synthesis of single-chain polystyrene nanoparticles using this strategy in 1996 [26]. In this work, linear polystyrene chains (M_w = 330 kDa) functionalised with chloromethylene groups were self-crosslinked by means of a $SnCl_4$ catalyst, obtaining hyper-crosslinked "nanosponges" of about 17 nm (in solution).

A few years later, Mecerreyes and co-workers presented the synthesis of unimolecular particles from copolymers based on (i) aliphatic polyesters (caprolactone-co-ε-caprolactone or L,L-lactide), (ii) poly(methyl methacrylate) and (iii) polystyrene [27]. The strategy that they used involved the synthesis of polymer backbones with pendant acrylate functionalities. Then, such macromolecules were intramolecularly crosslinked in ultradiluted solution using a radical initiator such as 2,2-azo-bis-isobutyronitrile (AIBN).

Thayumanavan and co-workers used a similar strategy to synthesise amine-functionalised polystyrene nanoparticles by AIBN induced radical cross-linking of styrene groups [28]. They demonstrated that the free pending amino groups were available for further functionalisation, and they proposed that the system could be useful for applications such as drug delivery.

One of the drawbacks of the strategies mentioned so far was that in order to prevent the competing and statistically favoured intermolecular cross-linking, the reactions needed to be carried out in ultra-dilute conditions (ca. 10^{-5}–10^{-6} M). This precludes the synthesis of such nanoparticles on a useful (multigram) scale. A very clever strategy to overcome this problem was introduced by Hawker and co-workers in 2002 [29]. The method consists of the continuous addition of the linear polymer to the reaction mixture. If the cross-linking reaction rate is faster than the addition rate, then the concentration of the reactive open-chain species will always be ultra-low, while the concentration of the unreactive nanoparticles will be constantly growing. Under these conditions, no intermolecular cross-linking reactions, leading to gelation or coupling of individual nanoparticles, are observed. To achieve this, Hawker chose the thermal-induced coupling of benzocyclobutene (BCB) units at 250°C. A series of BCB copolymers with styrene, methyl methacrylate, or *n*-butyl acrylate were used for this study.

Later on, Harth and co-workers reported the vinylbenzosulfone cross-linking monomer, which can be used as an alternative to BCB, and has the advantage of being easier to synthesise [30]. They copolymerized this precursor with styrene or benzyl acrylate. In the latter case, the subsequent deprotection of the benzyl ester groups resulted in the formation of SCPNs that were soluble in physiological conditions, and could therefore be envisaged as promising candidates for biomedical applications. In a subsequent work, the authors brilliantly demonstrated the usefulness of these nanoparticles as efficient nanocarriers for the intracellular delivery of peptide-based therapeutics [31].

Vinylbenzosulfone units were also used for the fabrication of SCPNs with single conducting polymers embedded in polystyrene, which resulted in a considerable increase in quantum efficiency [32].

Olefin cross-metathesis has also been used to induce the intramolecular cross-linking of polycarbonates with pending vinyl groups, as reported by Coates and co-workers [33]. The cross-linking was effected by the addition of a ruthenium catalyst into a dilute polymer solution. In this work, the formation of molecular nanoparticles was confirmed by atomic force microscopy (AFM) through visualisation of individual molecules at different stages of the cross-linking.

So far we have seen the fabrication of SCPNs by means of covalent cross-links between suitable pending groups of a polymer-chain. However, the collapse of polymer chains can also be accomplished through non-covalent interactions, such as hydrogen bonds, which leads to supramolecular single-chain nanoparticles. This is especially interesting from a biological point of view, due to the analogy with the folding of biomacromolecules. While synthetic copolymers are by no means as structurally complex as natural polymers, the continued development of these systems will lead to a better understanding of the processes of protein-folding. It is also expected to give rise to new synthetic systems capable of mimicking some of the structures and functions of nature's sophisticated machinery.

In recent work performed by the groups of Hawker and Kim [34], the synthesis of a random poly(methyl methacrylate) copolymers having dendritic self-complementary hydrogen-bonding units is described. The formation of intramolecular H-bonds between the dendritic units led to the collapse of the polymer coils, giving discrete and stable spherical SCPNs.

In a more recent work, Meijer and co-workers made use of 2-ureidopyrimidinone (Upy), a very efficient quadruple H-bond-forming unit, as the intramolecular cross-linking motif for the fabrication of poly(methyl methacrylate) supramolecular SCPNs [35]. In this elegant work, the polymer backbone was decorated with Upy units that were protected with a photo-cleavable group (Scheme 2.2). The irradiation with UV light released the protecting group, promoting the collapse of the chains and therefore, the formation of the nanoparticles.

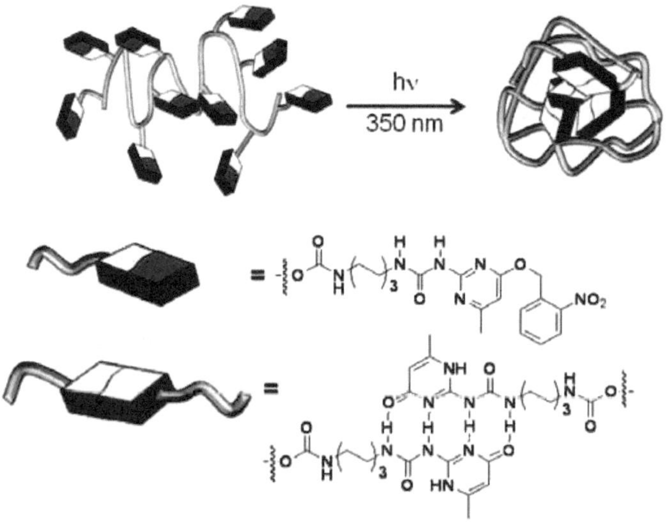

Scheme 2.2 UV irradiation induced collapse of a single polymer chain into a nanoparticle via the supramolecular cross-linking of the UPy-urethane side groups (nitrosoaldehyde side product omitted for clarity). Reproduced and adapted from ref. [35] with permission of ACS.

2.2.3 Hetero-Bifunctional Chain Collapse

Another strategy to synthesise SCPNs consists of decorating the polymer backbone with two different self-complementary motifs. Loinaz and co-workers have developed a strategy to produce poly(methyl methacrylate) SCPNs [36] at room-temperature by means of an intramolecular CuI-catalysed [3+2] cycloaddition, or "click" reaction, between azide and alkyne functional groups present in the same polymer backbone. Click chemistry [37, 38], and specifically the CuI-catalyzed [3+2] cycloaddition of alkynes and azides [39–41], is a selective and very efficient kind of reaction that can be performed under extremely mild conditions with high yields, good functional group tolerance and negligible by-products. The very mild conditions required for the chain-collapse makes this method ideal for the fabrication of SCPNs with polymers that are not stable at high temperatures.

In addition, the authors demonstrated the possibility of functionalising the resulting nanoparticles very easily with suitable biomolecules. To achieve that, an excess of azide groups was added to the polymer backbone. After the formation of the nanoparticle, an alkyne-containing molecule (propargylglycine) was attached to the surface by means of a second click reaction (Scheme 2.3).

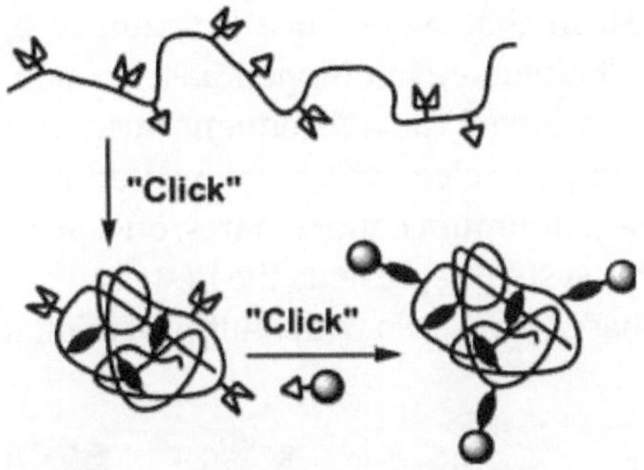

Scheme 2.3 Chain-collapse through intramolecular click cycloaddition and further functionalisation with a suitable biomolecule by means of a second click cycloaddition. Reproduced from ref. [36] with permission.

However, one of the major drawbacks of this method is the difficulty in the synthesis of the precursor copolymers, which need to have the two complementary reactive groups randomly distributed over the chain. This problem is solved by the use of a suitable difunctional cross-linker, as we will see in the following section.

2.2.4 Cross-Linker-Mediated Chain Collapse

The use of a difunctional cross-linker to force the collapse of a polymer chain is also a very efficient method to obtain SCPNs in a controlled and straightforward manner.

Hawker's group has developed a synthetic approach using this method, for the preparation of SCPNs under mild, room-temperature conditions. They make use of isocyanate functionalised acrylic polymers and a diamine cross-linker [42]. By varying the molecular weight and mole percentage of isocyanates of the starting linear copolymer, nanoparticles with diameters ranging from 8 to 20 nm were obtained. Interestingly, the analysis of the collapse reaction revealed that approximately 75% of the isocyanate groups along the backbone underwent cross-linking, the other 25% being available for further reactions with monofunctional amines, making them ideal for bioconjugation.

Pomposo and co-workers used an aliphatic dialkyne cross-linker to generate SCPNs from azide functionalised copolymers of diverse nature [43, 44]. The method consisted of adding a solution of the cross-linker very slowly to a solution of copolymer, by means of a syringe pump.

Similarly, Odriozola and co-workers prepared water soluble SCPNs from azide functionalised acrylic copolymers and a dialkyne cross-linker [45]. In that work, they introduced a gadolinium(III) chelating unit (diethylenetriaminepentaacetic acid, DTPA) into the cross-linker. This allowed the subsequent formation of Gd^{3+} loaded paramagnetic nanoparticles, which showed an increased relaxivity over their mono-gadolinium counterparts, on a per gadolinium basis (Scheme 2.4). This system represents the first example of potential MRI contrast agents based on SCPNs with multiple gadolinium centres.

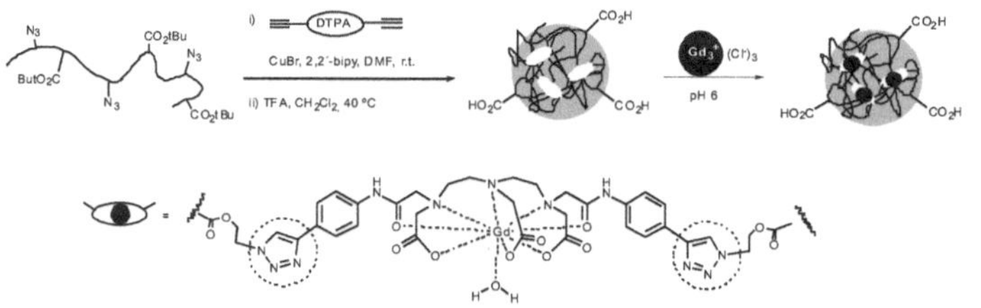

Scheme 2.4 Formation of single-chain PNPs and loading with Gd III. Dashed circles are used to highlight the newly formed 1,2,3-triazole rings during the click cycloaddition. Reproduced from ref. [46] with permission.

2.2.5 One-Block Collapse of Diblock or Triblock Copolymers

A unique polymer chain composed by more than one block can be designed to undergo selective collapse in only one of the blocks. If the starting chain is a diblock copolymer of type A-B, this results in the formation of nanoparticle-coil copolymers or molecular "tadpoles". This kind of structure is especially interesting from a biological point of view. Naturally occurring polymers such as peptides and proteins, often incorporate different architectures or conformations (i.e. globular, linear) into the same macromolecule, enabling the formation of discrete and unique nanoenvironments for catalysis and self-assembly [47, 48]. Recent developments in polymer therapeutics have seen the launch of several highly successful drugs with mixed globular-linear architecture, in which a globular protein is attached to a synthetic linear polymer such as poly(ethylene glycol) [49]. In these systems the synthetic linear-globular assembly showed vast performance enhancements over the natural globular protein on its own.

The first preparation and isolation of diblock tadpole molecules was published by Tao and Liu in 1997 [50]. They used a polystyrene-*block*-poly(2-cinnamoylethyl methacrylate) precursor, and they forced the intramolecular collapse by photo-cross-linking of the cinnamoyl units. However, their method only allowed the formation of tadpoles in very low yields. The process involved the tedious separation of the tadpoles from the nanospheres that were also formed in the reaction, using size-exclusion chromatography (SEC).

Hawker and co-workers described the synthesis of nanoparticle-coil structures from linear diblock copolymers of poly(ethylene glycol)-*block*-poly[styrene-*random*-(4-vinylbenzocyclobutene)] (Scheme 2.5) [29, 51]. The collapse was carried out by the slow addition of the precursor linear copolymer to a benzyl ether solution at 250°C. It is worth noticing that the linear block is water soluble, although the entire molecule was not in this case, probably due to the short dimension of the PEG fragment. A similar family of nanoparticle-coil copolymers were prepared by Pyun and co-workers having a poly(*n*-butyl acrylate) coil attached to the same styrenic nanoparticle [52].

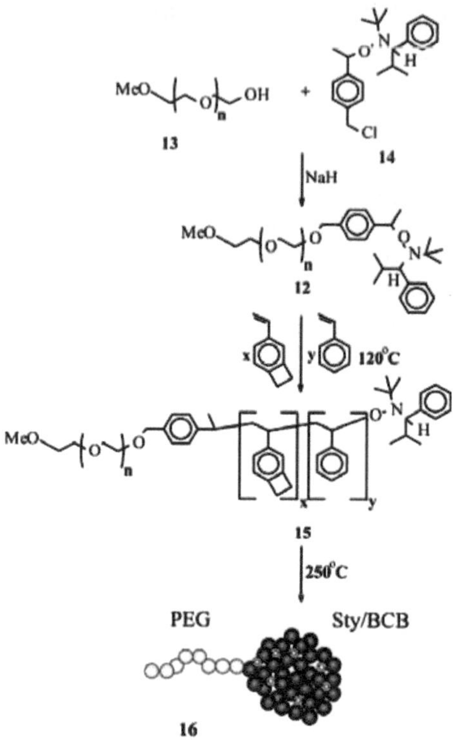

Scheme 2.5 Formation and intramolecular collapse of the PEG-b-PSt/BCB block copolymer, 15, to give a hybrid linear-nanoparticle copolymer, 16. Reproduced from ref. [29] with permission.

In a more recent paper, Liu and co-workers synthesise diblock copolymers of poly(*tert*-butyl acrylate)-*block*-poly(2-cinnamoyloxyethyl methacrylate) and poly(*tert*-butyl acrylate)-*block*-poly[(2-cinnamoyloxyethyl methacrylate)-*ran*-(2-hydrocinnamoyloxyethyl methacrylate)] [53]. The partial collapse of the cinnamoyl-containing blocks was carried out using the same photo-cross-linking strategy previously described [50]. Thus, the tadpoles were prepared by adding a diblock copolymer solution gradually into a solvent, under constant UV irradiation and stirring. One of the advantages of this method is that it is carried out at room-temperature, unlike Hawker's BCB-based systems which require very high temperatures.

Finally, an A-B-C type triblock copolymer can also be designed to undergo partial collapse of one of the blocks. In a recent example from Cheng and co-workers [54], coil-nanoparticle-coil systems are synthesised from a triblock copolymer precursor composed of polystyrene-*b*-poly(2-vinylpyridine)-*b*-poly(ethylene oxide). In this work, the middle block is collapsed by quaternisation of the pyridine rings using dibromobutane as the cross-linker.

2.3 Characterization and Physical Properties of SCPNs

As mentioned before, the synthesis of polymer nanoparticles with controlled characteristics has become an appealing research topic lately. The importance of obtaining nanoparticles with controlled size and a tailored arrangement of functional groups is increasing, due to the requirements of the specific potential applications. While the strategies used to prepare nanoparticles above 20 nm are generally successful, there is a trade off with respect to accessibility and desired size. Synthesis of nanoparticles less than 20 nm in size is invariably more difficult but yields particles of a more well-defined composition. Moreover, nanomedicinal applications seem to need structurally controlled delivery systems of less than 30 nm to avoid accumulation in the liver and spleen, as well as unwanted immunogenic reactions [31].

We have previously described that is essential to control the concentration of the linear-chain polymer in solution to favour intramolecular over intermolecular cross-linking. Intramolecular cross-linking dominates at very low concentrations, but as soon as the concentration increases polymer networks are generated due to intermolecular cross-linking. As described by Li *et al.* not only the concentration but the sizes of the linear precursors determine the reaction rates [55].

Most of the physical properties of polymers used to obtain SCPNs change once they have been converted into nanoparticles. There are several techniques that are utilized to study these properties. The molecular weight of the macromolecule is determined by gel permeation chromatography (GPC). Intramolecular cross-linking does not affect the molecular weight distribution of the polymer, but the properties related to polymer size, such as hydrodynamic volume and intrinsic viscosity, are affected [42]. As the GPC measurement is proportional to the hydrodynamic volume, when a random coil polymer collapses the retention time in the GPC increases compared to the one for the linear precursor. Thus, the nanoparticles show an apparent lower molecular weight, but what this really means is that intramolecular cross-linking took place (Figure 2.1a).

In case of intermolecular cross-linking the outcome is a polymer network with higher weight than the original polymer. The intrinsic viscosity also decreases in value when the coil polymer collapses, and according to Beck and co-workers, analogous nanoparticles display equivalent viscosities even if the molecular weights differ by 50% (Figure 2.1b).

This is due to the similarity between the nanoparticles and constant density spheres [26].

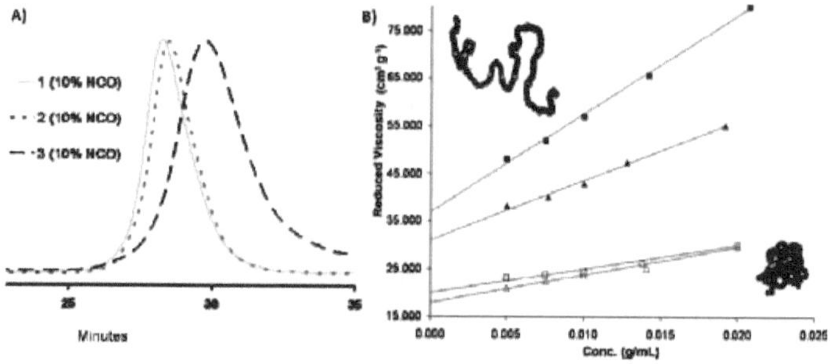

Figure 2.1 (A) Overlay of GPC traces for the starting copolymer 1, (Mn = 45,300), the corresponding linear control polymer 2 and nanoparticle 3 incorporating ca. 10 mol % NCO cross-linking functional groups. (B) Plot of reduced viscosity versus concentration for control copolymers 2 (■, 150 kDa; Δ, 100 kDa) and their analogous cross-linked nanoparticles 3 (□, 150 kDa; □, 100 kDa) in THF. Mol % NCO is 10 in this case. Reproduced from ref. [42] with permission.

Nuclear magnetic resonance (NMR) is also a useful technique to confirm the formation of SCNPs. There are signals that disappear once the linear polymer collapses to form the nanoparticle, as is clearly shown by Kim *et al.* [51]. When the particles are in solution, their radius can be measured by dynamic light scattering (DLS), even though the average sizes of this kind of nanoparticles are in the lower size limit of most of the commercial instruments. Also, if the SCNPs are dried on a surface, they can be analyzed by atomic force microscopy (AFM) and the dimensions of the collapsed coils can be visually studied. One of the most detailed studies of this type of nanoparticle has been carried out by Berda and co-workers, where they deduce the possible morphology of a collapsed supramolecular single molecule (Figure 2.2) [35]. Thermal characteristics also change after the formation of the SCPN [35, 51], and in some cases the solubility of the polymeric chain differs from the collapsed coil in certain solvents [34, 54].

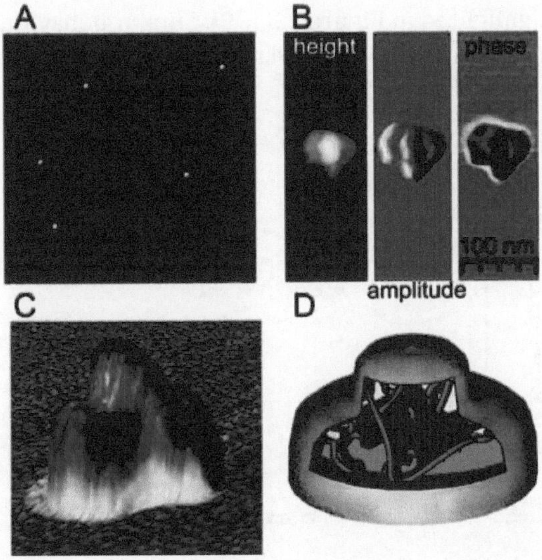

Figure 2.2 High-resolution AFM scan of individual SCNP: (A) Group of a few particles. (B) Height, amplitude, and phase images clearly indicating the complex geometry and raised core. (C) Three-dimensional height image with phase retrace overlay of this particle. (D) Cartoon depicting the possible particle morphology: 2-ureido-pyrimidinone (UPy)-urethane rich core (blue) immersed in a network of PMMA. Reproduced from ref. [35] with permission. See also Color Insert.

In relation to nanomedical applications, the feature that makes this type of nanoparticle so attractive is their small size. Up to now, the most successful nanocarriers, such as dendrimers, have had dimensions between 1 and 10 nm. That is one of the reasons why it would be desirable to obtain SCNPs with comparable proportions. As has been mentioned before, the size varies in relation to the molecular weight and chemical nature of the precursor polymer, as well as the amount of cross-links that are formed during the collapse. Depending on the major functional groups, the behaviour of the final nanoparticle varies when changing molecular weight and percentage of cross-linking units. The majority of SCNPs obtained so far in the literature are polystyrene based and covalently cross-linked. In this case, the size of the nanoparticle is basically proportional to the molecular weight and inversely proportional to the number of cross-links. Harth *et al.* carried out an extensive study about the relationship between these properties in polymers built on polystyrene (PS) cross-linked using benzocyclobutene (BCB) chemistry, highlighted in Figure 2.3 [29]. Similar behaviour has been identified in polymethyl methacrylate (PMMA) copolymers [36].

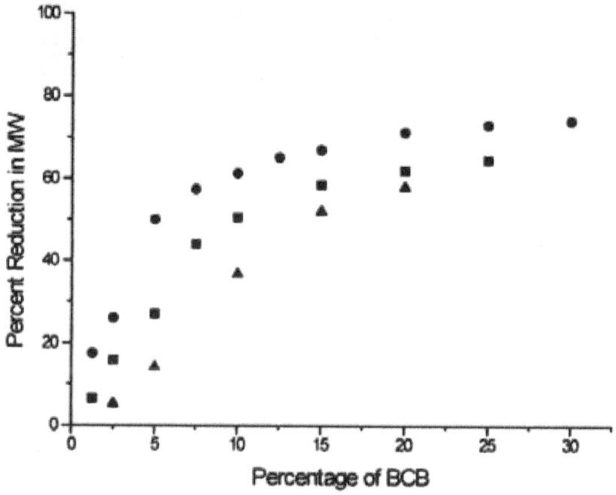

Figure 2.3 Variation in the percent reduction in molecular weight for the PS nanoparticles with the mol % of BCB units in the starting linear polymer for 44 K (•), 110 K (■), and 230 K (Δ) series. Reproduced from ref. [29] with permission.

The same tendency can be attributed to SNPCs formed from macromolecules with PMMA backbone and supramolecular cross-linking [34, 35]. It should be noted that these particles are larger than similar ones made through covalent cross-linking (around 10 nm in diameter), but additionally they are less dense [56]. In contrast, SCNPs obtained covalently from polymers with bulky side groups do not diminish in size when the number of links is raised, as is the case of PS-based nanoparticles that display *tert*-butyloxycarbonyl (BOC) protected amino moieties [28]. According to these results, it could be foreseen that macromolecules with charged side groups would also have the ability to form collapsed-coil polymers.

Nevertheless, the smallest SCPNs have been achieved using "click" chemistry through the cross-linker mediated collapse method [46], where the average diameter is around 1.5 nm in dry conditions. It is worth mentioning that Odriozola and co-workers obtained a reduction in the dimension by introducing gadolinium into the nanoparticle due to the chelating effect with the cross-linker (see Section 2.2.1.3).

2.4 Applications and Future Perspectives

Despite the advances shown in the previous sections, the application of SCPNs in nanomedicine is still in its infancy. However, it is clear to see that in forthcoming years, SCPNs will have a tremendous impact in that field and many new applications will emerge.

Hamilton and Harth have recently published a very nice example of SCPNs applied in nanomedicine. In this brilliant work, they describe the use of SCPNs conjugated with dendritic units for the intracellular delivery of peptide-based therapeutics [31]. The dendritic molecular transporters appeared to be critical for the delivery of the nanoparticle into 3T3 cells. The peptidic cargo was attached by means of disulfide linkages, which were cleaved intracellularly to release the therapeutic peptide. The intracellular uptake of the nanoparticles was monitored using fluorescent dyes (Figure 2.4).

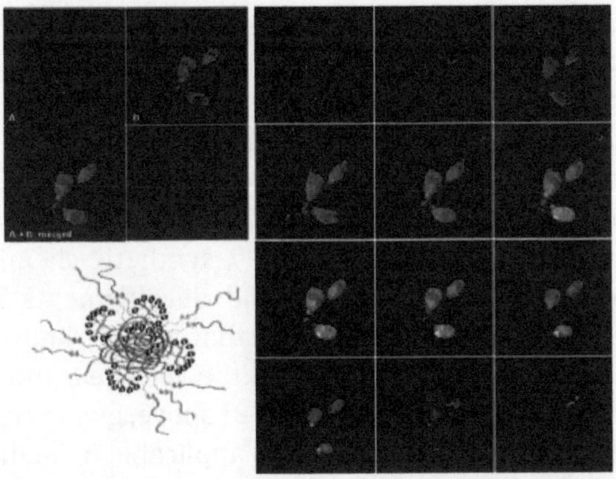

Figure 2.4 Cellular uptake experiments of nanoparticle transporter conjugate into NIH 3T3 cells investigated *via* confocal microscopy imaged for the fluorescence of the Alexa Fluor 568 dye (B) and the fluorescein (A), with complementing *z*-stack showing the presence of both fluorophores from the bottom (top, left) to the top of the cells (bottom, right). The cells were incubated for 30 min with a 37.2 μM solution of 15 in Hanks buffered saline solution (HBSS). Reproduced from ref. [31] with permission. See also Color Insert.

As already mentioned, Perez-Baena and co-workers have developed a new class of Gd-loaded paramagnetic SCNPs as potential contrast agents for MRI [46]. The novelty of this original approach relied on the insertion of the DTPA chelate in the form of a cross-linker instead of grafting it onto the polymeric chain in a conventional manner (Figure 2.5).

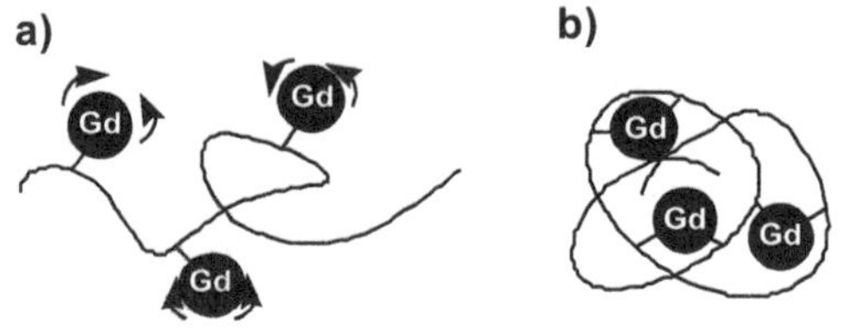

Figure 2.5 Schematic representation of a conventional Gd-grafted polymer (a) and a polymer intramolecularly cross-linked with Gd chelates (b). Reproduced from ref. [46] with permission.

This resulted in the formation of conformationally rigid systems in which the internal rotation of the Gd-DTPA moieties was restricted. This is very important, for it has been reported that non-rigid attachment of the Gd^{III} chelate to the macromolecule, or internal flexibility are often factors that limit the relaxivity of polymers containing multiple Gd^{III} centres.

The reader should have noticed that many of the nanoparticle systems described in this chapter are not soluble in organic solvents, which is not ideal as far as biomedical applications are concerned. This is due to the fact that historically, synthetic chemists find it easier to perform their syntheses and developments in organic media. Obviously one could envisage that all this knowledge will be extrapolated to aqueous systems in the very near future, as was the case for the two examples mentioned above, giving rise to a new class of powerful nanosystems directly applicable in medicine.

References

1. Minchin, R., *Sizing up targets with nanoparticles.* Nature Nanotechnology, 2008. **3**: p. 12–13.
2. Lewinski, N., Colvin, V., and Drezek, R., *Cytotoxicity of nanoparticles.* Small, 2008. **4**(1): p. 26–49.

3. Long, T.C., et al., *Titanium dioxide (P25) produces reactive oxygen species in immortalized brain microglia (BV2): implications for nanoparticle neurotoxicity.* Environmental Science & Technology, 2006. **40**(14): p. 4346–4352.
4. Dobrovolskaia, M.A., and McNeil, S.E., *Immunological properties of engineered nanomaterials.* Nature Nanotechnology, 2007. **2**: p. 469–478.
5. Shimada, A., Kawamura, N., Okajima, M., Kaewamatawong, T., Inoue, H., and Morita,T., *Translocation pathway of the intratracheally instilled ultrafine particles from the lung into the blood circulation in the mouse.* Toxicologic Pathology, 2006. **34**: p. 949–957.
6. Lockman, P.R., et al., *Nanoparticle surface charges alter blood–brain barrier integrity and permeability.* Journal of Drug Targeting, 2004. **12**(9–10): p. 635–641.
7. Gupta, U., and Jain, N.K., *Non-polymeric nano-carriers in HIV/AIDS drug delivery and targeting.* Advanced Drug Delivery Reviews. **62**(4–5): p. 478–490.
8. E. Soussan, S.C., Blanzat, M., and Rico-Lattes, I., *Drug delivery by soft matter: matrix and vesicular carriers.* Angewandte Chemie International Edition English, 2009. **48**: p. 274–288.
9. Doshi, N., and Mitragotri, S., *Designer biomaterials for nanomedicine.* Advanced Functional Materials, 2009. **19**: p. 3843–3854.
10. Sharma, P., and Garg, S., *Pure drug and polymer based nanotechnologies for the improved solubility, stability, bioavailability and targeting of anti-HIV drugs.* Advanced Drug Delivery Reviews. **62**(4–5): p. 491–502.
11. Wong, H.L., et al., *Nanotechnology applications for improved delivery of antiretroviral drugs to the brain.* Advanced Drug Delivery Reviews. **62**(4–5): p. 503–517.
12. Bharali, D.J., et al., *Nanoparticles and cancer therapy: a concise review with emphasis on dendrimers.* International Journal of Nanomedicine, 2009. **4**: p. 1–7.
13. Gaucher, G., Marchessault, R.H., and Leroux, J.C., *Polyester-based micelles and nanoparticles for the parenteral delivery of taxanes.* Journal of Controlled Release. **143**(1): p. 2–12.
14. Keller, M., *Nanomedicinal delivery approaches for therapeutic siRNA.* International Journal of Pharmaceutics, 2009. **379**(2): p. 210–211.
15. Santos-Magalhães, N.S., and Mosqueira, V.C.F., *Nanotechnology applied to the treatment of malaria.* Advanced Drug Delivery Reviews. **62**(4–5): p. 560–575.
16. Romero, E.L., and Morilla, M.J., *Nanotechnological approaches against Chagas disease.* Advanced Drug Delivery Reviews. **62**(4–5): p. 576–588.

17. Richard, C., et al., *Amphiphilic perfluoroalkyl carbohydrates as new tools for liver imaging.* International Journal of Pharmaceutics, 2009. **379**(2): p. 301–308.

18. Lammers, T., et al., *Polymeric nanomedicines for image-guided drug delivery and tumor-targeted combination therapy.* Nano Today. **5**(3): p. 197–212.

19. Motornov, M., et al., *Stimuli-responsive nanoparticles, nanogels and capsules for integrated multifunctional intelligent systems.* Progress in Polymer Science. **35**(1–2): p. 174–211.

20. Kumari, A., Yadav, S.K., and Yadav, S.C., *Biodegradable polymeric nanoparticles based drug delivery systems.* Colloids and Surfaces B: Biointerfaces, 2010. **75**(1): p. 1–18.

21. Wei, X., et al., *Biodegradable poly([var epsilon]-caprolactone)-poly(ethylene glycol) copolymers as drug delivery system.* International Journal of Pharmaceutics, 2009. **381**(1): p. 1–18.

22. Landfester, K., *Miniemulsion polymerization and the structure of polymer and hybrid nanoparticles.* Angewandte Chemie International Edition 2009. **48**: p. 4488–4508.

23. Anton, N., Benoit, J.P., and Saulnier, P., *Design and production of nanoparticles formulated from nano-emulsion templates — a review.* Journal of Controlled Release, 2008. **128**(3): p. 185–199.

24. Martin, J.E., and Eichinger, B.E., *Dimensions of intramolecularly crosslinked polymers. 1. Theory.* Macromolecules, 1983. **16**(8): p. 1345–1350.

25. Martin, J.E., and Eichinger, B.E., *Dimensions of intramolecularly crosslinked polymers. 2. Dilute solution thermodynamic parameters and photon correlation results on the polystyrene/cyclopentane system.* Macromolecules, 1983. **16**(8): p. 1350–1358.

26. Davankov, V.A., et al., *From a dissolved polystyrene coil to an intramolecularly-hyper-cross-linked "nanosponge".* Macromolecules, 1996. **29**(26): p. 8398–8403.

27. Mecerreyes, D., et al., *A novel approach to functionalized nanoparticles: self-crosslinking of macromolecules in ultradilute solution.* Advanced Materials, 2001. **13**(3): p. 204–208.

28. Jiang, J., and Thayumanavan, S., *Synthesis and characterization of amine-functionalized polystyrene nanoparticles.* Macromolecules, 2005. **38**(14): p. 5886–5891.

29. Harth, E., et al., *A facile approach to architecturally defined nanoparticles via intramolecular chain collapse.* Journal of the American Chemical Society, 2002. **124**(29): p. 8653–8660.

30. Croce, T.A., et al., *Alternative o-quinodimethane cross-linking precursors for intramolecular chain collapse nanoparticles.* Macromolecules, 2007. **40**(17): p. 6028–6031.

31. Hamilton, S.K., and Harth, E., *Molecular dendritic transporter nanoparticle vectors provide efficient intracellular delivery of peptides.* ACS Nano, 2009. **3**(2): p. 402–410.

32. Adkins, C.T., Muchalski, H., and Harth, E., *Nanoparticles with individual site-isolated semiconducting polymers from intramolecular chain collapse processes.* Macromolecules, 2009. **42**(15): p. 5786–5792.

33. Cherian, A.E., et al., *Formation of nanoparticles by intramolecular cross-linking: following the reaction progress of single polymer chains by atomic force microscopy.* Journal of the American Chemical Society, 2007. **129**(37): p. 11350–11351.

34. Seo, M., et al., *Polymeric nanoparticles via noncovalent cross-linking of linear chains.* Macromolecules, 2008. **41**(17): p. 6413–6418.

35. Berda, E.B., Foster, E.J., and Meijer, E.W., *Toward controlling folding in synthetic polymers: fabricating and characterizing supramolecular single-chain nanoparticles.* Macromolecules, 2010. **43**(3): p. 1430–1437.

36. Ruiz de Luzuriaga, A., et al., *Intramolecular click cycloaddition: an efficient room-temperature route towards bioconjugable polymeric nanoparticles.* Macromolecular Rapid Communications, 2008. **29**(12–13): p. 1156–1160.

37. Iha, R.K., et al., *Applications of orthogonal "click" chemistries in the synthesis of functional soft materials.* Chemical Reviews, 2009. **109**(11): p. 5620–5686.

38. Kolb, H.C., Finn, M.G., and Sharpless, K.B., *Click chemistry: diverse chemical function from a few good reactions.* Angewandte Chemie International Edition, 2001. **40**(11): p. 2004–2021.

39. Meldal, M., and C.W. Tornoe, *Cu-catalyzed azide-alkyne cycloaddition.* Chemical Reviews, 2008. **108**(8): p. 2952–3015.

40. Tornoe, C.W., Christensen, C., and Meldal, M., *Peptidotriazoles on solid phase: [1,2,3]-triazoles by regiospecific copper(I)-catalyzed 1,3-dipolar cycloadditions of terminal alkynes to azides.* The Journal of Organic Chemistry, 2002. **67**(9): p. 3057–3064.

41. Rostovtsev, V.V., et al., *A stepwise Huisgen cycloaddition process: copper(I)-catalyzed regioselective "ligation" of azides and terminal alkynes.* Angewandte Chemie International Edition, 2002. **41**(14): p. 2596–2599.

42. Beck, J.B., et al., *Facile preparation of nanoparticles by intramolecular cross-linking of isocyanate functionalized copolymers.* Macromolecules, 2009. **42**(15): p. 5629–5635.

43. Oria, L., et al., *A versatile "click" chemistry precursor of functional polystyrene nanoparticles.* Advanced Materials. (DOI: 10.1002/adma.201000243).
44. Ruiz de Luzuriaga, A., et al., *New route to polymeric nanoparticles by click chemistry using bifunctional crosslinkers.* Macromolecular Symposia. **in press**.
45. Perez-Baena, I., et al., *Single-chain polyacrylic nanoparticles with multiple Gd(III) centres as potential MRI contrast agents.* Journal of Materials Chemistry. **20**(33): p. 6916–6922.
46. Perez-Baena, I., et al., *Single-chain polyacrylic nanoparticles with multiple Gd(III) centres as potential MRI contrast agents.* Journal of Materials Chemistry, 2010(DOI: 10.1039/c0jm01025a).
47. Hartgerink, J.D., Beniash, E., and Stupp, S.I., Science, 2001. **294**: p. 1684.
48. Krejchi, M.T., et al., *Chemical sequence control of beta-sheet assembly in macromolecular crystals of periodic polypeptides.* Science, 1994. **265**: p. 1427–1432.
49. Reddy, K.R., et al., *Efficacy and safety of pegylated (40-kd) interferon α-2a compared with interferon α-2a in noncirrhotic patients with chronic hepatitis C.* Hepatology, 2001. **33**(2): p. 433–438.
50. Tao, J., and Liu, G., *Polystyrene-block-poly(2-cinnamoylethyl methacrylate) Tadpole Molecules.* Macromolecules, 1997. **30**(8): p. 2408–2411.
51. Kim, Y., et al., *The dramatic effect of architecture on the self-assembly of block copolymers at interfaces.* Langmuir, 2005. **21**(23): p. 10444–10458.
52. Pyun, J., et al., *Synthesis and direct visualization of block copolymers composed of different macromolecular architectures.* Macromolecules, 2005. **38**(7): p. 2674–2685.
53. Njikang, G., Liu, G., and Curda, S.A., *Tadpoles from the intramolecular photo-cross-linking of diblock copolymers.* Macromolecules, 2008. **41**(15): p. 5697–5702.
54. Cheng, L., et al., *Efficient synthesis of unimolecular polymeric Janus nanoparticles and their unique self-assembly behavior in a common solvent.* Macromolecules, 2008. **41**(21): p. 8159–8166.
55. Li, R., and McCoy, B.J., *Inter- and intramolecular crosslinking kinetics: partitioning according to number of crosslinks.* Macromolecular Rapid Communications, 2004. **25**(11): p. 1059–1063.
56. Foster, E.J., Berda, E.B., and Meijer, E.W., *Metastable supramolecular polymer nanoparticles via intramolecular collapse of single polymer chains.* Journal of the American Chemical Society, 2009. **131**(20): p. 6964–6966.

Chapter 3

Polyethylene Glycol Polyester Block Copolymers: Biocompatible Carriers for Nanoparticulate Drug Delivery

David S. Hart, Yunqi Zhao, and M. Laird Forrest
The University of Kansas 2095 Constant Ave. Lawrence, KS 66045, USA
mforrest@ku.edu

Poly (ethylene oxide) (PEO)-poly(ester) copolymers are biocompatible, biodegradable diblock polymers that spontaneously form core-shell nanoparticles (i.e., micelles) in water. The hydrophobic polyester core of these micelles can solubilize small, hydrophobic drug molecules that have shown promise in the treatment of cancer and infectious diseases. This core has undergone much development in recent years to improve the stability, drug loading capacity, and release rates of drugs. The PEO shell is well known to increase the circulatory lifetime of micelles with little or no immune response. This review will emphasize PEO-poly(ε-caprolactone) polymers as self-assembled nanocarriers in order to highlight recent advances in this area.

3.1 Introduction

Many of the more than 1,000 natural products that have been approved by FDA in the last 25 years for the treatment of cancer

Handbook of Harnessing Biomaterials in Nanomedicine: Preparation, Toxicity, and Applications
Edited by Dan Peer

ISBN 978-981-4316-46-0 (Hardback), 978-981-4364-27-0 (eBook)
www.panstanford.com

and infectious diseases have very poor water solubility [1]. This problem continues today in many pharmaceutical companies, as high throughput combinatorial screening frequently identifies drug targets with low water solubility [2–4]. Traditional techniques to improve aqueous solubility, such as chemical modifications and pH adjustments to form salts from ionizable groups often reduce or destroy these drugs' therapeutic activity. Thus unmodified drugs move on to become candidates and are so hydrophobic, they cannot be delivered via intravenous infusion, or without cytotoxic delivery vehicles such as Cremophor® EL, Tween, or harsh organic solvents such as ethanol and DMSO [5]. Therefore drug delivery vehicles that can solubilize and encapsulate high concentrations of these drugs are needed to formulate these prospective drug candidates. The polyester core of these micelles can encapsulate these hydrophobic drugs because alkane-rich (e.g., pentanes in poly-ε-caprolactones) segments between these esters increase the thermodynamic affinity of the drugs to the core. Polyester cores are biodegradable through esterases *in vivo*. There are three main ester monomers commonly used as cores: ε-caprolactone, $_{D,L}$-Lactic acid, and $_{D,L}$-Lactic acid-co glycolic acid. Recently, there have been many excellent reviews on the drug delivery from micelles of PEO-poly($_{D,L}$-Lactic acid) [6–10] and PEO-poly($_{D,L}$-Lactic acid-co glycolic acid) [11–13]. Therefore this review will focus on poly(ε-caprolactone) linear, star, and substituted cores in order to highlight recent developments in this area. These include improving stability, loading capacity, and tailoring release rates.

The poly(ethylene oxide) PEO portion of PEO-polyester micelles resides at the periphery of the micelle and is often referred to as the corona or shell. PEO has been deemed a "generally regarded as safe" molecule by the FDA and has little or no immunogenicity. When the micelles are less than approximately 200 nm in diameter, uptake by the reticuloendothelial systems (RES) of the liver and the spleen is limited. This lack of immune system recognition in conjunction with reduced RES uptake dramatically increases the circulatory lifetime of these micelles [14, 15]. In order for PEO- poly(ε-caprolactone) (PCL) micelles to be clinically effective, they need to have structural integrity *in vivo*, or low critical-micelle concentrations (CMC), and control the release of the target drugs. The molecular weights of the core and the shell can be designed to optimize micelle size, CMC, encapsulation efficiency, and rate of drug release. Understanding the thermodynamic affinity of a drug molecule for the micelle core is paramount to the design of future drug delivery systems. This understanding will allow researchers to foresee problems with encapsulation and attack those problems with substituted cores, additives to increase lipophilicity, or by simply adjusting the core block length. The synthesis of these micelles, encapsulation, and release characterizations of anticancer and immunosuppressive drugs, as well as drug models will be described. The assessment of the fate of these micelles *in vivo*, cell internalization studies, pharmacokinetics of drugs and micelles, and tissue distribution studies will conclude this review.

3.1.1 Synthesis of PEO-Poly(ε-Caprolactone)

PEO-poly(ε-caprolactone) (PCL) is typically synthesized by a ring-opening polymerization of ε-caprolactone from the terminal hydroxyl of PEO (Figure 3.1). Ring-opening polymerizations are generally catalyzed by stannous (II) octoate [16] or hydrochloric acid [17] but can be non-catalytically polymerized at high temperatures (160–200°C) for several days [18]. Other catalysts such as antimony compounds suffer from toxicity [19], whereas stannous octoate is FDA approved as a food additive, and HCl is commonly used in the formulation of pharmaceutics. The extent of polymerization is verified through comparison of characteristic peak shift intensities of PEO (3.39 and 3.64 ppm) and poly(ε-caprolactone) (1.38, 1.65, 2.31, and 4.06 ppm) through H1-NMR in CDCl3 (Figure 3.2).

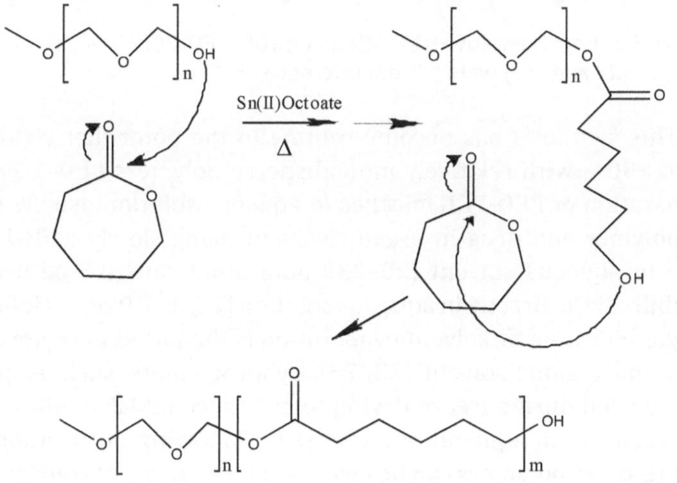

Figure 3.1 Catalyzed polymerization of PCL (m units) with methoxy PEO (n units).

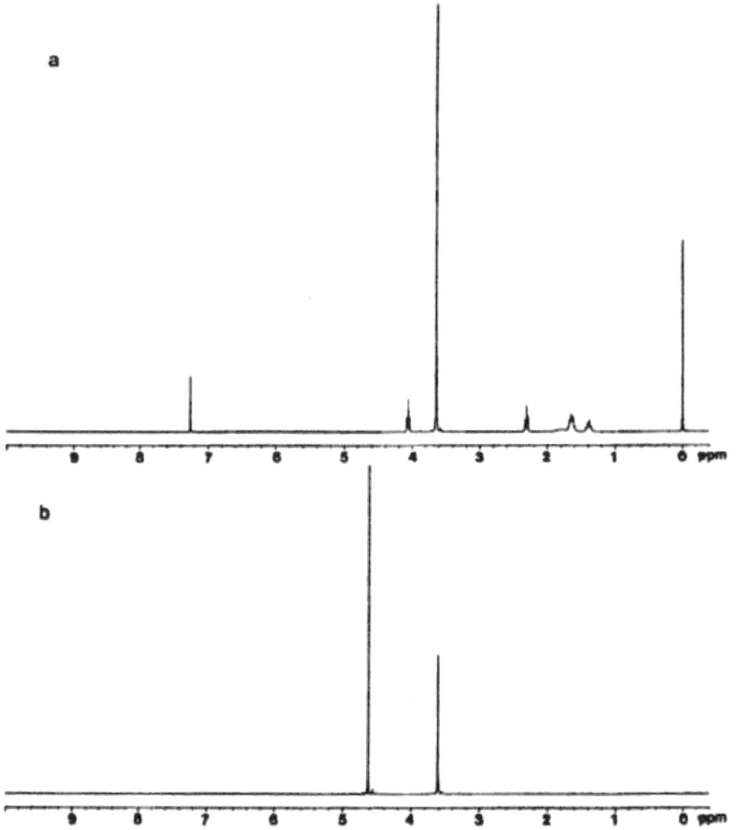

Figure 3.2 Representative H1-NMR spectra of a PEO-PCL triblock copolymer in (a) CDCl3 and (b) water. From reference [62].

This synthesis has become routine to the point that yields are often >90% with relatively monodisperse polymers (1.0–1.2). The preparation of PEO-PCL micelles in aqueous solution usually relies on polymer and drug in organic solvent being slowly added drop wise to aqueous solvent [20–23]. Sonication can also be used to solubilize PCL directly in aqueous solution [24, 25]. Dialysis followed by lyophilization or solvent evaporation is then used to remove free drug and organic solvent [22, 26]. Lyoprotectants, such as sugars can be used during freeze drying to ensure colloidal stability upon resuspension in aqueous solution [27]. Following purification and drying, these polymers can be evaluated by a variety of conventional solid characterization techniques.

3.1.2 Polymer Characterization of PEO-PCL

As PEO has been well characterized [28–30] as a polymer and in biological systems, the development of new PCL cores often warrants the copolymers characterization. PCL is a crystalline polymer, known to act as a rubber at room temperature since its glass transition temperature (T_g) is –60°C and its melting point (T_m) is 58.5°C when it is 21 kDa [31]. Thus its crystallinity is less affected through the addition of solutes into the PCL core of micelles compared with polylactic acid. Both the T_g and T_m are usually measured with DSC (differential scanning calorimetry). X-ray diffraction is also used to decipher the amorphorous or crystalline state of copolymers with or without drugs [32–34]. A variety of PEO-PCL copolymers have been developed for drug delivery: from conventional diblocks and triblocks to more exotic micelles with multi-arm stars, and substituted PCL blocks. Therefore, the following section will review the physical characterization of PEO-PCL micelles in aqueous solution.

3.1.3 Characterization of PEO-PCL Micelles

In the context of micelle-based drug delivery, encapsulation efficiency and release are irrevocably related to the equilibrium between unimers and micelles in aqueous solution. This equilibrium can be inferred indirectly from CMC measurements. The aggregation number (N_{agg}) determined from small angle neutron scattering (SANS) or fluorescent dye quenching techniques [35] provides a number average of unimers required to form a micelle. Self-diffusion coefficients of free PEO in solution obtained through NMR provide a relative scale to assess the presence of unimers in solution. This knowledge combined with the conformation and shape of the micelles provides a physical model of amphiphilic copolymer association on a thermodynamic and molecular basis. Understanding the discrete association of PEO-PCL copolymers may allow future block copolymers to be designed that do not require harsh conditions (e.g., organic solvents, sonication, or heating) to form micelles in aqueous solution. Jérôme and colleagues correlated SANS and small-angle x-ray scattering (SAXS) data with statistical mechanics models to more accurately describe the self association of PEO-PCL polymers in aqueous solution [36]. In order to dissolve the polymers directly in aqueous solution with heating a series of PEO-PCL polymers were synthesized with a constant

PEO block length of 5 kDa, and relatively short PCL blocks (0.35, 0.95, 1.5, 1.85, 2.2, and 3 kDa). The conformation of the PEO chains in the corona were determined to exist in a moderately extended geometry based on steric hindrance at the corona-core interface depicted by its low surface area. The surface area of this interface was calculated based on N_{agg}. Aggregation numbers ranged from 12 to 126 for PCL block lengths of 0.35–2.2 kDa. SANS and SAXS data were fit to various models to determine the conformation of core, which was depicted as a dense core of rods, based on the size and model. Micelle size was determined to be 20–25 nm in diameter for PCL block lengths of 0.95–2.2 kDa. Jérôme and coworkers have also shown that when micelles are formed from organic solvent and water, lower concentrations of copolymers lead to larger micelles, and depending on the solvent, the size can range from 30–100 nm [37]. The CMCs determined from surface tension data were on the order of 10^{-5}–10^{-6} M for PEO-PCL micelles with PCL block lengths ranging from 0.95–2.2 kDa. Using self-diffusion coefficients obtained from NMR, a higher content of unimers was present with smaller PCL blocks because their diffusion coefficients were very close to that of free PEO in solution. Transmission electron microscopy confirmed the spherical shape and monodispersity of the micelles. Stěpánek and coworkers characterized PEO-PCL micelles with larger PCL blocks (5, 13, and 32 kDa) at a constant PEO block length of 5 kDa with static (SLS) and dynamic light scattering (DLS) [23]. Scattering intensities and relaxation time distributions from DLS and SLS data do not indicate any dissociation dependence on concentration at low concentrations (i.e., kinetically frozen). The longer PCL blocks stabilize the micelles as is often evident through lower CMC values (Table 3.1). The geometry, block arrangement and functional groups substituted onto PCL also influence the CMC of micelles containing PEO and PCL blocks.

As expected, hydrodynamic radii and radii of gyration were comparable and thus indicative of a spherical shape. Average-density aggregation numbers (Z) were calculated from hydrodynamic radii to range from 2,300–10,900 for PCL blocks 5–32 kDa in length. These aggregation numbers were consistent with other micelles known to form vesicles at similar sizes. This implies that the inner core was liposome-like, or hollow. The diameter of these micelles increased from 80–200 nm across PCL blocks of 5–32 kDa as expected. Size distributions are normally characterized on many micelles.

Table 3.1 Influence of PCL block length, arrangement, geometry, and substitution on CMC

Copolymer	Block arrangement/ geometry	PCL Core MW range (kDa)	PEO MW (kDa)	CMC range (M)	Ref.
PEO-PCL	diblock	0.4–2.2	5.0	10^{-5}–10^{-6}	[36]
PEO-PVL	diblock	0.5–2.0	2.0	10^{-5}–10^{-6}	[53]
PEO-PVL	diblock	1.1–4.9	5.0	10^{-5}–10^{-6}	[53]
$(PEO)_6$-PVL	6-arm star	4.9–28.8[b]	11–22[b]	10^{-6}	[32]
PEO-PCCL	PCL-block w/ α-carboxylate	1.8	5.0	10^{-6}	[68]
PEO-PCL	diblock	2.5–4.0	5.0	10^{-7}	[22]
PEO-PCL	diblock	10.0	5.0	10^{-7}	[60]
PCL-PEO-PCL	triblock	4.8–7.5[a]	8.0	10^{-7}	[62]
PEO-PCL	diblock	18.0	5.0	10^{-8}	[60]
PEO-PCL	diblock	13.0–24.0	5.0	10^{-8}	[45]
PCL-PEO-PCL	triblock	15.8[a]	8.0	10^{-8}	[62]
PEO-$(PCL)_3$	3-arm star	14.2[b]	14.8	10^{-8}	[66]
PEO-$(PCL)_4$	4-arm star	20.4[b]	5.2	10^{-8}	[66]
PEO-PBCL	PCL-block w/ α-benzyl carboxylate	2.0	5.0	10^{-8}	[68]

[a]This MW is the sum of each block.

3.1.3.1 CMC measurements

Another common characterization is the CMC, or the lowest concentration of copolymer required to form a micelle, which indirectly describes the equilibrium and stability. This can be determined by measuring the fluorescent excitation intensity ratios of pyrene at 338–339 nm to 333–334 nm as a function of polymer concentration. As micelles form, pyrene preferentially localizes in the core of the micelles, and the ratio increases in this less polar environment. The CMC occurs at the onset of the increase in intensity as a function of polymer concentration.

3.1.3.2 Relative core microviscosity

As mentioned previously in Stěpánek's characterization, when the polymer concentration dependence of the longer PCL block micelles is absent at low concentration, the micelle is considered to be kinetically frozen. In this case, the equilibrium will ultimately shift to form unimers. However the core is so entangled and viscous with the larger PCL blocks, the time scale of the light scattering experiments cannot capture this. The relative core microviscosity of micelles can be estimated based the fluorescent emission intensity ratio of 1,3-bis-(1-pyrenyl)propane (dipyrene) and pyrene at 480 nm and 390 nm, respectively. Dipyrene forms an excimer when rotation is free around an alkyl chain between two pyrenes to change conformation and emits light at 480 nm (I_E). The emission of light from pyrene at 390 nm (I_M) (in competition with dipyrenes emission at 480 nm) is used as a reference to the excimer [38]. As the core becomes viscous, change in conformation is restricted, and the emission intensity at 480 nm decreases, and the ratio I_M/I_E increases. It should be noted that the I_M/I_E or I_E/I_M ratios are used interchangeably. These types of characterizations are useful in understanding release profiles of a model drug among a series of copolymers as well as the thermodynamic stability of micelles.

3.2 Drug Delivery from Diblock PEO-PCL Copolymer Micelles

In addition to knowledge of the thermodynamic stability of these micelles, understanding the thermodynamic affinity of a drug for the PCL core is also crucial for drug delivery. The impact of core length on release, biocompatibility, and efficacy *in vitro* in cell culture has been studied with a variety of lipophilic drugs, especially anti-cancer agents. Indomethacin, a hydrophobic non-steroidal anti-inflammatory drug (NSAID) was the first model drug encapsulated in diblock PEO-PCL micelles [39]. As expected, CMC's decreased with increasing hydrophobic chain length and were on the order of 10^{-7} M (Table 3.1). An encapsulation efficiency of 40% was achieved with indomethacin in PEO-PCL micelles with block molecular weights of 5 kDa and ~5.5 kDa. Release studies showed indomethacin to release in a Fickian profile over 12–14 days without a burst effect [40]. This work also showed that the micelle size increased when higher concentrations of drug were loaded, as has been seen with other drugs (fenofibrate and amiodarone) in PEO-PCL micelles [22, 41]. As shown in Table 3.2, the micelle size generally increases when the hydrophobic solute (drug) is retained in the core. This is expected as the PCL chains in the core will have a relatively small free volume (due to their crystallinity), and the inclusion of drug molecules will increase the core size, and thus the micelle size.

Table 3.2 Influence of encapsulated drug on PEO-PCL micelle size

PEO MW (kDa)	PCL MW (kDa)	Drug	Encapsulation efficiency (%)	Micelle size without drug (nm)	Micelle size with drug (nm)	Ref.
5.0	6.2	indomethacin	40	130	165	[40]
5.0	1.0	fenofibrate	29	19	22	[22]
5.0	2.5	fenofibrate	95	22	24	[22]
5.0	4.0	fenofibrate	92	33	41	[22]
5.0	5.0	CsA	52	88	100	[45]
5.0	13	CsA	64	79	99	[45]
5.0	24	CsA	50	100	102	[45]
2.0	2.0	DOX	n/a	17	25	[25]
5.0	2.5	DOX	n/a	30	23	[25]
5.0	5.0	DOX	n/a	41	37	[25]
5.0	8.5	DOX	n/a	57	84	[25]
5.0	25	DOX	n/a	86	105	[25]
5.0	6.0	rapamycin	24	31	48	[60]
5.0	6.0	rapamycin + 1:20 α-tocopherol	50	63	44	[60]
5.0	10	rapamycin	50	79	76	[60]
5.0	10	rapamycin + 1:20 α-tocopherol	73	109	107	[60]
5.0	18	rapamycin	31	40	46	[60]
5.0	18	rapamycin + 1:20 α-tocopherol	66	57	44	[60]

Allen *et al.* were first to study the biocompatibility of PEO_{44}-PCL_{20} micelles (subscripted numerals on PEO_{44}-PCL_{20} represent 44 ethylene glycol, and 20 ε-caprolactone units) with PC 12 (rat neuroendocrine tumor) and MCF-7 breast cancer cells [42]. PEO_{44}-PCL_{20} micelles with a PCL block length of 2.3 kDa, showed little cell death over a range of concentrations in the PC 12 and MCF-7 cell lines. Yet a PEO_{44}-PCL_{14} micelle with a PCL block length of 1.7 kDa induced 10–20% cell death over the same range of concentrations. This implies that the smaller micelle (PEO_{44}-PCL_{14}) may have internalized in the cell and disrupted essential metabolic functions. In the same study, *in vitro* release of FK506 (an immunosuppressive and neural outgrowth factor), and its synthetic analogue L-685,818 from the PEO_{44}-PCL_{20} micelles did not demonstrate enhanced differentiation in PC 12 cells without NGF (nerve growth factor) as was expected. Later work *in vivo* demonstrated PEO_{44}-PCL_{20} micelles containing FK506 promoted a faster recovery in Hanover-Wistar rats with crushed peripheral nerve lesions than simply injecting FK206 at the same concentration [43]. In comparison with the indomethacin loaded PEO-PCL micelles, the CMC of PEO_{44}-PCL_{20} was decreased to 10^{-8} M, and thus its *in vivo* stability was increased by increasing the length of PCL block relative to the PEO block. Dihydroxytestosterone (DHT), another highly lipophilic small molecule, was encapsulated with the PEO_{44}-PCL_{20} micelle to study its release and biological activity [44]. Similar to the release of indomethacin, DHT released in a Fickian manner and at a slower rate when the loaded concentration was increased. To assess the biological activity of DHT upon release, HeLa cells were co-transfected with MMTV-Luciferase and androgen receptor (AR). If DHT is still biologically active when it releases from the PEO_{44}-PCL_{20} micelles, then it will bind to AR and induce transcription of the luciferase gene and ultimately the translation of luciferase. This work demonstrated that the biological activity of free DHT and micelles containing DHT were equivalent in terms of luciferase expression. Therefore, the biological activity was retained upon release in cell culture.

The hydrophobic model drugs discussed until now utilized dialysis to remove free drug. This typically works for most model drugs and PEO-PCL micelles, however in the case of fenofibrate approximately 75% of the initially loaded model released during dialysis [22]. This can be overcome by loading polymer and fenofibrate in ACN, and approaching the azeotrope of water–ACN through the addition of water. The ACN can then be removed through solvent evaporation under vacuum. High loading efficiencies as great as 95% were achieved, and this efficiency was shown to have an optimal PCL block length. With constant PEO block length (5 kDa), the PCL block at 2.5 kDa loaded 95% fenofibrate, 4 kDa 90%, and 1 kDa only 30%. It would have been expected that the loading capacity would increase as the PCL block length increases. Thus the PCL block length should be optimized to obtain the highest encapsulation efficiency for each prospective drug.

Another instance of solvent evaporation in drug loading of PEO-PCL is cyclosporine A (CsA), an immunosuppressive agent with low water solubility [45]. Three different polymers were compared among loading capacity, release, and size, each with a constant PEO block molecular weight of 5 kDa, and PCL block molecular weights of 5, 13, and 24 kDa. Utilizing different solvents during solvent extraction, Aliabadi *et al.* were able to show that THF gave smaller micelles (40–86 nm in diameter) compared with acetone, which gave 80–100 nm-diameter micelles among the same series of PEO-PCL polymers. The release profile of CsA in PEO-PCL (13 kDa) was evaluated in comparison with the current formulation of CsA in Cremophor® EL (Sandimmune®) in phosphate-buffered saline (PBS) with 4% bovine serum albumin (BSA). The Cremophor® EL formulation depicted a burst-type release with approximately 80% of the drug cumulatively released at 12 h, while the PEO-PCL formulation showed a more sustained release: releasing only 10% over the same time frame. The PEO-PCL block copolymer had a lower CMC of 6×10^{-7} M compared with Cremophor® EL (4×10^{-5} M), and a lower relative micelle core viscosity, and thus diffusion of CsA was limited and the release was sustained. The same series of PEO-PCL polymers were investigated with respect to their ability to encapsulate and release the amphiphilic anti-anginal and anti-arrhythmic drug amiodarone (AMI). [41] Both a commercial formulation in the surfactant polysorbate 80 with benzyl alcohol and free AMI precipitate immediately upon dilution in aqueous milieu and induce red blood cell hemolysis. Increasing the length of the PCL block increased the loading amount of the amphiphilic drug AMI and reduced hemolysis in Sprague-Dawley rats. Only 20–40% of AMI in PEO-PCL (13 kDa) micelles precipitated after a 2× dilution into PBS at 37°C compared with 100% precipitation for free AMI. However, it should be noted that when 5 mg of AMI was loaded in PEO-PCL micelles, the amount precipitated nearly doubled compared with micelles loaded with 2 mg of AMI. PEO-PCL (13 kDa) micelles with 2 mg AMI induced 90% less hemolysis compared with equivalent free AMI over a two order magnitude concentration range. When this same micelle was loaded to 5 mg AMI, the extent of hemolysis was equivalent to free AMI. Thus, both the amount of drug loaded and the PCL block length should be optimized in preformulation of prospective drug candidates.

3.2.1 Drug Delivery of Anti-Cancer Agents from Diblock PEO-PCL Micelles

Since PEO-PCL micelles can protect from some unwanted drug side effects, it is useful to understand how they deliver cytotoxic, hydrophobic drugs often used in chemotherapy. One of the most widely used chemotherapeutic agents is doxorubicin (DOX), an anthracyline antibiotic that induces apoptosis in tumor-specific cells [46–49]. A series of PEO-PCL polymers were synthesized with varying PCL block lengths (2–24.7 kDa) to investigate the cytotoxicity of these micelles and their ability to load and release DOX [25]. Varying the PCL core length did not increase the loading capacity as seen with other model drugs, maximizing at 3–4% w/w DOX. However, no detectable hemolysis was induced at concentrations as high as 200 μg/mL DOX in PEO-PCL (5 and 24.7 kDa), compared with 11% hemolysis at the same concentration for free DOX. Dynamic light scattering showed substantial increases in polymer size with increases in PCL block length (22–100 nm in diameter). At pH 7.4, DOX was cumulatively released slightly faster (~15%) with a 24.7 kDa PCL block compared with a 5 kDa (~10%) over 35 days. At pH 5, the cumulative release was accelerated to 80% in the 24.7 kDa block, and to 60% in the 5 kDa block over the same time frame as pH 7.4. Slightly acidic conditions may have increased the rate of ester degradation in the core. However, it is more likely that the increase in release rate is due to the lowered octanol–water partition coefficient at reduced pHs (the Log Po/w of DOX is 5.1 at pH 7.4 and 0.2 at pH 5) [50]. The fact that the larger block length accelerated release at both pHs, suggests that the PCL core viscosity was reduced, potentially due to an increased volume of core. This unexpected release behavior will be analyzed further with respect to thermodynamic affinity. It is important to notice the increased rate of release at lower pH in relation to cancer therapy because tumor microenvironments are often slightly hypoxic.

Paclitaxel is a lipophilic small-molecule drug highly successful in the treatment of breast, ovarian, and lung cancers. Paclitaxel loading, cell culture release, and biocompatibility studies have been investigated with a series of PEO-poly(δ-valerolactone) (PVL) micelles by Allen and coworkers [53]. δ-Valerolactone is identical to ε-caprolactone except that the lactone ring contains only five carbons instead of six in ε-caprolactone; thus it is slightly less lipophilic. This slight reduction in lipophilicity may account for the higher CMC's 10^{-5}–10^{-6} M over a range of PVL block lengths (0.5–5 kDa) at two different PEO block lengths (2 and 5 kDa). The reason the reduction in lipophilicity may increase the CMC is because the micellization is based on the net difference in thermodynamic affinity between the water and PEO, and the difference of PVL and other PVL chains. The greater the affinity of the core chains for themselves induces a lower CMC. The PEO-PVL copolymer with both blocks being 2 kDa in molecular weight was found to retain the highest paclitaxel loaded concentration (9 mg/mL) following centrifugation and sterile filtration. This result was expected because all loaded micelles except this polymer had diameters on the order of magnitude of the filter. Thus filtration could have physically disrupted the micelle structure. These copolymers were shown to be biocompatible with a CHO-K1 cell line up to concentrations of 1 g/L. This micelle formulation increased paclitaxel aqueous solubility 9000-fold, and was found to biologically active upon release in MCF-7 breast and A2780 ovarian cancer cell lines. Although the loading potential of this class of micelles would only require 28 mL of a 10 wt% copolymer solution for ovarian cancer and Kaposi's sarcoma treatment, lesser administered volumes would be desired.

In order to potentially increase paclitaxel loading and decrease this administered volume, PEO-PCL polymers have been synthesized with a terminal maleic cap on the PCL end to crosslink the core [54]. This maleic-capped diblock was then activated with thionyl chloride, and subjected to radical polymerization with a potassium peroxodisulfate initiator. A series of diblock and triblock copolymers were synthesized with PEO block lengths of 2 and 5 kDa, and PCL blocks lengths ranging from 1.2–18 kDa. As the PCL block length increased, the paclitaxel loading efficiency increased as expected. As much as 85% of the loaded paclitaxel was encapsulated in a diblock

PEO (5 kDa)-PCL (18 kDa) copolymer. Although triblock copolymers will be covered in a following section, it is worthwhile to note that 72% of paclitaxel was loaded into the PEO (5 kDa)-PCL (18 kDa)-PEO (5 kDa). It is likely that a PCL (18 kDa)-PEO (5 kDa)-PCL (18 kDa) triblock would be superior in paclitaxel loading. However, this copolymer upon radical polymerization would likely phase separate from solution. Therefore, the diblock copolymer with the largest PCL core would remain the best option for a potential paclitaxel formulation. Aside from paclitaxel, there are some anticancer compounds that have a series of derivatives, which each have different levels of cytotoxicity.

Cucurbitacins, a family of STAT3 onco-signaling inhibitors, or have an interesting trend where derivatives' cytotoxicity is linearly related to hydrophobicity [55]. In this case, it may be feasible to utilize the same core with different block lengths for a series of derivatives. Molavi *et al.* investigated the release, and *in vitro* and *in vivo* activity of cucurbitacin I and B from PEO-PCL and poly(α-benzyl carboxylate ε-caprolactone)(PBCL)-PEO micelles. The addition of a benzylic carboxylate functional group to the PCL core increases the lipophilicity, and thus smaller block lengths compared with conventional PCL may facilitate similar thermodynamic affinities of the target drug to the core. A series of diblock copolymers employing a PEO block length of 5 kDa, PCL blocks of 5 or 24 kDa, or PBCL at 4.7 kDa were utilized to encapsulate cucurbitacin I and B. Cucurbitacin B differs only in an acetyl group in place of a hydroxyl at the 25′ position of cucurbitacin I [56]. Therefore cucurbitacin B has an axis of symmetric polarity, and is slightly more lipophilic than cucurbitacin I. The loading efficiency increases with PCL block length for both derivatives (~30–65%). However a substantial increase in efficiency occurs with cucurbitacin B in the 4.7 kDa PBCL core (92%) over cucurbitacin I (74%). This increase could be due to the greater lipophilicity of cucurbitacin B. All release profiles were Fickian, and the PEO-PCL (5 kDa) and PEO-PBCL (4.7 kDa) profiles were nearly identical for both derivatives. At 8 h, approximately all of the cucurbitacin I had been released, whereas 40–60% of cucurbitacin B was released. The sustained release of cucurbitacin B could be due to its lower polarity increased affinity for the non-polar core. Cucurbitacin I in PEO-PCL (24 kDa) was more potent (IC50 of 10 μM) than cucurbitacin B (IC50 of 50 μM) against a B16.F10 cell line (melanoma of C57/black origin) after 24 h. For both derivatives the IC50 of free cucurbitacin in methanol was approximately half of the IC50 of cucurbitacin released from PEO-PCL micelles. However, there was no statistical difference in terms of *in vivo* tumor volume upon treatment with free and PEO-PCL encapsulated cucurbitacin I as both virtually abolished growth. If a targeting moiety to the tumor (e.g., EGF [57], Her2/neu [58], PSMA [59]) was desired to cover the micelle and enhance *in vivo* activity, the micelle size may need to be reduced.

Additives may be used to improve encapsulation efficiency and potentially the release of the drug from the core while maintaining *in vivo* activity. Rapamycin, an inhibitor of cell proliferation in solid tumors, has been efficiently encapsulated into PEO-PCL micelle cores with the coaddition of α-tocopherol (Vitamin E) [60]. In this study, a series of PEO-PCL micelles with a constant PEO block length of 5 kDa and varying PCL block lengths of 6, 10, and 18 kDa were used to encapsulate and release rapamycin. α-Tocopherol is more lipophilic than a single unit of caprolactone, and will partition into the PCL core and provide greater thermodynamic affinity of rapamycin for the core; rapamycin is extremely lipophilic with an octanol–water partition coefficient of 5.8. As expected, the CMC of these micelles decreased with increasing PCL block length and were on the order of 10^{-7}–10^{-8} M. The addition of α-tocopherol in molar ratio of 1:10 and 1:20 to PEO-PCL demonstrated negligible increases in the CMC. However, addition of α-tocopherol beyond the ratio of 1:20 shifted the phase equilibria of the PEO-PCL-water system to precipitate as particles greater than 400 nm. Encapsulation efficiencies were increased with 1:20 molar ratios of α-tocopherol in each PEO-PCL micelle, with an apparent optimum PCL block length of 10 kDa resulting in 72% efficiency. The PEO-PCL micelles with 18 kDa PCL blocks encapsulated only 66%. As the reduction in efficiency compared with the 10 kDa block was unexpected, it foreshadowed precipitation in release studies. Thus the addition of rapamycin to PEO-PCL micelles loaded with α-tocopherol further shifted the phase equilibria of the PEO-PCL-water system to precipitate as seen with higher molar ratios (>1:20 α-tocopherol). The release of rapamycin in saline was not significantly impacted by α -tocopherol. However, in 4% BSA, α-tocopherol greatly improved the sustained release characteristics. This may be due to the improved affinity of rapamycin for the α-tocopherol-rich micelle core compared with BSA. In some cases, the addition of hydrophobic additives may not provide extended release or increased encapsulation. Also, the most efficient design of a core for natural product delivery is not always intuitive, as was the case of DOX in which a larger core actually accelerated the release. This trend was contrary to the release of other anticancer compounds with increased PCL block lengths. Since all of these compounds are usually polycyclic lipophilic compounds with a slight dipole, it is useful to resolve this disparity, and gain an understanding of drug-core affinity for future core designs.

3.2.2 Flory–Huggins Interaction Parameters Between Drugs and Polymeric Cores

Flory–Huggins interaction parameters have been employed to evaluate the thermodynamic affinity of geldanamycin prodrugs, among other anti-cancer agents for PCL cores [33]. Geldanamycin (GA) (Figure 3.3) is known to inhibit the ATP binding pocket of Hsp90, which reduces a cancer cells ability to refold essential proteins and eventually survive. The interaction parameter analysis facilitated the design of a novel type of prodrug, and illustrated how increasing lipophilicity of a target drug can increase the micelle loading capacity, and ultimately the aqueous solubility. Using functional group contributions of the drug and PCL chain, partial solubility parameters were estimated, and Flory–Huggins interaction parameter was calculated. When this interaction parameter approaches zero, the PCL chain is completely solvated with drug. A series of GA derivatives were synthesized with varying lengths of aliphatic chains at the 17′ position, and were evaluated with MCF-7 breast cancer cells to gauge the potency relative to GA. Most of these derivatives cytotoxicity was reduced at least an order of magnitude, however one bromoester derivative, 17-(ethylamino-2-bromododecȯnate)-17-demethoxygeldanamycin (GA 17′ C16Br) (Figure 3.3) IC50 reduced by only a factor of 5 (110 nM). As shown in Figure 3.3b, the ethylamine ester at the 17′ position will hydrolyze *in vivo* to activate the drug, and the addition of the electron withdrawing group (Br) increases the lability of the ester bond, decreasing the half-life.

GA was poorly soluble in PEO (5 kDa)-PCL (10 kDa) micelles, however GA 17′ C16Br's solubility was increased two orders of magnitude over GA and its loading efficiency approached 100% in the same micelle. Release studies of GA 17′ C16Br at physiological conditions demonstrated a Fickian sustained release over 2 weeks. The Flory–Huggins interaction parameter is a useful tool to understand thermodynamic affinity of a drug for a micelle core. As the interaction parameter would likely decrease with increased molecular weight of the PCL block[61], it is likely that DOX has a higher value interaction parameter than cucurbitacin with PCL.

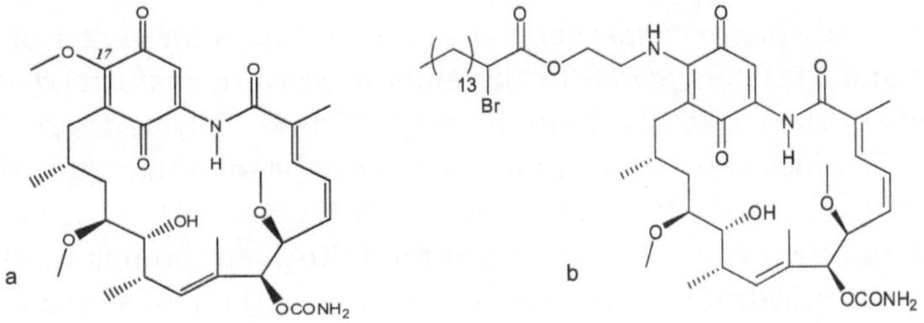

Figure 3.3 (a) Geldanamycin, and its (b) bromoester prodrug, GA 17′C16Br.

3.2.3 Drug Delivery from Triblock Copolymer Micelles of PEO and PCL Blocks

The first triblock PCL-PEO-PCL micelles used as a delivery vehicle were used to characterize the drug loading capacity and release of the model drug clonazepam [62]. Three triblock copolymers were investigated with each PCL chain being 2.4, 3.8, or 8.5 kDa and the PEO block of 8 kDa was constant among this series. The synthesis and preparation of the triblock copolymer micelles was similar to that of diblock PEO-PCL micelles, except the initiation of polymerization occurred on each end of the PEO chain. The loading efficiency of clonazepam was shown to range from 12–26% depending on the initial organic solvent. As expected the loading efficiency increased with PCL block length. Also similar to the diblock PEO-PCL micelles, these triblock micelles had CMC's on the order of 10^{-7}–10^{-8} M and were 20–30 nm in diameter. Clonazepam was released in a sustained Fickian manner over a period of 4 days. Similar release behavior has been seen in other triblock micelles of PEO, PCL, and PVL blocks with nimodipine [63], indomethacin [64], and 4′-demethylepipodophyllotoxin (DMEP) [65]. Although the triblock micelles have larger lipophilic cores, the drug loading efficiencies, capacities, and release behavior are not substantially improved compared with diblock PEO-PCL micelles. Therefore micelles with more dense lipophilic cores have been developed, such as substituted PCL blocks and star copolymers.

3.2.4 Drug Delivery from Star Copolymer Micelles of PEO and PCL

Three and Four arm star copolymers with PCL as the center of the star and PEO conjugated to the ends have were characterized in terms of their size distribution and CMC [66]. Polymerization for the PCL block was initiated off of pentaerythritol terminating with a hydroxyl, for the four-star copolymers (Figure 3.4). A carboxylic acid was then added to one end of the PEO chain through reacting succinic anhydride with a terminal hydroxyl. The PEO's carboxylic acid was then attacked by the hydroxyl of the four-star PCL block. For three-star armed copolymers, diblock PEO-PCL copolymers were conjugated to the 1,3,5-Benzenetricarboxylic acid (initiator) through PCL, after activating the initiator with thionyl chloride. The diblock PEO-PCL copolymers used for the three-star-armed copolymers had CMCs on the order of 10^{-7} M, and the CMC of the three- and four-star copolymers was sequentially lowered from 5×10^{-8} M to 2×10^{-8} M, respectively. This study demonstrated that effectively increasing the number of arms branched off of the core did increase the stability of the micelles through lower CMCs. It should be noted that when the ends of the star copolymers have PCL blocks with large enough molecular weights and the center is PEO; these polymers can gel and even phase separate in aqueous solution [67].

Another study evaluated the drug delivery potential of four-arm PCL-PEO star copolymers with all-trans-retinoic acid (*at*RA) [34]. This work characterized a four-arm center block of PCL (19.6 kDa) with 2 kDa PEO conjugated to each end. Micelles were formed by drop-wise precipitation from organic solvent into water, or by sonicating a polymer and drug suspension in water. Sonication produced larger micelles (144 nm in diameter compared with 77 nm) and had higher loading efficiencies (10% compared with 6%). Additionally, micelles produced by sonication extended the cumulative release of *at*RA to 40% at 170 h, compared with the complete release of *at*RA in drop wise prepared micelles over the same time frame. To further increase the stability of these micelles, Allen and colleagues developed six-arm-star copolymers, using

PVL in the center of the star with PEO at the terminal ends [32]. Polymerization of PVL was initiated off of dipentaerythritol and PEO was coupled to the PVL ends. These micelles had somewhat lower CMC's on the order of 10^{-6} M than the diblock PEO-PVL micelles. As much as star copolymers have contributed to our knowledge of the range of copolymer block geometries that will form micelles, the development to this point has only slightly increased their stability. Therefore, PEO-PCL diblock copolymers with functional groups coupled to the PCL were developed.

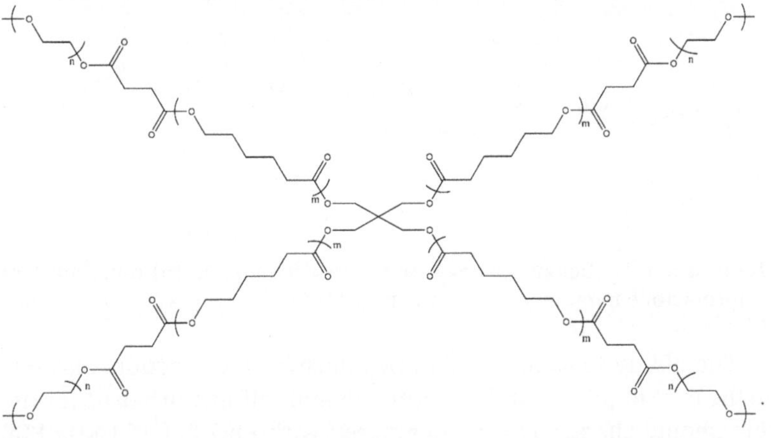

Figure 3.4 Structure of (a) four-arm star PEO-PCL block copolymer. From reference [66].

3.2.5 Drug Delivery from Substituted Diblock PEO-PCL Copolymer Micelles

Lavasanifar and coworkers synthesized α-substituted ε-caprolactone monomers (Figure 3.5) with functional substituents of benzyl carboxylate or carboxylic acid to produce PEO-poly(α-benzyl carboxylate ε-caprolactone) (PBCL) and PEO-poly(α-carboxylate ε-caprolactone) (PCCL) [68]. Also, functional groups such as hydroxyls, carboxylic acids and epoxides can be grafted onto the PCL chain post-post polymerization via atom transfer radical addition reactions or Michael-type additions [69–71].

The addition of benzyl carboxylate or carboxylic acid demonstrated how the CMC can be tuned within a PEO-PCL copolymer with nominally the same block lengths. A 5 kDa PEO block was used for each copolymer prepared. With a PBCL block length of 2 kDa, the CMC was 8 × 10^{-8} M, whereas a typical PEO-PCL diblock with a PCL block length of 5 kDa has a CMC twice that. Conversely, the addition of a carboxylic acid functional group to a slightly smaller PCL block (1.8 kDa) increased the CMC of the PEO-PCL diblock by two orders of magnitude. It should be noted that the addition of the benzyl carboxylate function group increased the micelle size to 60 nm over the typical PEO-PCL (5 kDa) diblock (40 nm).

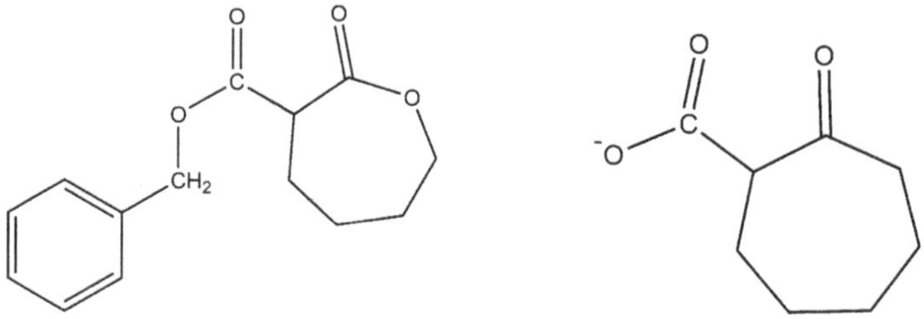

(a) (b)

Figure 3.5 (a) α-benzyl carboxylate ε-caprolactone and (b) α-carboxylate ε-caprolactone monomers. From reference [68].

The ability to tune the CMC by adjusting the functional groups on the core implies that the thermodynamic affinity of a drug for the core should change as well. Compared with PEO-PCL (24 kDa PCL block), a PEO-PBCL micelle with one-fifth of the PCL block length increased the encapsulation efficiency of cucurbitacin B almost 30%. However, the cumulative release from the PBCL core was slightly faster than the 24 kDa PCL core. Nonetheless, the increases in stability and encapsulation efficiency for some drugs are superior to typical diblock PEO-PCL copolymers.

3.3 Characterization of Cellular Uptake and Pre-Clinical Efficacy *in vivo*

As a first step in understanding what happens to these micelles *in vivo*, the micelle-cell interaction was studied extensively *in vitro* in multiple cell lines. It is well known that when PEO chains reside at the corona, they impart negative zeta potentials on the micelles [72–74]. A smaller PEO chain would increase the magnitude of this negative zeta potential because the layer of bound water is smaller than that of micelles with larger PEO chains. Negative zeta potential increases the micelles' uptake by macrophages of the mononuclear phagocyte system [74, 75].

3.3.1 Cellular Internalization of PEO-PCL Micelles

As this macrophage uptake would represent one mode of the micelles clearance *in vivo*, it is also important to understand how these micelles interact with other cells. This question has typically been addressed through the use of fluorescent dyes or radioactive compounds. Both of these approaches were used to demonstrate that the cellular uptake of PEO_{44}-PCL_{20} micelles in a PC 12 cell line was temperature and pH dependent [76] in a manner indicative of endocytosis uptake mechanisms. Mahmud *et al.* studied the uptake of various PEO-PCL micelles with different PCL block lengths in MCF-7 breast cancer cells [21]. These micelles were loaded with a lipophilic fluorescent dye, DiI, and the mechanism of endocytic uptake was investigated with chlorpromazine and cytochalasin B. An optimal PCL block length of 13 kDa, and PEO block length of 5 kDa demonstrated the highest cellular uptake. Chlorpromazine is known to inhibit clathrin-mediated endocytosis by reducing clathrin-coated pit formation at the cellular membrane, while cytochalasin B inhibits phagocytosis through disruption of microfilament bundles at the cell membrane. Both endocytosis inhibiting agents reduced uptake at the optimal block lengths of PEO and PCL. Incubation of MCF-7 cells at 4°C in the absence of these agents also reduced uptake. This suggests an energy-dependent uptake mechanism, which further supports both clathrin-mediated endocytosis and phagocytosis.

3.3.2 Cellular Distribution of PEO-PCL Micelles

Further work investigated the cellular distribution of PEO_{45}-PCL_{23} micelles with tetramethylrhodamine-5-carbonyl azide (TMRCA) conjugated to the end of the PCL block in PC 12 and NIH 3T3 cell lines [77]. Although PEO is known prevent protein adsorption, and had been shown to reduce uptake of PEO:PLGA nanoparticles in human monocytes [78], not all of the PEO-PCL micelles were excluded from these cell lines. Using a series of organelle and nuclear selective dyes, it was found that PEO-PCL was primarily taken up into cytoplasmic organelles, specifically the Golgi apparatus and mitochondria. Shuai *et al.* also saw DOX with PEO-PCL micelles localized to the cytoplasm, as opposed to free DOX localized in the nucleus [25]. Cisplatin, another anti-cancer agent was encapsulated with 73% efficiency into PEO-PCL micelles and was taken up into SKOV-3 ovarian cancer cells [72]. However its localization to endocytic vesicles in the cytoplasm retarded its potential cytotoxicity compared with pH-sensitive micelles localizing the drug in the nucleus. Thus PEO-PCL micelles are endocytosed into a variety of cell lines, and typically localize in endocytic vesicles in the cytoplasm. Although the majority of the drug is likely be released independent of cellular internalization, if the drug requires localization in the nucleus, there may be reduced efficacy *in vivo*.

3.3.3 Efficacy and Stability of PEO-PCL Micelle Drug Delivery *in vivo*

Micelles of PEO-PCL have demonstrated sustained release, improved solubilization, and good efficacy *in vitro*. Lavasanifar and coworkers examined the pharmacokinetics and biodistribution of CsA released from PEO-PCL micelles in Sprague-Dawley rats compared with the current formulation in Cremophor® EL [79]. The PEO-PCL micelles with PCL block lengths of 5 and 13 kDa both encapsulated approximately 30% of the drug and were nominally 100 nm in saline. These micelles increased both the blood and plasma CsA concentrations approximately 6-fold and reduced the volume of distribution and clearance 10- and 8-fold, respectively. The pharmacokinetics of these micelles imposed lower concentration distributions of CsA in all organs except the heart. Most paramount, the PEO-PCL micelles reduced the concentration in the kidneys, the primary site of toxicity.

Rapamycins pharmacokinetics and tissue distribution in rats was investigated upon release from PEO-PCL micelles with and without α-tocopherol, compared with the current solution formulation of Tween 80/PEO400/*N,N* dimethylacetamide [80]. The blood and plasma concentrations were not significantly increased with the PEO-PCL micelles with or without α-tocopherol. However, the micelles with α-tocopherol had a reduced volume of distribution and clearance. Additionally, the organ distribution of rapamycin was significantly reduced in PEO-PCL micelles with α-tocopherol liver, kidney, spleen, brain, lung, and heart. PEO-PCL micelles optimally reduced rapamycin distribution compared with micelles with α-tocopherol and the control formulation. As rapamycin demonstrates acute neurotoxicity, it is worthwhile to note its significant decrease in the brain with PEO-PCL micelles. Also important to the administration of micelle-delivered drugs is the fate of the micelle.

3.3.3.1 Fate of PEO-PCL micelles *in vivo*

To prevent a burst release *in vivo*, it is important that the micelles are stable. The equilibrium between unimers and micelles *in vivo* as well as the CMC are necessary to understand the proper polymer concentration administered. Liu *et al.* have evaluated this equilibrium for PEO-PCL micelles in Balb/C mice [17]. Three PEO-PCL micelles with a constant PCL block length of 5 kDa and PEO block lengths of 2, 5, 10 kDa were evaluated. The PEO-PCL with a PEO block length of 5 kDa was the most stable retaining a monomodal size distribution according to DLS at physiological conditions with 4.5% BSA over 10 days. PEO-PCL copolymers were incubated with mouse plasma for 5 h and 37°C at concentrations an order of magnitude below the CMC. No significant interactions between the plasma and micelles were found. Tritium labeled [^{3}H] PEO-PCL micelles were injected into the tail vein of Balb/C mice and samples were analyzed via a scintillation counter. At copolymer concentrations 70-fold above the CMC (250 mg/kg, upon dilution in the mice), 74% of the micelles were intact in the plasma after 24 h according to gel filtration chromatography. At copolymer concentrations 2-fold below the CMC (2 mg/kg upon dilution), 55% of the micelles remained intact after 24 h. The tissue distribution of PEO-PCL at 250 mg/kg and 2 mg/kg remained at approximately 10% of the initial dose for each concentration in the liver through 48 h. Other tissue distribution studies of PEO-PCL micelles have noted the increased uptake in the liver due to their size being less than 70 nm [81]. Between 1% and 5% of the initial dose was retained in the heart, kidney, spleen, and lung through 48 h for the same doses. However when 0.2 mg/kg PEO-PCL was administered, the accumulation in the liver rose from 10% of the initial dose to approximately 40% through 48 h. Between 5% and 10% of the initial dose remained in the heart, kidney, spleen, and lung through 48 h. The higher retention of this dose (0.2 mg/kg) in organs may be a reflection of the pharmacokinetics. At 0.2 mg/kg, the PEO-PCL micelle was rapidly cleared from the plasma in approximately 12 h. However, the 2 mg/kg dose wasn't cleared from the plasma until 50 h, and the 250 mg/kg dose had 20% of the initial dose retained in the plasma over the same time frame. Also, the volumes of distribution were quite high (four times the total blood volume of the mouse). This indicates a broad tissue distribution likely resulting from the amphiphilic nature of the PEO-PCL copolymer. Thus, the optimization of the block lengths of PEO for stability *in vitro* translated over to stability *in vivo* based on the pharmacokinetics and thermodynamic stability.

3.3.3.2 Stability of PEO-PCL micelles *in vivo*

Another approach to evaluating *in vivo* stability utilizes conjugated fluorescent dyes to PEO_{45}-PCL_{21} copolymers [82]. A derivative of 5-fluorescein cadaverine (F-5-CADA) was conjugated to the terminal end of the PCL chain to investigate the stability of the PEO_{45}-PCL_{21} micelles in PBS with 5% fetal bovine serum (FBS). F-5-CADA is not fluorescent, but becomes fluorescent upon hydrolytic cleavage in water. Through 48 h only 2% of the dye was fluorescent from the micelle solution. Thus these micelles were stable, because the intact micelles displayed virtually no fluorescence and the free dye emitted 33% fluorescence through 48 h and at the same conditions. The reason the free dye emitted only 33% is due to the slow partial hydrolytic activation in PBS. In RPMI-1640 cell culture medium with and without FBS, the micelles were less stable. Through 48 h in RPMI without serum, the PEO-PCL micelles had 13% activation, compared with 83% for free dye. The presence of serum drastically reduced the stability of the micelles as RPMI with 5% FBS, and FBS without RPMI activated 64% and 74% respectively. The free dye was fully activated in FBS without RPMI, while 83% of the free dye was activated in RPMI with 5% FBS. These results demonstrate that FBS is an excellent screening agent for the stability of micelles since the equilibrium between micelles and unimers is media dependent. The stability of the micelles in FBS at 10 and 100 times the CMC depicted modest increases in stability (10–12%) with similar activations of F-5-CADA to those already mentioned. When these micelles were incubated with T24 human bladder carcinoma cells, an increase in fluorescence due to disruption of PEO_{45}-PCL_{21}-F-5-CADA micelles was seen with time in lysed cells and was substantial at 18 h (approx 70% of maximum). Intravenous bolus injections of PEO_{45}-PCL_{21}-F-5-CADA micelles showed accumulation in the bladder of hairless SKH-1 mice. This implies that the filtration in the kidneys disrupted these micelles. Both subcutaneous and intramuscular injections showed an increase in fluorescence signal at the site of injection after 1 h. These results suggest that subcutaneous and intramuscular injection provide a means for micelles to simply solubilize a drug and then be site-injected to a target organ or a solid tumor that is inoperable. Alternatively, if blanket coverage of the circulatory system needs to be to be treated as is the case in metastatic cancers, intravenous injection of the micelles would be the preferred route. Conjugated fluorescence dyes to PEO-PCL micelles *in vitro* and *in vivo* will play an important role in pre-clinical evaluation of micelle delivered drugs.

Although stability of the micelles *in vivo* is an important factor to consider, sometimes micelles need to protect the drug from degradation. This is the case with curcumin, a anti-cancer agent known to down regulate genes associated with angiogenesis of tumors [83]. PEO-PCL micelles with a PEO block length of 5 kDa and PCL with a block length of 13 kDa were used to deliver curcumin to investigate the pharmacokinetics in Sprague-Dawley rats [84]. In this study, the micelle formulation of curcumin was compared with a solubilized formulation employing dimethylacetamide, PEG 400, and isotonic dextran. High-performance liquid chromatography (HPLC) was used to analyze curcumin in plasma. Since curcumin is rapidly hydrolytically degraded, the soluble formulation had a half-life of only 0.5 h, while the PEO-PCL formulation increased this half-life approximately 120-fold. After 2 h, HPLC wasn't able to detect curcumin from the soluble formulation, whereas curcumin from the PEO-PCL micelle formulation was detectable for 2 days. Not only did the PEO-PCL micelles protect curcumin from degradation, it also increased the solubility several orders of magnitude.

Another anticancer agent, 10-hydroxycamptothecin (HCPT), is a powerful antitumor drug against lung, ovarian, breast, and stomach cancers. Yet it is limited therapeutically due to its poor water solubility and a short half-life *in vivo*. PEO-PCL micelles were used to encapsulate HCPT and were injected into Wistar rats and S_{180} tumor bearing mice to evaluate the pharmacokinetics and tissue distribution [73]. A series of PEO-PCL micelles with variations in the hydrophilic PEO block length and lipophilic PCL block length were shown to have CMC's on the order of 10^{-7}–10^{-8} M. Radiolabeled ^{125}I-HCPT had greater tumor specificity and increased half-life in micelles with PEO block lengths of 10 kDa, compared with 2 or 5 kDa PEO blocks. Thus not only should the PCL block be optimized in preclinical studies, but so should the PEO block.

3.4 Concluding Remarks

PEO-PCL micelles have many advantages many harsh traditional pharmaceutical excipients (e.g., Cremophor® EL or Tween 80) for poorly water soluble drugs. They have been shown to be biocompatible with multiple cell lines, can provide extended release, and can retain a drugs biological activity *in vitro* and *in vivo*. One important factor in the design of future PEO-PCL cores is the achievement of the lowest possible CMC's (Table 3.1) to maximize micelle stability. In terms of drug solubilization, increasing PCL block length with very poorly water soluble or lipophilic drugs usually increases encapsulation efficiency due to the lowered core polarity and increased viscosity. In addition to optimizing core block length, it is possible to crosslink the core and use very lipophilic additives such as α-tocopherol to improve drug solubility. Increasing the number of core chains relative to the corona through use of triblocks or star copolymers, though a viable alternative to diblocks, does not significantly improve the stability of these micelles nor increase the encapsulation efficiency. Micelles stability does improve with increased PCL chain length or by adding highly lipophilic substituent functional groups such as α-benzyl carboxylate (Table 3.1). Conversely, the CMC will increase with the addition of hydrophilic functional groups such as carboxylic acids. Once the micelle structure has been optimized for *in vitro* solubility and release, it is then relevant to evaluate the delivery vehicle in cell culture and *in vivo*. A certain percentage of PEO-PCL micelles can enter cells through a combination of clathrin-mediated endocytosis and phagocytosis. Once the micelles have entered the cells they tend to localize in cytoplasmic organelles, specifically the Golgi apparatus and mitochondria. PEO-PCL micelles have been shown to enhance the pharmacokinetics of drugs *in vivo* by increasing their circulatory half-life and altering their tissue distribution. Micelles can also protect red blood cell hemolysis upon injection. During *in vivo* studies, optimization of the PEO block length can increase the half-life of some drugs. With the development of new PCL core chemistries, core stability may be increased with new substituents or new exotic geometries.

References

1. Clardy, J., and Walsh, C. (2004). Lessons from natural molecules. *Nature* 432: 829–837.

2. Gordon, E. M., Barrett, R. W., Dower, W. J., Fodor, S. P., and Gallop, M. A. (1994). Applications of combinatorial technologies to drug discovery. 2. Combinatorial organic synthesis, library screening strategies, and future directions. *J Med Chem* 37: 1385–1401.

3. Stockwell, B. R. (2004). Exploring biology with small organic molecules. *Nature* 432: 846–854.

4. Lipinski, C. A., Lombardo, F., Dominy, B. W., and Feeney, P. J. (2001). Experimental and computational approaches to estimate solubility and permeability in drug discovery and development settings. *Adv Drug Deliv Rev* 46: 3–26.

5. Pawar, R., Shikanov, A., Vaisman, B., and Domb, A. J. (2004). Intravenous and regional paclitaxel formulations. *Curr Med Chem* 11: 397–402.

6. Nahar, M., *et al.* (2006). Functional polymeric nanoparticles: an efficient and promising tool for active delivery of bioactives. *Crit Rev Ther Drug Carrier Syst* 23: 259–318.

7. Yasugi, K., Nagasaki, Y., Kato, M., and Kataoka, K. (1999). Preparation and characterization of polymer micelles from poly(ethylene glycol)-poly(D,L-lactide) block copolymers as potential drug carrier. *J Control Release* 62: 89–100.

8. Croy, S. R., and Kwon, G. S. (2006). Polymeric micelles for drug delivery. *Curr Pharm Des* 12: 4669–4684.

9. Kataoka, K., Harada, A., and Nagasaki, Y. (2001). Block copolymer micelles for drug delivery: design, characterization and biological significance. *Adv Drug Deliv Rev* 47: 113–131.

10. Aliabadi, H. M., and Lavasanifar, A. (2006). Polymeric micelles for drug delivery. *Expert Opin Drug Deliv* 3: 139–162.

11. Avgoustakis, K. (2004). Pegylated poly(lactide) and poly(lactide-co-glycolide) nanoparticles: preparation, properties and possible applications in drug delivery. *Curr Drug Deliv* 1: 321–333.

12. Yoo, H. S., and Park, T. G. (2001). Biodegradable polymeric micelles composed of doxorubicin conjugated PLGA-PEG block copolymer. *J Control Release* 70: 63–70.

13. Moghimi, S. M., Hunter, A. C., and Murray, J. C. (2001). Long-circulating and target-specific nanoparticles: theory to practice. *Pharmacol Rev* 53: 283–318.

14. Harris, J. M., Martin, N. E., and Modi, M. (2001). Pegylation: a novel process for modifying pharmacokinetics. *Clin Pharmacokinet* 40: 539–551.

15. He, X. H., Shaw, P. C., and Tam, S. C. (1999). Reducing the immunogenicity and improving the *in vivo* activity of trichosanthin by site-directed pegylation. *Life Sci* 65: 355–368.

16. Pitt, C. G. (1990). Poly(ε-caprolactone) and its copolymers. In *Biodegradable Polymers as Drug Delivery Systems* (M. Chasin and R. Langer, Eds.). Marcel Dekker, New York, NY.
17. Liu, J., Zeng, F., and Allen, C. (2007). *In vivo* fate of unimers and micelles of a poly(ethylene glycol)-block-poly(caprolactone) copolymer in mice following intravenous administration. *Eur J Pharm Biopharm* 65: 309–319.
18. Cerrai, P., Tricoli, M., Andruzzi, F., Paci, M., and Paci, M. (1999). Polyether-polyester block copolymers by non-catalysed polymerization of of ε-caprolactone with poly(ethylene glycol). *Polymer* 30: 338–343.
19. Choi, E. J., and Park, J. K. (1993). Microstructure of L-Lactide/ε-caprolactone Copolymer using Antimony(III) Oxide As a Catalyst. In *The Polymer Society of Korea*, p. 10.
20. Luo, L., Tam, J., Maysinger, D., and Eisenberg, A. (2002). Cellular internalization of poly(ethylene oxide)-b-poly(epsilon-caprolactone) diblock copolymer micelles. *Bioconjug Chem* 13: 1259–1265.
21. Mahmud, A., and Lavasanifar, A. (2005). The effect of block copolymer structure on the internalization of polymeric micelles by human breast cancer cells. *Colloids Surf B Biointerfaces* 45: 82–89.
22. Jette, K. K., Law, D., Schmitt, E. A., and Kwon, G. S. (2004). Preparation and drug loading of poly(ethylene glycol)-block-poly(epsilon-caprolactone) micelles through the evaporation of a cosolvent azeotrope. *Pharm Res* 21: 1184–1191.
23. Sachl, R., Uchman, M., Matejicek, P., Prochazka, K., Stepanek, M., and Spirkova, M. (2007). Preparation and characterization of self-assembled nanoparticles formed by poly(ethylene oxide)-block-poly(epsilon-caprolactone) copolymers with long poly(epsilon-caprolactone) blocks in aqueous solutions. *Langmuir* 23: 3395–3400.
24. Gou, M. L., *et al.* (2007). Preparation and characterization of magnetic poly(epsilon-caprolactone)-poly(ethylene glycol)-poly(epsilon-caprolactone) microspheres. *J Mater Sci Mater Med* 19:1033–1041.
25. Shuai, X., Ai, H., Nasongkla, N., Kim, S., and Gao, J. (2004). Micellar carriers based on block copolymers of poly(epsilon-caprolactone) and poly(ethylene glycol) for doxorubicin delivery. *J Control Release* 98: 415–426.
26. Aliabadi, H. M., Elhasi, S., Mahmud, A., Gulamhusein, R., Mahdipoor, P., and Lavasanifar, A. (2007). Encapsulation of hydrophobic drugs in polymeric micelles through co-solvent evaporation: the effect of solvent composition on micellar properties and drug loading. *Int J Pharm* 329: 158–165.
27. Layre, A. M., Couvreur, P., Richard, J., Requier, D., Eddine Ghermani, N., and Gref, R. (2006). Freeze-drying of composite core-shell nanoparticles. *Drug Dev Ind Pharm* 32: 839–846.

28. Yu, D. M., Amidon, G. L., Weiner, N. D., and Goldberg, A. H. (1994). Viscoelastic properties of poly(ethylene oxide) solution. *J Pharm Sci* 83: 1443–1449.

29. Gref, R., *et al.* (1997). Poly(ethylene glycol)-coated nanospheres: potential carriers for intravenous drug administration. *Pharm Biotechnol* 10: 167–198.

30. Israelachvili, J. (1997). The different faces of poly(ethylene glycol). *Proc Natl Acad Sci USA* 94: 8378–8379.

31. Zhu, K. J., *et al.* (2005). Preparation, characterization and *in vitro* release properties of ibuprofen-loaded microspheres based on polylactide, poly(epsilon-caprolactone) and their copolymers. *J Microencapsul* 22: 25–36.

32. Zeng, F., Lee, H., Chidiac, M., and Allen, C. (2005). Synthesis and characterization of six-arm star poly(delta-valerolactone)-block-methoxy poly(ethylene glycol) copolymers. *Biomacromolecules* 6: 2140–2149.

33. Forrest, M. L., Zhao, A., Won, C. Y., Malick, A. W., and Kwon, G. S. (2006). Lipophilic prodrugs of Hsp90 inhibitor geldanamycin for nanoencapsulation in poly(ethylene glycol)-b-poly(epsilon-caprolactone) micelles. *J Control Release* 116: 139–149.

34. Quaglia, F., *et al.* (2006). Nanoscopic core-shell drug carriers made of amphiphilic triblock and star-diblock copolymers. *Int J Pharm* 324: 56–66.

35. Winnik, F. M., and Regismond, S. T. A. (1996). Fluorescence methods in the study of the interactions of surfactants with polymers. *Colloids Surf A Physicochem Eng Aspects* 118: 1–39.

36. Vangeyte, P., Leyh, B., Heinrich, M., Grandjean, J., Bourgaux, C., and Jerome, R. (2004). Self-assembly of poly(ethylene oxide)-b-poly(epsilon-caprolactone) copolymers in aqueous solution. *Langmuir* 20: 8442–8451.

37. Vangeyte, P., Gautier, S., and Jerome, R. (2004). About the methods of preparation of poly(ethylene oxide)-b-poly(ε-caprolactone) nanoparticles in water: Analysis by dynamic light scattering. *Colloids Surf A* 242: 203–211.

38. Winnik, F. M., Winnik, M. A., Ringsdorf, H., and Venzmer, J. (1991). Bis (1-pyrenylmethyl) Ether as an Excimer-Forming Probe of Hydrophobically Modified Poly(*N*-isopropylacrylamides) in Water. *J Phys Chem* 95:2583–2587.

39. Shin, I. G., Kim, S. Y., Lee, Y. M., Cho, C. S., and Sung, Y. K. (1998). Methoxy poly(ethylene glycol)/epsilon-caprolactone amphiphilic block copolymeric micelle containing indomethacin. I. Preparation and characterization. *J Control Release* 51: 1–11.

40. Kim, S. Y., Shin, I. G., Lee, Y. M., Cho, C. S., and Sung, Y. K. (1998). Methoxy poly(ethylene glycol) and epsilon-caprolactone amphiphilic block copolymeric micelle containing indomethacin. II. Micelle formation and drug release behaviours. *J Control Release* 51: 13–22.

41. Elhasi, S., Astaneh, R., and Lavasanifar, A. (2007). Solubilization of an amphiphilic drug by poly(ethylene oxide)-block-poly(ester) micelles. *Eur J Pharm Biopharm* 65: 406–413.

42. Allen, C., Yu, Y., Maysinger, D., and Eisenberg, A. (1998). Polycaprolactone-b-poly(ethylene oxide) block copolymer micelles as a novel drug delivery vehicle for neurotrophic agents FK506 and L-685,818. *Bioconjug Chem* 9: 564–572.

43. Allen, C., Eisenberg, A., Mrsic, J., and Maysinger, D. (2000). PCL-b-PEO micelles as a delivery vehicle for FK506: assessment of a functional recovery of crushed peripheral nerve. *Drug Deliv* 7: 139–145.

44. Allen, C., Han, J., Yu, Y., Maysinger, D., and Eisenberg, A. (2000). Polycaprolactone-b-poly(ethylene oxide) copolymer micelles as a delivery vehicle for dihydrotestosterone. *J Control Release* 63: 275–286.

45. Aliabadi, H. M., Mahmud, A., Sharifabadi, A. D., and Lavasanifar, A. (2005). Micelles of methoxy poly(ethylene oxide)-b-poly(epsilon-caprolactone) as vehicles for the solubilization and controlled delivery of cyclosporine A. *J Control Release* 104: 301–311.

46. Emens, L. A., Kennedy, M. J., Fetting, J. H., Davidson, N. E., Garrett, E., and Armstrong, D. K. (2002). A phase I toxicity and feasibility trial of sequential dose-dense induction chemotherapy with doxorubicin, paclitaxel, and 5-fluorouracil followed by high dose consolidation for high-risk primary breast cancer. *Breast Cancer Res Treat* 76: 145–156.

47. Tsutani, Y., Saeki, T., Aogi, K., Ohsumi, S., and Takashima, S. (2005). Toxicity of doxorubicin and cyclophosphamide (60 mg/600 mg/m^2) in adjuvant chemotherapy for breast cancer. *Gan To Kagaku Ryoho* 32: 809–813.

48. Kosugi, S., Kanda, T., Nakagawa, S., Ohashi, M., Nishimaki, T., and Hatakeyama, K. (2005). Efficacy and toxicity of fluorouracil, doxorubicin, and cisplatin/nedaplatin treatment as neoadjuvant chemotherapy for advanced esophageal carcinoma. *Scand J Gastroenterol* 40: 886–892.

49. Suzuki, F., *et al.* (2005). Induction of tumor-specific cytotoxicity and apoptosis by doxorubicin. *Anticancer Res* 25: 887–893.

50. Formariz, T. P., Sarmento, V. H., Silva-Junior, A. A., Scarpa, M. V., Santilli, C. V., and Oliveira, A. G. (2006). Doxorubicin biocompatible O/W microemulsion stabilized by mixed surfactant containing soya phosphatidylcholine. *Colloids Surf B Biointerfaces* 51: 54–61.

51. Fitzpatrick, F. A., and Wheeler, R. (2003). The immunopharmacology of paclitaxel (Taxol), docetaxel (Taxotere), and related agents. *Int Immunopharmacol* 3: 1699–1714.
52. Blagosklonny, M. V., and Fojo, T. (1999). Molecular effects of paclitaxel: myths and reality (a critical review). *Int J Cancer* 83: 151–156.
53. Lee, H., Zeng, F., Dunne, M., and Allen, C. (2005). Methoxy poly(ethylene glycol)-block-poly(delta-valerolactone) copolymer micelles for formulation of hydrophobic drugs. *Biomacromolecules* 6: 3119–3128.
54. Shuai, X., Merdan, T., Schaper, A. K., Xi, F., and Kissel, T. (2004). Core-cross-linked polymeric micelles as paclitaxel carriers. *Bioconjug Chem* 15: 441–448.
55. Molavi, O., *et al.* (2007). Polymeric micelles for the solubilization and delivery of STAT3 inhibitor cucurbitacins in solid tumors. *Int J Pharm.*
56. Chen, J. C., Chiu, M. H., Nie, R. L., Cordell, G. A., and Qiu, S. X. (2005). Cucurbitacins and cucurbitane glycosides: structures and biological activities. *Nat Prod Rep* 22: 386–399.
57. Zeng, F., Lee, H., and Allen, C. (2006). Epidermal growth factor-conjugated poly(ethylene glycol)-block-poly(delta-valerolactone) copolymer micelles for targeted delivery of chemotherapeutics. *Bioconjug Chem* 17: 399–409.
58. Di Lorenzo, G., *et al.* (2004). HER-2/neu receptor in prostate cancer development and progression to androgen independence. *Tumori* 90: 163–170.
59. Aggarwal, S., Singh, P., Topaloglu, O., Isaacs, J. T., and Denmeade, S. R. (2006). A dimeric peptide that binds selectively to prostate-specific membrane antigen and inhibits its enzymatic activity. *Cancer Res* 66: 9171–9177.
60. Forrest, M. L., Won, C. Y., Malick, A. W., and Kwon, G. S. (2006). *In vitro* release of the mTOR inhibitor rapamycin from poly(ethylene glycol)-b-poly(epsilon-caprolactone) micelles. *J Control Release* 110: 370–377.
61. Eliassi, A., and Modarress, H. (1999). Measurement of Activity of Water in Aqueous Poly(ethylene glycol) Solutions (Effect of Excess Volume on the Flory–Huggins χ-Parameter). *J Chem Eng Data* 44: 52–55.
62. Ryu, J., Jeong, Y. I., Kim, I. S., Lee, J. H., Nah, J. W., and Kim, S. H. (2000). Clonazepam release from core-shell-type nanoparticles of poly(epsilon-caprolactone)/poly(ethylene glycol)/poly(epsilon-caprolactone) triblock copolymers. *Int J Pharm* 200: 231–242.
63. Ge, H., *et al.* (2002). Preparation, characterization, and drug release behaviors of drug nimodipine-loaded poly(epsilon-caprolactone)-poly(ethylene oxide)-poly(epsilon-caprolactone) amphiphilic triblock copolymer micelles. *J Pharm Sci* 91: 1463–1473.

64. Lin, W. J., Juang, L. W., and Lin, C. C. (2003). Stability and release performance of a series of pegylated copolymeric micelles. *Pharm Res* 20: 668–673.

65. Zhang, Y., and Zhuo, R. X. (2005). Synthesis and *in vitro* drug release behavior of amphiphilic triblock copolymer nanoparticles based on poly (ethylene glycol) and polycaprolactone. *Biomaterials* 26: 6736–6742.

66. Kim, K. H., Cui, G. H., Lim, H. J., Huh, J., Ahn, C. H., and Jo, W. H. (2004). Synthesis and Micellization of Star-Shaped Poly(ethylene glycol)-block-Poly(ε-caprolactone). *Macromol Chem Phys* 205: 1684–1692.

67. Lu, C., Guo, S., Zhang, Y., and Yin, M. (2006). Synthesis and aggregation behavior of four types of different shaped PCL-PEG block copolymers. *Polym Int* 55: 694–700.

68. Mahmud, A., Xiong, X. B., and Lavasanifar, A. (2006). Novel Self-Associating Poly(ethylene oxide)-block-poly(ε-caprolactone) Block Copolymers with Functional Side Groups on the Polyester Block for Drug Delivery. *Macromolecules* 39: 9419–9428.

69. Riva, R., Lenoir, S., Jerome, R., and Lecomte, P. (2005). Functionalization of poly(ε-caprolactone) by pendant hydroxyl, carboxylic acid and epoxide groups by atom transfer radical addition. *Polymer* 46: 8511–8518.

70. Rieger, J., Van Butsele, K., Lecomte, P., Detrembleur, C., Jerome, R., and Jerome, C. (2005). Versatile functionalization and grafting of poly(epsilon-caprolactone) by Michael-type addition. *Chem Commun (Camb)*: 274–276.

71. Riva, R., Schmeits, S., Jérôme, C., Jérôme, R., and Lecomte, P. (2007). Combination of Ring-Opening Polymerization and "Click Chemistry": Toward Functionalization and Grafting of Poly(ε-caprolactone). *Macromolecules* 40: 796–803.

72. Xu, P., *et al.* (2006). Anticancer efficacies of cisplatin-releasing pH-responsive nanoparticles. *Biomacromolecules* 7: 829–835.

73. Shi, B., C., F., You, M. X., Zhang, Y., Fu, S., and Pei, Y. (2005). Stealth MePEG-PCL micelles: effects of polymer composition on micelle physicochemical characteristics, *in vitro* drug release, *in vivo* pharmacokinetics in rats and biodistribution in S_{180} tumor bearing mice. *Colloids Polym Sci* 283: 954–967.

74. Yamamoto, Y., Nagasaki, Y., Kato, Y., Sugiyama, Y., and Kataoka, K. (2001). Long-circulating poly(ethylene glycol)-poly(D,L-lactide) block copolymer micelles with modulated surface charge. *J Control Release* 77: 27–38.

75. Gref, R., *et al.* (2000). 'Stealth' corona-core nanoparticles surface modified by polyethylene glycol (PEG): influences of the corona (PEG chain length and surface density) and of the core composition on phagocytic uptake and plasma protein adsorption. *Colloids Surf B Biointerfaces* 18: 301–313.

76. Allen, C., Yu, Y., Eisenberg, A., and Maysinger, D. (1999). Cellular internalization of PCL(20)-b-PEO(44) block copolymer micelles. *Biochim Biophys Acta* 1421: 32–38.

77. Savic, R., Luo, L., Eisenberg, A., and Maysinger, D. (2003). Micellar nanocontainers distribute to defined cytoplasmic organelles. *Science* 300: 615–618.

78. De Jaeghere, F., Allemann, E., Feijen, J., Kissel, T., Doelker, E., and Gurny, R. (2000). Cellular uptake of PEO surface-modified nanoparticles: evaluation of nanoparticles made of PLA:PEO diblock and triblock copolymers. *J Drug Target* 8: 143–153.

79. Aliabadi, H. M., Brocks, D. R., and Lavasanifar, A. (2005). Polymeric micelles for the solubilization and delivery of cyclosporine A: pharmacokinetics and biodistribution. *Biomaterials* 26: 7251–7259.

80. Yanez, J. A., Forrest, M. L., Ohgami, Y., Kwon, G. S., and Davies, N. M. (2007). Pharmacometrics and delivery of novel nanoformulated PEG-b-poly(epsilon-caprolactone) micelles of rapamycin. *Cancer Chemother Pharmacol* 61:133–144.

81. Lin, W. J., Chen, Y. C., Lin, C. C., Chen, C. F., and Chen, J. W. (2006). Characterization of pegylated copolymeric micelles and *in vivo* pharmacokinetics and biodistribution studies. *J Biomed Mater Res B Appl Biomater* 77: 188–194.

82. Savic, R., Azzam, T., Eisenberg, A., and Maysinger, D. (2006). Assessment of the integrity of poly(caprolactone)-b-poly(ethylene oxide) micelles under biological conditions: a fluorogenic-based approach. *Langmuir* 22: 3570–3578.

83. Thangapazham, R. L., Sharma, A., and Maheshwari, R. K. (2006). Multiple molecular targets in cancer chemoprevention by curcumin. AAPS J 8: E443–449.

84. Ma, Z., Shayeganpour, A., Brocks, D. R., Lavasanifar, A., and Samuel, J. (2007). High-performance liquid chromatography analysis of curcumin in rat plasma: application to pharmacokinetics of polymeric micellar formulation of curcumin. Biomed Chromatogr 21: 546–552.

Chapter 4

Recent Progress in Polymer Therapeutics as Nanomedicines

Hemda Baabur-Cohen,* Liora Omer,* and Ronit Satchi-Fainaro
Department of Physiology and Pharmacology, Sackler School of Medicine, Tel Aviv University, Tel Aviv 69978, Israel
ronitsf@post.tau.ac.il

The term Polymer Therapeutics is defined as water-soluble biocompatible polymers that can function as bioactive nanomedicines, or as nanocarriers conjugated with therapeutic agents, i.e., low-molecular-weight drugs, proteins or nucleic acids. The therapeutic agent is loaded onto the polymeric nanocarrier either by conjugation or by supramolecular complexation. Here we present an overview of polymer therapeutics with a focus on the components and structure of these nanoscale delivery systems. Examples of their utilization in cancer and other angiogenesis-dependent diseases treatment are given.

4.1 Introduction

In 1975, Helmut Ringsdorf presented his idea regarding the use of polymers as targetable drug carriers [1]. He foresaw the basic

* These authors contributed equally.

Handbook of Harnessing Biomaterials in Nanomedicine: Preparation, Toxicity, and Applications
Edited by Dan Peer

ISBN 978-981-4316-46-0 (Hardback), 978-981-4364-27-0 (eBook)
www.panstanford.com

architecture of polymer–drug conjugates: a polymeric spacer, drug attached via a hydrolytically or enzymatically cleavable spacer and a targeting group complementary to a receptor/antigen at the target cell. Since then, most of the polymer–drug conjugates have been designed and developed according to Ringsdorf's model (Figure 4.1A). Most of the earlier systems rarely advanced beyond *in vitro* testing. However, over the last 15 years, a growing number of polymer therapeutics have been synthesized and characterized. In particular, PEG–protein conjugates have reached the market, and polymer–drug conjugates and polymeric micelles entered clinical trials mainly as anti-cancer agents.

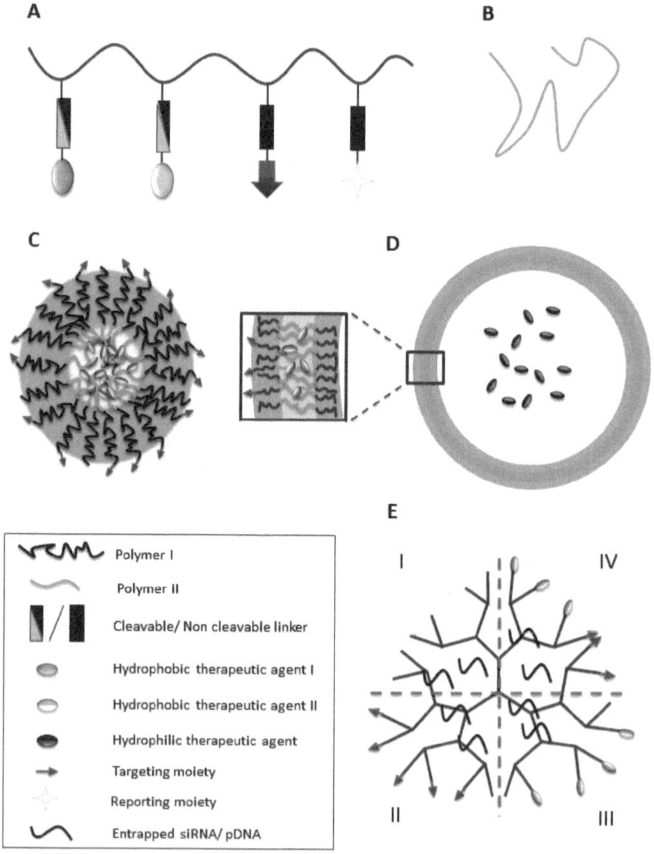

Figure 4.1 Structures of polymer therapeutics: (A) Modified Ringsdorf's model, (B) polymeric drug, (C) polymeric micelle, (D) polymersome, and (E) dendrimer. See also Color Insert.

Polymer therapeutics in the sense of nanocarriers for low-molecular-weight precursors (e.g., drugs, proteins, nucleic acids) possess several advantages: (i) protection of the precursor from degradation and preservation of its activity during circulation, (ii) an increased circulation half-life, (iii) a reduction in antigenic activity of the drug or the active entity leading to a weaker immunological body response, (iv) an increase in water solubility of low soluble or insoluble drugs, (v) the ability to provide passive or active targeting specifically to the site of action, (vi) promoting cellular up-take and appropriate intracellular trafficking, and (vii) the possibility to form an advanced complex drug delivery system. All these properties improve the pharmacokinetic and pharmacodynamic profiles of the therapeutic agent, leading to increased efficacy and reduced toxicity, and may enable easier administration and increased patient compliance.

Many of the above advantages arise from the size of the polymer therapeutic. The high-molecular-weight therapeutic can only enter cells via endocytosis, resulting in longer circulation of the conjugate in the bloodstream compared with the free drug. In contrast, low-molecular-weight therapeutic agents pass rapidly through cell membranes and will non-selectively penetrate most tissues. Moreover, the work by Maeda and co-workers [2, 3] has established that cancerous tissue is characterized by impaired leaky vasculature and poor lymphatic drainage. This phenomenon was termed by them as the enhanced permeability and retention (EPR) effect. Macromolecules as opposed to low-molecular-weight compounds do not extravasate through the capillaries of normal tissues. However, the capillaries in tumors are fenestrated and leaky; so macromolecules selectively reach the malignant tissue and are subsequently retained there due to poor lymphatic drainage, resulting in passive targeting and accumulation of macromolecules in the tumor site. Targeting of macromolecules through leaky vascular bed is possible also in other angiogenesis-dependent diseases, such as arthritis, macular degeneration, diabetic retinopathy, and sites of inflammation. Most of the work with polymer therapeutics has been done in the field of cancer research and treatment, and it will also be the focus of this chapter. For other targets, the reader is referred to a recent review [4].

Usually the Mw range of 20–200 kDa is used to avoid rapid renal excretion and to take advantage of the EPR effect. Particle size range of 20–100 nm was found as an optimum for prolonged circulation, accumulation in tumor tissue, and enhanced diffusion within tissue [5–7]. The uptake to most cells is through fluid phase pinocytosis, where the size limit is 150 nm. A different way of internalization is through receptor-mediated endocytosis, in which macromolecules bind to complementary receptors on the cell surface and enter the cell as receptor-macromolecule complex in clathrin-coated vesicles. This process increases the efficiency of internalization of particular macromolecules more than 1000-fold compared with ordinary pinocytosis [8]. The macromolecule, which enters the cell through either process, finds itself in the interior of the endosome, where the environment is kept acidic (pH 5–6) and many receptors release their bound cargo. From the endosome the molecules proceed to the digestive lysosome, in which about 40 types of hydrolytic enzymes are active at the acidic pH [8]. Many strategies use the acidic pH or the proteolytic enzymes for the release of the therapeutic agent from the polymeric nanocarrier. However, care must be taken that the hostile environment of the lysosome will not hamper the structure and activity of the therapeutic agent.

In order to design a polymeric nanocarrier, one should pay a careful attention to each one of the different components; the polymer backbone, linker, targeting moiety if it exists, and obviously the therapeutic agent itself should be chosen after taking into consideration the (i) stability of the polymer-therapeutic attachment during circulation and transport, (ii) adequate loading capacity in relation to the potency of the therapeutic agent being carried, and (iii) ability to target the diseased cell or tissue by an active or a passive mechanism. In the next sections, we first elaborate on the different components, and then we will review the different families of polymer therapeutics with stimulating examples from research and clinical trials.

4.1.1 Polymeric Backbone

The choice of polymeric backbone for the conjugate has great implications on the pharmacokinetics and pharmacodynamics of the drug. The polymer characteristics, such as molecular weight, polydispersity, architecture, charge, and hydrophilicity, impose the drug solubility, its biodistribution, body excretion, and the interaction with the immune system. The polymeric backbone of the conjugate can be synthetic, natural, or semi-natural. Copolymerization enhances design versatility by allowing systematic variation of the distribution of active units along a polymer chain. Thus, copolymers can be tailor-made in order to vary hydrophilicity or lipophilicity of the entire molecule or of single domains (block systems), or to introduce various functional groups. Properties of the microenvironment in a polymer coil differ drastically from those of the bulk solution and are dictated mainly by monomers composition.

Since our final goal is to use these materials as carriers for pharmaceuticals, some criteria must be met: The polymeric nanocarriers should be biocompatible and non-toxic, and they should avoid interaction with the immune system (unless it is the target), to enable repeated administration. In addition, biodegradable polymers are favored for better clearance from the body. Finally, many groups choose to work with FDA-approved polymers, to facilitate the approval for clinical use of their system. In any way, all polymer therapeutics are considered new chemical entities (NCE) from the regulatory point of view. The most common polymers used in the field of polymer therapeutics are listed in Table 4.1. We will focus on several polymers, which are in early clinical trials as polymeric nanocarriers for anti-cancer agents [9].

For a suitable conjugation to chemical and biopharmaceutical drugs, many polymers have been proposed as carriers, including N-(2-hydroxypropyl)methacrylamide (HPMA) copolymers, poly(ethyleneimine) (PEI), linear polyamidoamines, polyvinylpyrrolidone (PVP), polyglutamic acid (PGA), polyacrylamide (PAAm), polydimethylacrylamide (PDAAm), polyvinyl alcohol (PVA), chitosan, and dextrin. It is important to note that polyethylene glycol (PEG) has significant contribution specifically in the field of polymer–protein conjugates, as will be discussed later on. PEGylation has been proven to be one of the most straightforward procedures for enhancing the therapeutic and biotechnological potential of peptides and proteins [10].

The different types of polymer backbones can be divided into two sub-groups according to the feature of biodegradability in the main chain.

4.1.2 Degradable Polymers Backbone

PGA is synthesized by ring-opening co-polymerization of the corresponding N-carboxyanhydrides (NCA), initiated by amines or nucleophilic agents. PGA is water soluble, non-toxic, and biodegradable. Cysteine proteases, particularly cathepsin B, play key role in the lysosomal degradation of PGA. In addition, PGA has a γ-carboxyl group in each repeating unit of $_L$-glutamic acid that offers multivalent attachment to drugs. Those features make PGA an attractive drug carrier, and indeed PGA-PTX (OPAXIO™, former names XYOTAX and CT-2103) is the most progressed polymer–drug conjugate in the pipeline for market approval [11, 12].

Several polysaccharides are being used as polymeric carriers [13, 14]. Among natural and semi-synthetic polysaccharides, hyaluronic acid, chitosan, and dextran have been largely investigated for drug bioconjugation [13]. Dextran is a natural polysaccharide containing monomers of simple sugar glucose. This polyglucose biopolymer is characterized by a-1,6 linkages, with hydroxylated cyclohexyl units [14]. Dextran has been particularly popular owing to its clinical approval for use as a plasma expander. Dextran is a water-soluble biopolymer, but it can also dissolve in some organic solvents, such as dimethyl sulfoxide (DMSO), N,N-dimethylformamide (DMF) formamide, ethylene glycol, and glycerol. Dextran is biocompatible and biodegradable in blood and in the gastrointestinal (GI) tract. However, it is not degraded in lysosomes. Dextran possesses multiple primary and secondary hydroxyl groups that can be used for binding drugs or proteins directly or via spacers [23].

Pullulan is another interesting natural, non-ionic, and linear homopolysaccharide, formed by repeated units of maltotriose condensed through α-1,6 linkage (α-1,4-linked glucose molecules, polymerized by α-1,6-linkages to the terminal glucose) [24]. Owing to its excellent biological and physicochemical features, namely biodegradability, low immunogenicity, and polyfunctionality together with its fair solubility in aqueous and few organic solvents, pullulan has become an attractive ingredient for many pharmaceutical applications and chemical manipulations [25]. There are several examples in the literature for the use of pullulan as a carrier, in which the drug is conjugated to the primary hydroxyl groups via ester bonds or through lysosomal-sensitive peptide spacers [26].

4.1.3 Non-Degradable Polymer Backbone

PEG has good water solubility, but it can also dissolve in many organic solvents. This feature together with its biocompatibility has made

Table 4.1 Polymeric backbone

Polymer backbone	PEG	HPMA copolymer	PGA	Dextran	PEI
Monomer	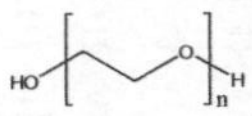	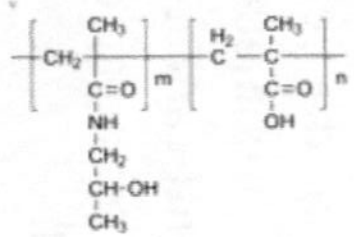	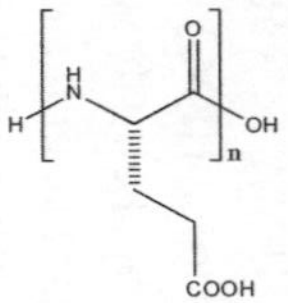	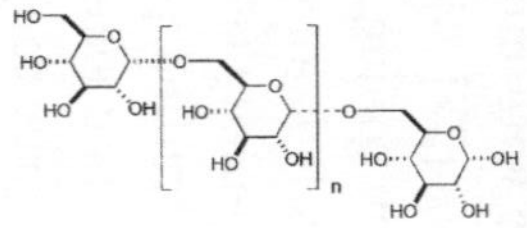	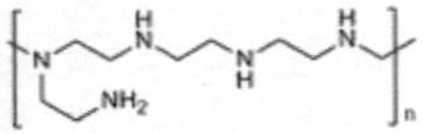
Biodegradability	X	X	√	√	X
Immunogenicity	X	X	X	√	
Toxicity	X	X	X	X	√
Maximal loading	2	n	n	3n	Charge matching
Clinical status	Approved	Phase II (PK2)	Phase III, (OPAXIO)	Approved*	*in vivo*
Reference	[15]	[16, 17]	[18]	[13, 19, 20]	[21, 22]

PEG: poly(ethylene glycol); HPMA: N-(2-hydroxypropyl)methacrylamide; PGA: poly(glutamic acid), PEI: polyethyleneimine.
*As a plasma expander.

it a versatile carrier in polymer therapeutics. PEG is commercially available with either one or two attachment points. It can be produced as a linear or branched polymer. The functional hydroxyl group at the chain termini can be conjugated with drugs or other functional groups. The lack of multivalency is one of the limitations of this polymer; it limits the loading capacity and the potential use of PEG as a backbone. To overcome this limitation, additional reactive groups can be added by reaction of the OH^- groups with multifunctional compounds, such as glutamic acid dendron [27]. While PEG is mostly common in the field of polymer–protein conjugates, it is also extensively used in the polymer therapeutics field in general, as a drug carrier or as stabilizing and as immunogenicity reducer.

HPMA copolymers are one of the most studied platforms for polymer–drug conjugates; they have been studied extensively over the last 30 years [17]. Most of HPMA polymer–drug conjugates were developed for the treatment of cancer, with a special focus on the site-specific delivery of anti-cancer drugs. HPMA is water soluble, neutral, biocompatible, and non-immunogenic. HPMA copolymer conjugated to DOX via a peptidyl linker Gly-Phe-Leu-Gly was the first synthetic polymer-based anti-cancer conjugate to enter clinical trial in 1994 [28] (i.e., PK1) and has been the breakthrough that led to the exponential growth of interest in the field of polymer therapeutics. Although PK1 is a promising cancer treatment, the polymer is not biodegradable; so there are issues as to how it is metabolized and cleared from the body. Since then, five other anti-cancer compounds and two gamma camera imaging agents conjugated to HPMA copolymer have been evaluated clinically [16].

In recent years, living free radical polymerization methods, including atom transfer radical polymerization (ATRP) and reversible addition-fragmentation chain transfer (RAFT), have been used for the synthesis of HPMA copolymers with narrow molecular weight distributions. Matyjaszewski's laboratory was the first to report on polymerization of HPMA by ATRP method [29, 30]. It was reported that the polymerization was difficult to control and the yield was low in some cases. McCormick and coworkers were the first to report on the polymerization of HPMA using the RAFT method [31]. They presented conditions that facilitate the direct controlled RAFT polymerization of this copolymer. This living polymerization method allows the addition of further amounts of monomers during the reaction. Using the RAFT technique, several HPMA copolymer–drug conjugates were designed, synthesized, and characterized [32, 33].

HPMA, PGA, and dextran are most commonly used as a backbone for polymer–drug conjugates.

4.1.4 Linker

One aspect in utilizing polymeric nanocarriers for therapeutics is the specific release of the original form of the active agent at the target site. Thus, the choice of linker between the active agent and the polymer backbone has a significant role in achieving this aim. Furthermore, the linker should be stable in the bloodstream and the extracellular interstitium in physiological pH. For some medical applications, the drug is essentially biologically inert when attached by a linker to the polymer. So a drug that would otherwise cause side effects can exist in the bloodstream as a conjugate and will not harm the patient.

In the case of cancer, the unique pathophysiology of tumors, such as the acidic, neoplastic supporting microenvironment is being used. It has been found to overexpress specific proteases that are active in the acidic conditions of the tumor. The drug is selectively released to its target by linking it with a spacer cleavable by hydrolysis at low pH or by lysosomal or tumor-associated overexpressed enzymes. Thus, the linkers in the polymer therapeutics field are either enzymatically cleavable [34, 35] or pH-sensitive [36–38]. The release of the free drug can occur extra- or intra-cellularly.

Disulfide linkers that are cleaved by reduction have also been proposed as alternative, but it has not been progressed beyond an experimental stage [39]. Many different classes of enzymes, including nucleases, proteases, phosphatases, lipases, etc., are present in the lysosomes. Since water-soluble polymer–drug conjugates enter the cell via endocytosis and then continue to the lysosomes, the presence of an enzymatically cleavable linker between the backbone and the drug enables selective targeting.

A common example is the oligopeptide spacers, terminated with a drug and susceptible to enzymatically catalyzed hydrolysis in the lysosomes, specifically by cathepsin B and K. The cathepsin B-cleavable tetrapeptide Gly-Phe-Leu-Gly was extensively used in HPMA copolymer for delivery of several anti-cancer drugs, since cathepsin B is overexpressed in many tumor cells and tumor endothelial cells [40]. This spacer is cleaved intracellularly in the lysosome and therefore is used for drug release to the cytosol. Another common enzymatically cleavable tetrapeptide is the Gly-Gly-Pro-Nle spacer, which is cleaved by cathepsin K. Cathepsin K is involved in bone resorption (osteoporosis, osteoarthritis and bone neoplasms), and overexpressed in bone metastases. In contrast to cathepsin B, it is localized and active in the tumor microenvironment. Cathepsin K-cleavable peptide has been used in polymer–drug conjugates to deliver drugs to bone tissues for the treatment of calcified diseases. It should be noted that there are further peptide sequences, which are known to be cleaved by cathepsin B, K and others, such as Phe-Lys or Val-Arg by cathepsin B [41] and Phe-Arg by cathepsin B and L [42].

Other proteases, which are overexpressed in tumors and play a critical role in tumor progression, tumor angiogenesis and metastasis, were studied. For example, the lysosomal proteases legumain [43, 44] and the matrix metallopreoeinases (MMPs), i.e., MMP2 and MMP9 [45], which are active intracellularly and extracellularly, respectively.

Because the enzymes that are used for pro-drug activation are also present in normal cells, activation of an enzymatically cleavable pro-drug can be observed in healthy tissue too. Thus, there is a growing demand for improving tumor uptake through active or passive targeting and to study the overexpression of those enzymes in the individual tumor clinically.

The acid-labile spacers are extensively used in the field of polymer–drug conjugates. There is a significant drop in the pH value from the physiological pH 7.2–7.4 in the blood or extracellular space to pH 4.0–6.5, in the various intracellular compartments [46]. In addition, the fact that the extracellular pH surrounding tumor tissue is also slightly lower than that of normal tissue also supports the rationale for the corporation of these spacers.

Typical examples of acid-sensitive bonds are *N*-cis-aconityl, hydrazone and carboxylic-hydrazone bonds, acetal, imine and trityl bonds. While *N*-cis-aconityl and hydrazone linkers are the most studied ones, several pro-drugs with acid-labile acetal bonds have also been investigated [36, 46]. Careful attention should be given to the choice of suitable linkers. The chosen chemical bond effect the pH-dependent stability of the pro-drug, as well as the molecular weight of the carrier and the site attachment on the carrier.

Another interesting sub-group of acid-labile linkers are pH-sensitive bonds that incorporate in the backbone of the polymeric carrier. Recently, a number of reports on linear polymers were published in which the monomer units were linked by ketal, acetal, and *cis*-aconityl bonds [46]. By doing so, the polymer backbone undergoes a breakdown under the acidic conditions after cellular uptake and thus has the benefit of being biodegradable. This strategy still suffers from several disadvantages, such as low Mw and absence of functional groups for attaching drugs, and thus requires further optimization.

Recently, a novel class of polymer backbone in which the drug and the polymer backbone are connected via a non-covalent, biologically inspired binding motif was proposed [47]. This linker consists of a pair of complementary peptides that are wound around each other in a super-helical fashion to form a tertiary structural motif that is referred to as coiled coil. In order to form the non-covalent polymer therapeutics, the polymeric carrier functionalized with one peptide is mixed in an aqueous solution with the drug of interest, which is functionalized with the complementary sequence to the peptide. The drug will be intracellularly released when the conjugate will be exposed to the relatively low pH of the endosomal compartments. This innovative coiled coil-based peptide linkers may be useful to form different compound libraries, depending on the pool of carriers and drugs that we create.

4.1.5 Targeting Moiety

As mentioned above, passive targeting of polymeric nanocarriers is obtained by utilizing the EPR effect. However, there are several limitations to this approach, including variable vascular hyperpermeability among different tumor types and different areas of the heterogenic tumor tissue. In addition, low cellular uptake of nanocarriers after extravasation can be another limitation, reducing the actual drug concentration within the tumor cells due to the stagnation around the tumor tissue. Thus, a targeting moiety can be used in order to direct the molecule of interest to the target in a more specifically way, and basically overcome those limitations.

Already back in the 1900s, Paul Ehrlich foresaw the concept of the direct targeting of drugs to specific molecular cancer targets [48]. Following his vision, active targeting combined with passive targeting became dominant in the design of drug delivery systems. Active targeting is expected to lead higher and faster intra-tumor accumulation and, in the case of targeting with internalizing ligands, to increase intracellular concentrations of the drug.

Active targeting to the tumor can be achieved by molecular recognition of cancer cells either via ligand-receptor, antibody–antigen interactions, or by targeting through aptamers [49]. A successful targeting moiety should have high affinity and specificity of binding to cell surface receptors and should be well suited to chemical modification due to conjugation considerations. When nanocarriers are targeted to the extracellular portion of transmembrane tumor antigens, a different mechanism of uptake is occurred. The nanocarrier is taken up by cancer cells through receptor-mediated endocytosis. Since the receptor is internalized with the ligand, the system is becoming saturated and uptake will decline until receptors are recycled to the surface.

In general, there are two approaches for targeted delivery to cancer tissues. The first main approach is aimed to target the tumor cells themselves. The second one utilizes the process of angiogenesis by targeting the proliferating tumor endothelial cells (TEC). There are several cases in which the targets are expressed at the same level on tumor cells and normal cells (e.g., CD19) [50].

Targeting the tumor cells themselves offers a direct killing of the cells and thus aims to cause eradication of the tumor. Anti-cancer therapy is basically specific to the tumor cells and is not supposed to harm healthy tissues. In contrast, the anti-angiogenic therapy, physiological processes of angiogenesis (e.g., wound healing, female reproductive cycle, and organ and tissue regeneration) are susceptible to the treatment as well. However, tumor cells suffer from genetic instability, which leads to treatment's resistance, and indeed this is one of the major drawbacks of targeting the tumor cells.

Several receptors that are overexpressed in tumor cells were used as targets in the field of polymer therapeutics and are apparent in Figure 4.2 and listed in Table 4.2.

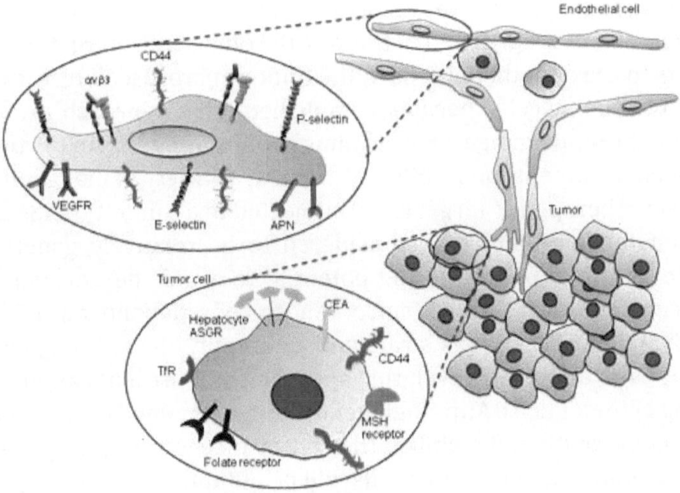

Figure 4.2 Molecular targets on tumor cells and on tumor endothelial cells. See also Color Insert.

Table 4.2 Targeting moieties and their targets

	Target	Targeting moiety	Ref.
Endothelial cells	Integrin $\alpha v\beta 3$	RGD motif	[51–55]
	Integrin $\alpha v\beta 5$	RGD motif	[54, 55]
	Aminopeptidase N (CD13)	NRG motif	[56]
	VEGFRs	Pegaptanib	[57]
	EGFR	EGFR-peptide	[58]
	E-selectin	Ebsp, Synthetic analog of sLex	[59, 60]
	HA receptor/CD44	HA	[61]
Tumor cells	Folate receptor	Folic acid	[62–67]
	TfR	Transferrin	[6, 68, 69]
	LHRH receptor	LHRH analog peptide	[70–73]
	HA receptor/CD44	HA	[61]
	MSH receptor	MSH	[74]
	Hepatocyte ASGR	Galactosamine	[75, 76]
	CEA	Anti CEA half-antibody	[77]

EGFR: epidermal growth factor receptor; Ebsp: E-selectin-binding-peptide; HA: hyaluronic Acid; TfR: Transferrin receptor; LHRH: Luteinizing hormone-releasing hormone; MSH: melanocyte-stimulating hormone; ASGR: asialoglycoprotein receptor; CEA: Carcinoembryonic antigen.

Since angiogenesis was recognized as a significant process in the formation and progression of tumors, the objective of targeting toxic agents to the endothelial cells in the tumor microvasculature, rather than the tumor cells, became established. This approach presents mainly three advantages: First, killing proliferating TEC in the tumor microenvironment can be effective against a variety of malignancies, since the therapeutic target is not subjected to a tumor type. Second, anti-angiogenic therapy is considered to be relatively genetically stable and thus possesses the potential to avoid the development of drug resistance. Third, since cancer cells depend on TEC for survival and growth, this strategy may amplify the anti-angiogenic therapeutic effect. However, this approach still presents an indirect killing of tumor cells. Anti-angiogenic therapy is aimed to cause delay of tumor growth and stabilize the cancer disease. In this approach, limited eradication of tumor cells will be obtained. In addition, since usually lower concentration of the drug is being used, the duration of the treatment will be longer. But, it is important to note that fewer side effects will be expected from the same reason. Representative examples of molecular markers of the angiogenic blood vessels of tumors are presented in Figure 4.2 and listed in Table 4.2.

4.2 Polymeric Drugs

Unlike polymer–protein and polymer–drug conjugates, examples of intrinsically bioactive polymers are relatively scarce [78]. However, a careful examination of the characteristics of polymers reveals that they offer a number of features that are not present in traditional small molecule therapies. For examples, when ingested orally, high Mw characteristics of polymers limit their absorption through the gastrointestinal (GI) tract. In this way, we can limit these functional polymers to the GI or other areas and avoid systemic exposure. Furthermore, polymeric drugs as active pharmaceutical ingredients offer more simplicity, since the polymer itself serves as the drug and complicated synthesis of polymer conjugates is avoided. Finally, the ability to incorporate a variety of binding sites and large amount of ligands along the polymer chain can lead to multivalent interaction with target ligands and thus offers higher binding constant than with smaller molecular weight drugs.

A wide range of novel functional polymers have been synthesized during the last three decades, in which the role of polymers in biomedicine has seen significant growth [79]. Polymeric drugs offer selective recognition and sequestration of molecular and macromolecular species. The presence of detrimental substances in the human GI beyond a certain concentration has been implicated as the causative agent for different diseases. The well-established and FDA-approved polymeric drugs are specified to other diseases than cancer. However, it is inevitable that further research will be carried out regarding treatment of cancer by polymeric drugs.

One family of polymeric drugs has been found to be effective in removing those undesired agents from the body at acceptable therapeutic doses and has shown therapeutic benefits in various human diseases. For the treatment of cardiovascular diseases, several cholesterol-lowering agents were developed [80–86], which have also showed efficiency in the control of hyperglycemia [87–89]. Welchol® is a cholesterol-binding polymer, which was approved in 2000 for the reduction of elevated LDL-C and in 2008 for the reduction of glucose type-2 diabetes. For the treatment of renal diseases, amines containing cationic hydrogels or cross-linked polymers were designed and synthesized. These polymers act as safe and effective phosphate binders, and their discovery led to the development and approval of Renagel® in 1998 [90–94]. Similarly, this family offers several iron chelators in the case of iron overload disorders [95–99] and polymeric sequestrants of *C. difficile* toxins, such as Tolevamer, which has shown efficacy in human clinical trials [100].

Another family of polymeric drugs is based on chemically modified biomedical polymers as treatments for osteoarthritis [101–103]. The onset of this disease is characterized by degradation of hyaluronan (HA), which is an anionic biopolymer that provides the viscoelastic properties for the normal function of the joints. A variety of HA and chemically cross-linked HA have been approved as visco-supplements for patients with osteoarthritis (i.e., Artz®, Hyalgan®, and Synvisc®). In addition, HA-based products are also used in the area of reducing the extent and severity of post-surgical adhesion [104–106].

The design and synthesis of functional polymers showed inherent therapeutic efficacy. In spite of the progress in this area (Table 4.3), there are some underlying concerns attributed to polymers as new chemical entities for therapeutic applications, including the issue of broad molecular weight distribution and compositional and structural heterogeneity. These features were considered to impede drug development and regulatory approval. The topic of polymeric drugs was reviewed lately by Dhal et al. [78].

Table 4.3 Examples of polymeric drugs in the market

Company	Application	Trade name	Polymer
Teva Pharmaceutical Industries Ltd.	Multiple sclerosis	Copaxone®	Random copolymer composed of L-alanine, L-lysine, L-glutamic acid, and L-tyrosine
Genzyme Corporation	Chronic kidney disease	Renagel®	Poly(allylamine)
Sanofi-aventis	Osteoarthritis	Hyalgan®	Hyaluronan
Daiichi-Sankyo	Cardiovascular disease	Welchol	Cross-linked poly(allylamine hydrochloride)

4.3 Polymer–Drug Conjugates

In this section, we will present the basic concepts and innovations in the field of polymer–drug conjugates and will demonstrate how Ringsdorf's vision became and is still becoming a reality.

Polymer–anti-cancer drug conjugates typically comprise a minimum of three components: a water-soluble polymeric carrier, a biodegradable polymer-drug linkage, and the bioactive agent. Polymer–drug conjugates progressing through clinical trials, as anti-cancer agents are, in fact, macromolecular pro-drugs.

From the synthetic point of view, a successful bioconjugation depends on the chemical structure, molecular weight, steric hindrance, and the reactivity of the biomolecule as well as the polymer. In order to synthesize a bioconjugate, both chemical entities need to possess a reactive or functional groups such as –COOH, –OH, –SH, or $-NH_2$. However, the presence of multiple reactive groups complicates the synthesis, since it will involve protection or deprotection of those groups. Many of the most commonly used strategies involve the use of both coupling agents such as dicyclohexyl carbodiimide (DCC), 1-Ethyl-3-(3-dimethylaminopropyl)carbodiimide (EDC), and *N,N*-diisopropylcarbodiimide (DIC) or the use of *N*-hydroxysuccinimide (NHS) esters.

Most anti-tumor drugs in clinical use act on metabolic pathways related to cell growth and high mitotic activity. In addition, many anti-cancer agents are low-molecular-weight compounds that readily gain access to all cells. These highly non-specific effects cause serious damage to healthy tissues while treating the tumor, thus leading to dose-limiting side effects and impaired quality of life. Chemotherapeutic treatment is often restricted by dose limiting systemic toxicity, or by the appearance of drug resistance. Moreover, the formulation of poorly soluble drugs may cause additional side effects. Therefore, there is much to gain by conjugating such drugs to polymeric carrier for anti-neoplastic therapy. The most commonly used polymer conjugated drugs are camptothecin, paclitaxel, doxorubicin, and platinum. Examples of polymer–drug conjugates in the pipeline are listed in Table 4.4.

The first polymer–drug conjugate to enter clinical trials was PK1, a HPMA copolymer–doxorubicin conjugate [107]. Doxorubicin (DOX) is the most commonly used anthracycline anti-tumor antibiotics. It has a wide range of anti-tumor activity, and is effective in the treatment of carcinomas of the breast, lung, thyroid, ovary, and soft tissue sarcomas. However, anthracycline therapy is associated with significant general organ toxicities, especially myelosuppression, mucositis, and cardiac toxicity. PK2, which is the relative conjugate of PK1, possesses an additional targeting residue — a galactosamine group that is the ligand for asialoglyoprotein. PK2 was designed with the aim of improving treatment of primary hepatocellular carcinoma and metastatic liver disease. In early phase I/II clinical trials, both PK1 and PK2 displayed reduced twofold to fivefold anthracycline toxicity, and the dose-limiting toxicities were typical of the anthracyclines, which included febrile neutropenia and mucositis. Despite high cumulative doses of DOX, no cardiotoxicity was observed. Furthermore, no signs of immunogenicity or polymer related toxicity were observed [107, 108]. Phase II study of PK1 for the treatment of breast and colorectal carcinomas and non-small cell lung cancer (NSCLC) confirmed these results. No activity against colorectal cancer, and activity restricted to anthracycline-naive patients in breast cancer were observed. However, the activity of PK1 against NSCLC was encouraging with 11.5% response rate, even though DOX is known to have minor effect in NSCLC [109]. DOX was also conjugated to dextran and tested clinically (phase I) [23]. However, this study was not continued, probably due to the reduced biodegradability of the conjugated dextran [110].

Table 4.4 Examples of polymer–drug conjugates in clinical trials

Company	Application	Trade name (clinical status)	Polymer
Pfizer, Inc.	Lung, breast and colorectal cancer	PK1, FCE28068 (phase II)	HPMA copolymer-doxorubicin
Pfizer, Inc.	Hepatocellular carcinoma	PK2, FCE2806 (phase I)	HPMA copolymer-doxorubicin-galactosamine
Access Pharmaceuticals, Inc	Ovarian and colorectal cancer	ProLindac™ (AP5346) (phase II)	HPMA copolymer-diaminocyclohexaneplatinum
Mersana Therapeutics, Inc.	Non-small cell lung cancer and other cancers	XMT-1001 (phase I)	Poly(1-hydroxymethylene hydroxylmethyl formal) (PHF)- Camptothecin (CPT)
Cerulean Pharma Inc.	Ovarian cancer and other cancers	CRLX-101(IT-101) (phase I/II)	Cyclodextrin-Camptothecin (CPT)
Cell therapeutics, Inc.	Colorectal and ovarian cancer	CT-2106 (phase I/II)	PGA-Camptothecin (CPT)
Cell therapeutics, Inc.	Non-small cell lung cancer and ovarian cancer	OPAXIO™ (paclitaxel poliglumex, CT-2103; XYOTAX) (phase III)	PGA-Paclitaxel
Nektar	Opioid bowel dysfunction (OBD), and opioid-induced constipation (OIC).	NKTR-118 (phase II)	PEG-naloxol

Paclitaxel is a drug commonly used for the treatment of advanced breast, prostate, and ovarian cancers. It is a very potent cytotoxic drug, although it is hydrophobic and causes side effects such as neutropenia, neuropathies, and hypersensitivity (due to the solubilizing Cremophor EL). Paclitaxel was conjugated with high loadings to PGA (paclitaxel poliglumex, OPAXIO; Cell Therapeutics, Inc.) Although paclitaxel is conjugated to PGA via an ester bond, the polymer backbone is generally stable in the circulation [111]. OPAXIO is currently being evaluated in phase III clinical trials against particularly non-small-cell lung cancer, ovarian cancer as a single agent or in combination therapy with carboplatin. Retrospective analysis of clinical data suggests that OPAXIO's anti-tumor activity may be modulated by estrogen levels. Recent *in vivo* studies indicate that OPAXIO metabolism by some cancer cells is enhanced in the presence of estrogen, which leads to increased levels of paclitaxel in tumor tissue and greater anti-tumor effects [112–115].

Cisplatin is another major chemotherapeutic drug, used in combination with a wide range of other drugs in treatment of various cancers. Its use is restricted due to severe dose-limiting side effects, such as nephrotoxicity, neurotoxicity, ototoxicity, and myelosuppression, which arise from the indiscriminate uptake of the drug into all rapidly dividing cells and the body's attempt to excrete the drug through the kidneys. In addition, the limited doses enable the tumor to develop resistance to the treatment. Therefore, the improvement of platinum-based anti-cancer drugs either by reduced side effects or by overcoming the resistance to this drug is the goal of many studies [116]. Many low-molecular-weight derivatives have been suggested, and some got clinically approved (carboplatin, oxaliplatin). Two HPMA copolymer–platinum conjugates were clinically assessed by Access Pharmaceuticals, namely AP5280 and AP5346. In these two conjugates, the diamine or a diaminocyclohexane (DACH) moiety is bound to a dicarboxylate ligand that is coupled to the polymer. Although phase I clinical trial of AP5280 was promising [117], they chose to focus on AP5346, now named ProLindac™. ProLindac phase II has been completed with the results of excellent tolerability and equivalent efficacy, if not superior to oxaliplatin. Recently, a combination study of ProLindac with paclitaxel has been started in the second-line treatment of pre-treated advanced ovarian cancer [118].

Camptothecin (CPT) is a potent anti-neoplastic agent with activity against a broad range of cancer types. Unmodified CPT has low solubility, high levels of protein binding, and rapid activation through lactone ring hydrolysis [119]. CPT was recently conjugated to the polymeric backbone Fleximer (poly[1-hydroxymethylene hydroxymethyl formal]), which is also called PHF. This polymeric prodrug derivative of CPT, named XMT-1001, is a hydrophilic, biodegradable 40–70 kDa conjugate. Release of CPT from intravenously administered XMT-1001 involves a dual-phase release mechanism, in which CPT is first released in plasma as the lipophilic prodrugs CPT-SI (a succinimidoglycinate derivative) and CPT-SA (a succinamidoyl glycinate derivative), which are then hydrolyzed in tissues to release the lactone active form of CPT. The release of prodrugs to the blood is thought to lower bladder toxicity, due to lower levels of active CPT in the urine. XMT-1001 showed enhanced efficacy and safety in animal models and is currently undergoing phase I clinical trials in cancer patients [119]. Another conjugated form of CPT is CRLX-101 (former name IT-101). CRLX-101 is a conjugate of CPT based on a cyclodextrin polymer. CPT is attached to the polymer at the 20-OH position, which inhibits the ring opening of CPT, so it remains in its active lactone form [120]. CRLX-101 is currently undergoing clinical trials for various types of cancers. So far evidence of function with low side effects was found [121].

Another anti-neoplastic approach is anti-angiogenic therapy, first proposed in 1971 by Judah Folkman [122]. This approach has been since extensively developed, and it is well accepted now that the process of angiogenesis has a strategic role in cancer [123]. The microvasculature endothelial cells, recruited by a tumor, have become an important second target in cancer therapy. However, the vast majority of the anti-angiogenic agents are low-molecular-weight compounds exhibiting poor pharmacokinetic profile with short half-life in the bloodstream and high overall clearance rate [10].

In preclinical studies, caplostatin, an HPMA copolymer conjugate of the anti-angiogenic agent TNP-470, which is a low-molecular-weight analog of fumagillin, has been shown to effectively inhibit tumor progression, and no drug-related toxicities were observed [39,41]. Another anti-angiogenic approach involves specific targeting to tumor endothelial of chemotherapeutics. Polyak et al. used a PEG–DOX conjugate with an RGD peptidomimetic targeting moiety. This conjugate targets endothelial and tumor cells overexpressing $\alpha_v\beta_3$ integrin, thus dual targeting is achieved [52].

4.4 Polymer–Protein Conjugates

Among the different types of polymer therapeutics, polymer–protein conjugates are the most abundant one in clinics (Table 4.5). More than that, the first polymer therapeutic products were the polymer–protein conjugates Zinostatin Stimaler® and Adagen® approved in 1990 for routine clinical use. Proteins as therapeutic agents, like antibodies, cytokines, growth factors and enzymes, are limited in their clinical application. They suffer from instability toward degrading enzymes, short plasma half-life, and immunogenicity. Thus, the coupling of proteins or peptides to polymer carriers could overcome these limitations.

In the field of polymer–protein conjugates, PEG is the most popular option since the clinical value of PEGylation is well established. Besides PEG, only one more polymer conjugate has entered the market. Maeda and co-workers synthesized SMANCS (Zinostatin Stimaler®) by coupling two styrene maleic anhydride (SMA) polymer chains with the anti-tumor protein neocarzinostatin (NCS). During the preclinical trials they noticed that SMANCS was passively accumulating at the tumor site. This phenomenon was defined as the well-known now EPR effect [124]. SMANCS was approved in Japan in 1990 for hepatocellular carcinoma.

PEG has been widely used for conjugation due to its good safety profile, its hydrophilicity and the relative ease of conjugation to proteins. PEGylation as delivery technology differs from the traditional formulations, in which the drug is not released from the formulation and in fact is classed as a new active pharmaceutical ingredient.

The market entry of PEG–protein conjugates was a landmark achievement that advanced the whole field of polymer therapeutics. PEGylation proved to be effective in shielding sensitive sites at the protein surface, as well as prolonging the drug's half-life by decreasing the kidney clearance, suggesting that PEGylated proteins could markedly impact drug behavior *in vivo*. In addition, the decrease in side effects with less frequent dosing has enabled PEGylated protein therapeutics to serve as significant part of the protein therapeutics platform [125]. Several proteins with therapeutic relevance, such as (i) antibodies, (ii) cytokines, (iii) growth factors, and (iv) enzymes, have been conjugated to PEG. In here, an example of each group will be presented.

(i) In the case of cancer and related conditions, most of the investigated proteins are monoclonal antibodies. Certolizumab pegol (CDP870, Cimzia®) is an engineered humanized anti-TNF-α antibody Fab′ fragment that is conjugated to PEG. Clinical studies have demonstrated efficacy in the treatment of moderate-to-severe active Crohn's disease [126]. In 2009 the U.S. FDA-approved Cimzia® for the treatment of adult patients with moderately to severely active rheumatoid arthritis (RA).

Table 4.5 Examples of polymer–protein conjugates and their clinical status

Company	Application	Trade name (clinical status)	Polymer
Yamanouchi pharmaceuticals Co., Ltd.	Hepatocellular carcinoma	Zinostatin Stimalmer® (approved)	Styrene-maleic acid copolymer conjugated to neocarcinostatin
Enzon Pharmaceuticals Inc.	SCID	ADAGEN® (approved)	PEG-adenosine deaminase (ADA)
Enzon Pharmaceuticals Inc.	Acute lymphoblastic leukemia	Oncaspar® (approved)	PEG-L-asparaginase
Roche	Hepatitis C	PEGASYS (approved)	PEG-Interferonα2a (IFNα2a)
Schering-Plough	Hepatitis C	PEG-INTRON® (approved)	PEG-Interferonα2b (IFNα2b)
Amgen	Neutropenia	Neulasta (Pegfilgrastim) (approved)	PEG-Granulocyte colony-stimulating factor (GCSF)
Nektar	Rheumatoid arthritis (Filed for approval US) and Chron's disease (Approved US)	Cimzia® (approved)	PEG-anti TNF alpha antibody fragment
UCB pharma	Non-small cell lung cancer	CDP 791 (phase II)	PEGylated-anti VEGFR2 Fab fragments

Another example is the PEG-antibody fragment angiogenesis inhibitor (CDP791) which is now in phase II clinical study in combination with carboplatin and paclitaxel chemotherapy in first-line non-small cell lung cancer (NSCLC) [127].

(ii) Interferons (IFNs) are multifunctional regulatory cytokines involved in the control of cell function and replication. PEGylation of IFN delays its clearance and reduces its immunogenicity [128]. In addition, two PEG–interferon-α conjugates, IFN-α-2a (PEGASYS®) and IFN-α-2b (PEG-INTRON®), have been approved as treatments for hepatitis B and C [129]. These days, several clinical studies are evaluating the effectiveness of PEG-INTRON® as adjuvant therapy in certain anticancer protocols. This conjugate is now in phase II study for resected stage III melanoma. In the case of PEGASYS®, the coupling of IFN-α-2a to a branched PEG 40 kDa enables the prolongation of the *in vivo* half-life, although a reduction in the *in vitro* activity occurs. This conjugate serves as a good example for the benefits and limits of PEGylation [15].

(iii) PEG 20 kDa conjugated to the granulocyte colony stimulating factor (G-CSF) showed an improved pharmacokinetic profile as consequence to reduced kidney excretion. The PEG–G-CSF conjugate (Neulasta®) was approved for human use in 2002 for the treatment of febrile neutropenia [130].

(iv) Delivering depleting enzymes to the tumor area will cause to degradation of essential amino acids, and eventually to the inhibition of the tumor growth. PEG-asparaginase (Oncaspar®) was the first anti-tumor PEGylated conjugate/enzyme to be approved for clinical use in 1994 as treatment of patients with lymphoblastic leukaemia (ALL). Asparaginase converts asparagine into aspartate and ammonia, thus can treat cancer cells, which rely on the serum supply of asparagine, like the leukemic lymphoblasts cells. This approach of amino acid depleting anti-cancer therapy yielded additional PEG–enzyme conjugates, which are presently under clinical trials [15]. A different example is the PEG-adenosine deaminase, which was the first PEGylated protein to enter the market in 1990. It is used to treat adenosine deaminase deficient X-linked severe combined immunodeficiency disease (SCID)[131].

PEGylation is a mature and effective delivery technology for improving the therapeutic index of proteins. The growing interest in PEGylation is clearly demonstrated by the number of PEG–protein conjugates reaching the market or under clinical trials. Today, polymer–protein conjugates are used routinely as anti-cancer therapeutics, as an adjunct to chemotherapy, and are also being developed as components for combination therapy [132].

4.5 Defined-Shape Polymeric Nanocarriers

4.5.1 Self-Assembled Polymers

Self-assembling aggregates, such as micelles and vesicles, can be used as delivery vehicles for therapeutics. Most self-assembling structures are composed of amphiphilic molecules containing hydrophobic and hydrophilic domains. In aqueous environment, the amphiphilic molecules associate through non-covalent interactions forming supra-molecular structures. The hydrophilic domains of the amphiphilic molecules face the aqueous solvent, and the hydrophobic domains are shielded from the solvent in a bulk hydrophobic volume core. Usually drugs are encapsulated in the hydrophobic region of the aggregate and released by passive diffusion, or on the disassembly or the degradation of the aggregate. Self-assembled aggregates can be designed to release their payload in response to environmental changes in pH, temperature, and redox potential, as reviewed by Branco and Schneider [133]. The self-assembly process is spontaneous, and when conducted in the presence of small drugs, easy loading is achieved [133, 134].

Lipids were the first self-assembled materials used for drug delivery, mainly in the form of micelles and liposomes (lipid-based vesicles). Such systems have been extensively investigated, bearing fruit in a significant number of commercially available drug formulations, and many undergoing clinical trials. Self-assembling polymers have been used in a similar manner to lipid systems holding few advantages over them. Self-assembled polymeric vehicles have enhanced stability compared with lipid aggregates, leading to a better control over drug release [134]. In addition, polymeric aggregates' size and shape can be tailor-made by suitable choice of monomers type and sequence and molecular weight of the polymer. Moreover, using polymers, bigger micelles can be achieved than with low-molecular-weight lipids and surfactants (usually 20–200 nm for polymeric micelles as opposed to up to few nanometers for lipid micelles).

There are several aggregates structures used for drug delivery. Here we will briefly discuss the common ones (Figures 4.1C and D). Frequently encountered structure is the micelle. Diblock and triblock copolymers are commonly used to construct micellar assemblies, where the hydrophilic block constitutes the shell of the micelle that interacts with the aqueous surroundings and the hydrophobic block forms the micellar core. The hydrophobic core can serve as a depot for small non-soluble drugs. Usually PEG (also referred to in this field as PEO, polyethyleneoxide) is used as the hydrophilic block. Polycaprolactone (PCL) and polylactic acid (PLA) are typical hydrophobic blocks, but other hydrophobic polymers, peptide segments, or fatty acids are used as well. The incorporation of other functions such as targeting and increased cellular uptake can be achieved by attaching functional moieties to the hydrophilic block, thus placing them in the solvent exposed shell of the micelle. For example, Wu et al. [135] prepared targeted pH-responsive micelles by mixing AP peptide, that has a specific affinity to IL-4 receptors of atherosclerotic plaques and breast tumor tissue, conjugated to PEG-PLA copolymer, with pH-responsive methyl ether poly(ethylene glycol) (MPEG)-poly(β-amino ester) (PAE) block copolymer (MPEG-PAE). The mixed block copolymers were self-assembled forming 150 nm-diameter micelles, which disassemble at pH below 6.8. The micelles were loaded with doxorubicin. This system showed efficient delivery and excellent anti-cancer therapeutic efficacy in MDA-MB231 human breast tumor-bearing mice (compared with free doxorubicin and doxorubicin encapsulated in equivalent micelles without the AP targeting). There are many more studies in progress, and some are viewed in recent reviews [133, 136]. Some polymeric micellar systems are already in clinical trials (Table 4.6), such as Genexol-PM, methoxypoly(ethylene glycol)-block-poly(D,L-lactide) (mPEG-PDLLA) polymeric micelles used for the formulation of paclitaxel. These micelles were successfully tested in phase II for the treatment of metastatic breast cancer [137], advanced or metastatic pancreatic cancer [138], and advanced non-small-cell lung cancer in combination with cisplatin [139].

Another structure commonly in use is the vesicle. Polymeric vesicles are termed polymersomes (similarly to lipid vesicles-liposomes) and are composed of polymeric membrane closing on itself to form a sphere around an aqueous core (Figure 4.1D). These structures hold great advantage since the water-filled core allows additional encapsulation of hydrophilic therapeutics, thus making polymersomes an attractive vehicle for combination therapy. The release of drugs from the aqueous core is achieved by slow diffusion through the vesicle membrane or when the vesicle degrades and its content is spilled. Like in micelles, the release can be environmentally triggered by pH, temperature or redox changes. Ahmed et al. [140] mixed inert PEG-polybutadiene diblock copolymer with biodegradable PEG-PLA diblock copolymer (75:25 % respectively) to form vesicles. Hydrophobic paclitaxel was encapsulated in the thick polymeric membrane, while hydrophilic doxorubicin was trapped in the aqueous core of the polymersomes, thus ensuring simultaneous delivery. These polymersomes rapture at the endolysosome and were shown to cause shrinkage of MDA-MB231 tumors in mice, while the free drugs only slowed tumor growth [140]. Although this approach is very elegant and promising, only few studies demonstrated drug delivery using polymersomes.

Table 4.6 Examples of polymeric micelles and polymer-nucleic acid complexes

Company	Application	Trade name (clinical status)	Polymer
		Polymeric micelles	
Samyang	Breast, pancreatic and advanced non-small-cell lung cancer	Genexol-PM (phase II)	mPEG-poly(D,L-lactide) encapsulating paclitaxel
NanoCarrier	Advanced solid tumors	NK105 (Marketed in Asia)	PEG-poly(aspartic acid) block copolymer-paclitaxel
NanoCarrier	Advanced solid tumors	NC-6004 (Marketed in Asia)	PEG-poly(glutamic acid) block copolymer-cisplatin

Supratek Pharma Inc.	Carcinoma of the oesophagus, Adenocarcinoma of the upper gastrointestinal tract	SP1049C (phase II)	Pluronic-doxorubicin
	Polymer-nucleic acid complexes		
Eyetech Pharmaceuticals, Inc./Pfizer, Inc.	Macular degeneration (wet AMD)	Pegaptanib, Macugen (approved)	PEGylated neutralizing RNA aptamer for vascular endothelial growth factor (VEGF)
Calando Pharmaceuticals	Various solid tumors	CALAA-01 (phase I)	siRNA against RRM2 complexed with cyclodextrin adamantine-PEG/ transferrin complexes

4.5.2 Dendrimers

Although self-assembling aggregates show many advantages as drug delivery vehicles, they often suffer from low stability under shear force and dilution, which are important environmental effects in drug administration. An interesting alternative is the use of dendrimers that are practically unimolecular micelles. A typical dendrimer comprises a multifunctional central core, branched units and surface groups, all covalently attached. The repeated layers are termed "generations" (G) and are related to the number of steps in the synthesis, i.e., the number of brunching points between the core and the surface (Figure 4.1E). Dendrimers are monodisperse, and their size can be set between 5 and 20 nm [141] depending on choice of components and number of generations. Small hydrophobic drugs can be encapsulated at the inner cavity of the dendrimers, while combination of drugs, DNA/RNA, targeting, solubilizing, or imaging moieties, can be attached to the surface groups covalently or electrostatically.

Their stability, monodispersity, and, especially, multivalency make the dendrimers attractive candidates for drug delivery. Although there is a massive research in that direction, this field is still in a preliminary stage and only few *in vivo* studies have been reported. Well-known commercialized dendrimers are polypropyleneimine (PPI) and polyamido amine (PAMAM), both carrying cationic surface groups. Cationic dendrimers are attractive mainly as nucleic acids carriers, as will be discussed later. However, cationic dendrimers interact non-specifically with negatively charged biological membranes, which results in toxicity. Conversely, anionic or neutral dendrimers are non-toxic [142, 143]. Most current efforts are focused at lowering the toxicity and utilizing dendrimers as therapeutic nano-carriers either by developing biocompatible and biodegradable dendrimers, or by surface modifications of dendrimers. Various biocompatible dendrimers have been developed such as citric acid dendrimers [144], phosphate dendrimers [145], and lysine dendrimers [146]. Biodegradable dendrimers such as polyester dendrimers [147], polyether dendrimers [148] and triazine dendrimers [149] have also been examined. Another promising approach is modifying the surface of dendrimers with various functional groups, thus masking the cationic charge of the dendrimers and gaining functionality. Examples for surface functionality are targeting and enhanced cellular internalization moieties, drug or DNA/RNA complexation or conjugation, improved pharmacokinetic properties by PEGylation, etc. Singh et al. [150] used 4G PAMAM dendrimers conjugated to folic acid through PEG spacer and loaded them with anti-cancerous drug 5-fluorouracil (5-FU). Their results indicated that this dendrimer conjugate is significantly safer and more effective in tumor targeting compared with free drug and non-PEGylated formulation. Another interesting utilization of dendrimers is for imaging, as was explored by Zhang et al. [151]. 5G PAMAM dendrimers were radiolabeled with ^{99m}Tc that were similarly conjugated to PEG and folic acid, and successfully used in micro-SPECT (single photon emission computed tomography) imaging of KB tumor bearing nude mice, showing specific accumulation in tumors.

4.5.3 The Influence of Shape on Performance

Although the elegance of dendritic and micellar systems aesthetically appeals to us, we should ask ourselves what the true advantages of these systems are. The most striking advantage is their surface multivalency. In addition, these systems are relatively monodisperse and are of defined shape, usually globular. Geng et al. [152] studied filomicelles (long filamentous stable diblock copolymeric micelles of PEG–polyethylethylene or PEG–polycaprolactone) and showed that filament structures persist in circulation after intravenous injection considerably longer than rigid rods (λ-phages) and flexible spheres ("stealth" polymersomes). Filomicelles of varied length loaded with paclitaxel shrank A549 tumors in nude mice, with greater efficacy for longer filomicelles (up to 8 μm). They attributed this to the nanoparticles behavior under flow; spherical and short filaments are readily taken up by cells, while flexible long filaments are extended by the flow and flow past the cells. Under static conditions, long filaments are relaxed and internalized by cells. Thus the elongated filament shape, as well as filament flexibility, makes it a better delivery system. These *in vitro* experiments were conducted under flow velocity similar to that in the spleen. It should be interesting to conduct similar experiments under conditions resembling the sluggish flow of tumor vasculature. This may shed more light on physical mechanisms leading to the EPR effect. Saad et al. [153] conducted a comparative efficacy study of various drug nanocarriers. They used 30 nm linear PEG polymer, 5 nm PAMAM dendrimer, and 100 nm liposome to deliver paclitaxel to H69 and A549 lung cancer cells and tumors on nude mice. All nanocarriers were marked with Cy5.5 and a synthetic analog of LHRH peptide was attached for targeting. They found that all nanocarriers showed enhanced efficacy compared with the free drug. Without the targeting LHRH peptide, dendrimeric nanocarrier was the least effective, while PEG polymer nanocarrier was the most effective in suppressing tumor growth. This result correlates well with Geng et al. [152] theorem of better efficacy for long flexible filaments as nanocarriers. The most surprising result of Saad et al. [153] was received when adding targeting moieties to these nanocarriers. Targeting with LHRL peptide significantly enhanced anti-tumor activity of all nanocarriers and leveled down the differences between them. This suggests that when using effective targeting, nanocarriers can be selected based on parameters such as type of therapeutic, solubility, electric charge, ease of preparation, etc., rather than architectural parameters such as size and shape.

4.6 Polymer–DNA/RNA Complexes

Nucleic acids are the focus of massive therapeutic studies (46,505 hits on PubMed for "gene therapy") for gene delivery (pDNA) and gene silencing (siRNA, ODNs). Both DNA and RNA molecules have an anionic phosphodiester backbone and can interact with cationic agents. For therapeutic effect, pDNA has to reach cell nucleus, while the siRNA molecules need to enter the cytosol. Nucleic acids, and especially RNA, suffer from enzymatic degradation. In addition, even if they reach their target cell, their negative charge and the uncondensed pDNA size hinder cell internalization. Therefore, nucleic acids have a true need for a carrier, a need well met by cationic polymers.

The complexes of nucleic acids with their polymeric nanocarriers, termed polyplexes, are usually formed by electrostatic interactions; thus, polycations such as poly(L-lysine) (PLL) and PEI have been extensively used for *in vitro* delivery. After cell internalization, the polyplexes should escape the endosome. This escape is achieved by disrupting the endosomal membrane either by conjugation to a membrane disruptive protein, or by swelling and bursting of the endosome through protonation of excess amine groups on the polymer itself. This "proton-sponge" effect causes an influx of chloride ions followed by osmotic swelling and a disruption of the endosome [154]. PEI has been considered the gold standard in many *in vitro* and *in vivo* assays in terms of transfection efficiency, due to favorable characteristics of DNA protection, cell binding and uptake, endosomal escape, and release from the carrier. Its main drawbacks are the significant cytotoxicity both *in vivo* and *in vitro*, at least for the high-molecular-weight forms of the polymer. The limited degradability of PEI excludes repeated systemic therapeutic use [22]. Its and other polymers' toxicity is a result of a net excessive positive surface charge, promoting non-specific interactions with negatively charged biological membranes and serum proteins. Various approaches were pursued to overcome this hurdle. Many reports describe analogous biodegradable polymers, which decompose to smaller metabolites of lowered toxicity [155]. Self-assembled structures, such as micellar structures composed of diblock copolymers, have been used as well. The nucleic acids are bound to the cationic inner core, while usually PEG provides the neutral steric protecting outer shell. Kataoka and coworkers prepared such system with PEG block and polycation block carrying ethylenediamine side chains as a nanocarrier for reporter genes (luciferase and FLAG pDNAs) transfection to rabbit carotid artery with induced neointimal lesions. These polyplexes showed reduced cytotoxicity and thrombogenicity, and appreciable gene transfer *in vivo* [156]. Dendrimers are also frequently used. Ofek et al. [157] examined polyglycerol-based core with amine shell dendrimers for the delivery of siRNA. They evaluated the dendrimers as nanocarriers for gene silencing using luciferase-based model *in vitro* and *in vivo*. The luciferase siRNA loaded dendrimers were found to be biocompatible and showed efficient inhibition of luciferase expression in luciferase-expressing tumors in mice [157].

Davis et al. [158] have been conducting a phase I clinical trial of siRNA systemic delivery system to patients with solid cancers. They use IV-administrated 70 nm self-assembled nanoparticles. The siRNA electrostatically binds to a linear cyclodextrin-based polymer (CDP), which is a short copolymer of cyclodextrin and amide charge centers. Adamantane (AD) strongly associates with cyclodextrin to form inclusion complexes. This property was used to introduce surface cyclodextrin modifications of the nanoparticles; AD-PEG was added for the steric stabilization of the surface by PEG, and AD-transferrin protein (AD-Tf) was added as a targeting ligand to transferrin receptors (TfR) on cancer cells. Imidazole end group was attached to the linear CDP to provide escape from endocytic vesicles and nanoparticle release of the nucleic acid into the cytoplasm. Each of the delivery components is sufficiently small to enable kidney clearance when the nanoparticle disassembles into individual components. Using this platform, a potent siRNA against RRM2 (ribonucleotide reductase subunit 2), which exhibits significant anti-proliferative activity in a broad spectrum of cancer types of human, mouse, rat, and monkey, is currently delivered in humans [6, 158].

A few systems have progressed beyond pre-clinical trials (Table 4.6). For efficient nucleic acid delivery, the polymeric carriers have to fulfill many complicated demands. They need to stabilize the nucleic acid against degradation but release it at its biological site of action. They need to penetrate the cell membrane without harming them, to escape the endosome, and to release and target their cargo intracellularly. These challenging demands require sophisticated carriers for effective gene therapy.

4.7 Combination Therapy

A great advantage of the polymeric delivery system is the ability to tailor different compounds with controlled loading percentage on the polymeric backbone (Figure 4.1). The concomitant targeted delivery of two agents that act synergistically allows the administration of lower concentrations of each agent, increasing their combined anti-tumor efficacy and decreasing their toxicity. This direction has been explored lately by many. Here we will give a few examples. The reader is referred to a thorough review about combination therapy in polymer therapeutics [159].

DOX and the aromatase inhibitor aminoglutethimide (AGM) were conjugated to HPMA copolymer by Vicent et al. [160]. This conjugate was the first to combine endocrine therapy and chemotherapy on one polymeric backbone. It exhibited increased anti-tumor activity *in vitro* on breast cancer cells. Santucci et al. [161] conjugated both epirubicin and nitric oxide (NO) agents on PEG. The combination of these two agents is synergistic. Furthermore, NO displays cardioprotective action that could counterbalance the cardiotoxicity induced by epirubicin. The resulting conjugate induced higher cytotoxic effect on Caco-2 cells than free epirubicin. Moreover, NO presented a protection effect against epirubicin-mediated cardiotoxicity in adult cardiomyocytes [161]. In another combination study, HPMA copolymer was conjugated to DOX and anti-inflammatory drug dexamethason through pH-sensitive linker. The release of the drugs was examined *in vitro* [162]. Bae et al. [163] conjugated DOX and a phosphatidylinositol-3 kinase inhibitor wortmannin (WOR) to poly(ethylene glycol)-poly(aspartate hydrazide) block copolymers through a hydrazone bond. These polymer–drug conjugates assembled into less than 100 nm micelles in which the drug mixing ratios between DOX/WOR were precisely controlled. Cytotoxicity assay against a human breast cancer MCF-7 cell line showed enhanced cytotoxic activity.

Combining bone-targeting moiety and a drug on a polymeric backbone is also attracting much attention, aiming to target bone-related diseases actively. Work done in our laboratory recently presented two HPMA copolymer conjugates based on the bone-targeting anti-angiogenic bisphosphonate alendronate. On one HPMA copolymer paclitaxel and alendronate were conjugated. This conjugate exhibited a binding capacity to hydroxyapatide, antiproliferative, anti-angiogenic properties [41]. The anti-angiogenic agents TNP-470 and alendronate were also conjugated with HPMA copolymer using the RAFT technique [32]. The combination of these two agents showed to have a synergistic anti-angiogenic effect. Therefore, the conjugation of both TNP-470 and alendronate with HPMA copolymer could serve both as an efficient bone drug delivery system and as a potent anti-cancer combination therapy.

Another fascinating direction is the combined delivery of a drug with DNA or RNA. For example, Wang et al. [164] designed a biodegradable cationic amphiphilic copolymer, composed of poly(*N*-methyldietheneamine sebacate) (PMDS) cationic main chain and cholesterol side chains. This copolymer self-assembles in aqueous solution forming a hydrophobic cholesterol core and a cationic shell. Paclitaxel was encapsulated in the hydrophobic core, while IL-12-encoded plasmid was used as therapeutic gene electrostatically attached to the cationic shell. These polymeric micelles were delivered into 4T1 mouse breast tumors, showing a significantly reduced growth rate of the tumors. *In vitro* examination of paclitaxel and Bcl-2-targeted siRNA combination using these polymeric micelles showed synergistic effect as well [164].

As demonstrated in the examples above, polymeric systems are the ideal platform for true combination therapy, where the therapeutics are given simultaneously in one injection and share the same pharmacokinetic profile. This exciting field holds great promise and is rapidly evolving.

4.8 Summary and a Look into the Future

There is a growing number of polymer therapeutics entering clinical trials. As we can see in this chapter, the literature is full of studies on polymer–drug conjugates, polymer–protein conjugates, defined-shape polymer architectures, and polyplexes. However, only few polymeric nano-carriers have reached the market. One obstacle is the regulatory issue. All polymer therapeutics are considered new chemical entities (NCEs) [165], since the drug is covalently bound to the polymeric carriers, as opposed to the conventional drug delivery systems, in which the drug is entrapped. The heterogeneity of the polymer product, molecular weight, and biodegradability of the polymer backbone are important parameters that influence the human safety for any new polymeric nanomedicine. Furthermore, there is still a need to improve the characterization of these NCEs, in order to facilitate their entry to clinical trials. There are still challenges to ensure the safe and rapid translation of polymer therapeutics into routine clinical use.

A big step forward was the discovery and utilization of the EPR effect for passive targeting. Unquestionably, it is one of the main factors that have promoted the field of polymer therapeutics [166]. However, there is still a need to gain more information regarding the individual tumor types and metastases in humans, for improved efficiency and specificity of the pro-drugs.

Nevertheless, the field of polymer therapeutics has seen a significant progress with the entry of PEGylated proteins into the market [15], together with the flourish in all polymer therapeutics studies in recent years. The implementation of targeting moieties and combinations of therapeutics on the same polymeric nanocarrier may take us the extra step toward a smart therapeutic system, which holds a true advantage over existing therapies. The desirable goal of specific and controlled drug release, with minimal side effects, is coming into being. The use of polymers as carriers together with the innovations in the polymer chemistry area and further understanding of cell biology (i.e., mechanism of binding and uptake of the polymers, biodistribution, etc.), will eventually result in the rational design of effective drug delivery systems and their extensive use in cancer and other related diseases, such as angiogenesis-dependent ones.

References

1. Ringsdorf, H., *Structure and properties of pharmacologically active polymers.* J. Polym. Sci. Symp., 1975. **51**: p. 135–153.
2. Matsumura, Y. and H. Maeda, *A New Concept for Macromolecular Therapeutics in Cancer-Chemotherapy — Mechanism of Tumoritropic Accumulation of Proteins and the Antitumor Agent Smancs.* Cancer Research, 1986. **46**(12): p. 6387–6392.
3. Maeda, H., et al., *Tumor vascular permeability and the EPR effect in macromolecular therapeutics: a review.* J Control Release, 2000. **65**(1–2): p. 271–284.
4. Sanchis, J., et al., *Polymer-drug conjugates for novel molecular targets.* Nanomedicine (London). **5**(6): p. 915–935.

5. Alexis, F., et al., *Factors affecting the clearance and biodistribution of polymeric nanoparticles.* Mol Pharm, 2008. **5**(4): p. 505–515.
6. Davis, M.E., *The first targeted delivery of siRNA in humans via a self-assembling, cyclodextrin polymer-based nanoparticle: from concept to clinic.* Mol Pharm, 2009. **6**(3): p. 659–668.
7. Perrault, S.D., et al., *Mediating tumor targeting efficiency of nanoparticles through design.* Nano Lett, 2009. **9**(5): p. 1909–1915.
8. Alberts B., B.D., Johnson A., Lewis J., Raff M., Roberts K., Walter P., *Essential Cell Biology*. 1998, New York: Garland Publishing. 472–477.
9. Pan H. and K. J., *Multifunctional Water-Soluble Polymers for Drug Delivery*, in *Multifunctional Pharmaceutical Nanocarriers*, M. Ferrari, Editor. 2008, Springer. p. 81–142.
10. Satchi-Fainaro, R., R. Duncan, and C.M. Barnes, *Polymer therapeutics for cancer: Current status and future challenges*, in *Polymer Therapeutics II: Polymers as Drugs, Conjugates and Gene Delivery Systems.* 2006, Springer-Verlag Berlin: Berlin. p. 1–65.
11. Markman, M., *Improving the toxicity profile of chemotherapy for advanced ovarian cancer: a potential role for CT-2103.* J Exp Ther Oncol, 2004. **4**(2): p. 131–136.
12. Langer, C.J., *CT-2103: a novel macromolecular taxane with potential advantages compared with conventional taxanes.* Clin Lung Cancer, 2004. **6 Suppl 2**: p. S85–S88.
13. Pawar, R., et al., *A. Polysaccharides as carriers of bioactive agents for medical application.* Natural-Based Polymers for Biomedical Applications, ed. R.L.E. Reis. 2008, New York: Woodhead Pub. 50.
14. Caliceti, P., S. Salmaso, and S. Bersani, *Polysaccharide-base anticancer prodrugs.* Macromolecular Anticancer Therapeutics, ed. P.E. Harivardhan R.L.; Couvreur. 2010, New York: Humana Press. 163–220.
15. Pasut, G. and F.M. Veronese, *PEG conjugates in clinical development or use as anticancer agents: an overview.* Adv Drug Deliv Rev, 2009. **61**(13): p. 1177–1188.
16. Duncan, R., *Development of HPMA copolymer-anticancer conjugates: clinical experience and lessons learnt.* Adv Drug Deliv Rev, 2009. **61**(13): p. 1131–1148.
17. Kopecek, J. and P. Kopeckova, *HPMA copolymers: origins, early developments, present, and future.* Adv Drug Deliv Rev, 2010. **62**(2): p. 122–149.
18. Chun, L., *Poly(L-glutamic acid)-anticancer drug conjugates.* Adv Drug Deliv Rev, 2002. **54**: p. 695–713.

19. Bisht, S. and A. Maitra, *Dextran-doxorubicin/chitosan nanoparticles for solid tumor therapy.* Wiley Interdiscip Rev Nanomed Nanobiotechnol, 2009. **1**(4): p. 415–425.

20. Baldwin, A.D. and K.L. Kiick, *Polysaccharide-modified synthetic polymeric biomaterials.* Biopolymers, 2010. **94**(1): p. 128–140.

21. Grzelinski, M., et al., *RNA interference-mediated gene silencing of pleiotrophin through polyethylenimine-complexed small interfering RNAs in vivo exerts antitumoral effects in glioblastoma xenografts.* Human Gene Ther, 2006. **17**(7): p. 751–766.

22. Schaffert, D. and E. Wagner, *Gene therapy progress and prospects: synthetic polymer-based systems.* Gene Ther, 2008. **15**(16): p. 1131–1138.

23. Danhauser-Riedl, S., et al., *Phase I clinical and pharmacokinetic trial of dextran conjugated doxorubicin (AD-70, DOX-OXD).* Invest New Drugs, 1993. **11**(2–3): p. 187–195.

24. Singh, R.S., G.K. Saini, and J.F. Kennedy, *Pullulan: microbial sources, production and applications.* Carbohyr Polym, 2008. **73**: p. 515–531.

25. Leather, T.D., *Production and applications of pullulan.* Appl. Microbiol Biotechnol, 2003. **62**: p. 468–473.

26. Kim, S., et al., *Insulinotropic activity of sulfonylurea/pullulan conjugate in rat islet microcapsule.* Biomaterials, 2003. **24**(26): p. 4843–4851.

27. Clementi, C., et al., *Dendritic Poly(ethylene glycol) bearing Paclitaxel and Alendronate for targeting bone neoplasms.* Mol Pharm, 2011. **8**(4): p. 1063–1072.

28. Vasey, P.A., et al., Phase I clinical and pharmacokinetic study of PK1 [*N*-(2-hydroxypropyl)methacrylamide copolymer doxorubicin]: first member of a new class of chemotherapeutic agents-drug-polymer conjugates. Cancer Research Campaign Phase I/II Committee. *Clin Cancer Res*, 1999. **5**(1): p. 83–94.

29. Teodorescu, M. and K. Matyjaszewski, *Atom transfer radical polymerization of (meth)acrylamides.* Macromolecules, 1999. **32**: p. 4826–4831.

30. Teodorescu, M. and K. Matyjaszewski, *Controlled polymerization of (meth)acrylamides by atom transfer radical polymerization.* Macrol. Rapid Commun., 2000. **21**: p. 190–194.

31. Scales, C.W., et al., Direct, controlled synthesis of the nonimmunogenic, hydrophilic polymer, poly(*N*-(2-hydroxypropyl)methacrylamide) via RAFT in aqueous media. *Biomacromolecules*, 2005. **6**(4): p. 1846–1850.

32. Segal, E., et al., *Targeting angiogenesis-dependent calcified neoplasms using combined polymer therapeutics.* PLoS One, 2009. **4**(4): p. e5233.

33. Chytil, P., et al., *N*-(2-Hydroxypropyl)methacrylamide-based polymer conjugates with pH-controlled activation of doxorubicin for cell-specific or passive tumour targeting. Synthesis by RAFT polymerisation and physicochemical characterisation. *Eur J Pharm Sci*, 2010. **41**(3–4): p. 473–482.

34. Ulbrich, K., et al., *Polymeric conjugates of drugs and antibodies for site-specific drug delivery.* Macromol Symp, 1996. **103**: p. 177–192.

35. Putnam, D. and J. Kopecek, *Polymer conjugates with anticancer activity.* Biopolymers II, 1995. **122**: p. 55–123.

36. Ulbrich, K. and V. Subr, *Polymeric anticancer drugs with pH-controlled activation.* Adv Drug Deliv Rev, 2004. **56**(7): p. 1023–1050.

37. Kratz, F., U. Beyer, and M.T. Schutte, *Drug-polymer conjugates containing acid-cleavable bonds.* Crit Rev Ther Drug Carrier Syst, 1999. **16**(3): p. 245–288.

38. Rodrigues, P.C.A., et al., Correlation of the acid-sensitivity of polyethylene glycol daunorubicin conjugates with their *in vitro* antiproliferative activity. Bioorg Med Chem, 2006. **14**(12): p. 4110–4117.

39. Meng, F.H., W.E. Hennink, and Z. Zhong, *Reduction-sensitive polymers and bioconjugates for biomedical applications.* Biomaterials, 2009. **30**(12): p. 2180–2198.

40. Kopeček, J., et al., *Synthetic polymeric drugs*, U.S. Patent, Editor. 1991.

41. Miller, K., et al., *Targeting bone metastases with a bispecific anticancer and antiangiogenic polymer-alendronate-taxane conjugate.* Angew Chem Int Ed Engl, 2009. **48**(16): p. 2949–2954.

42. Dubowchik, G.M., et al., *Cathepsin B-labile dipeptide linkers for lysosomal release of doxorubicin from internalizing immunoconjugates: model studies of enzymatic drug release and antigen-specific in vitro anticancer activity.* Bioconjug Chem, 2002. **13**(4): p. 855–869.

43. Liu, C., et al., *Overexpression of legumain in tumors is significant for invasion/metastasis and a candidate enzymatic target for prodrug therapy.* Cancer Res, 2003. **63**(11): p. 2957–2964.

44. Stern, L., et al., *A novel antitumor prodrug platform designed to be cleaved by the endoprotease legumain.* Bioconjug Chem, 2009. **20**(3): p. 500–510.

45. Kratz, F., et al., *Development and in vitro efficacy of novel MMP2 and MMP9 specific doxorubicin albumin conjugates.* Bioorg Med Chem Lett, 2001. **11**(15): p. 2001–2006.

46. Kratz, F., et al., *Prodrug strategies in anticancer chemotherapy.* ChemMedChem, 2008. **3**(1): p. 20–53.

47. Apostolovic, B., et al., *Hybrid polymer therapeutics incorporating bioresponsive, coiled coil peptide linkers.* Biomacromolecules, 2010. **11**(5): p. 1187–1195.

48. Strebhardt, K. and A. Ullrich, *Paul Ehrlich's magic bullet concept: 100 years of progress.* Nat Rev Cancer, 2008. **8**(6): p. 473–480.

49. Parveen, S. and S.K. Sahoo, *Polymeric nanoparticles for cancer therapy.* J Drug Target, 2008. **16**(2): p. 108–123.

50. Ishida, T., et al., *Targeted delivery and triggered release of liposomal doxorubicin enhances cytotoxicity against human B lymphoma cells.* Biochim Biophys Acta, 2001. **1515**(2): p. 144–158.

51. Ryppa, C., et al., *In vitro and in vivo evaluation of a paclitaxel conjugate with the divalent peptide E-[c(RGDfK)2] that targets integrin alpha v beta 3.* Int J Pharm, 2009. **368**(1–2): p. 89–97.

52. Polyak, D., et al., *Development of PEGylated doxorubicin-E-[c(RGDfK)2] conjugate for integrin-targeted cancer therapy.* Polym. Adv. Technol., 2011. **22**: p. 103–113.

53. Kaneshiro, T.L. and Z.R. Lu, *Targeted intracellular codelivery of chemotherapeutics and nucleic acid with a well-defined dendrimer-based nanoglobular carrier.* Biomaterials, 2009. **30**(29): p. 5660–5666.

54. Oba, M., et al., *Cyclic RGD peptide-conjugated polyplex micelles as a targetable gene delivery system directed to cells possessing alphavbeta3 and alphavbeta5 integrins.* Bioconjug Chem, 2007. **18**(5): p. 1415–1423.

55. Arnaout, M.A., S.L. Goodman, and J.P. Xiong, *Coming to grips with integrin binding to ligands.* Curr Opin Cell Biol, 2002. **14**(5): p. 641–651.

56. Adar, L., et al., *Pro-apoptotic peptide-polymer conjugates to induce mitochondrial-dependent cell death.* Polym Adv Technol, *in press,* 2010.

57. Gragoudas, E.S., et al., *Pegaptanib for neovascular age-related macular degeneration.* N Engl J Med, 2004. **351**(27): p. 2805–2816.

58. Milane, L.J., Z. Duan, and M.M. Amiji, *Development of EGFR-targeted polymer blend nanocarriers for Paclitaxel/Lonidamine delivery to treat multi-drug resistance in human breast and ovarian tumor cells.* Mol Pharm, 2010. **8**(1): p. 185–203.

59. Shamay, Y., et al., *E-selectin binding peptide-polymer-drug conjugates and their selective cytotoxicity against vascular endothelial cells.* Biomaterials, 2009. **30**(32): p. 6460–6468.

60. Kneuer, C., et al., *Selectins — potential pharmacological targets?* Drug Discov Today, 2006. **11**(21–22): p. 1034–1040.

61. Park, K., et al., *Target specific tumor treatment by VEGF siRNA complexed with reducible polyethyleneimine-hyaluronic acid conjugate.* Biomaterials, 2010. **31**(19): p. 5258–5265.
62. Canal, F., et al., *Relevance of folic acid/polymer ratio in targeted PEG-epirubicin conjugates.* J Control Release, 2010. **146**(3): p. 388–399.
63. Pinhassi, R.I., et al., *Arabinogalactan-folic acid-drug conjugate for targeted delivery and target-activated release of anticancer drugs to folate receptor-overexpressing cells.* Biomacromolecules. **11**(1): p. 294–303.
64. Pasut, G., et al., *Antitumoral activity of PEG-gemcitabine prodrugs targeted by folic acid.* J Control Release, 2008. **127**(3): p. 239–248.
65. Yang, X., et al., Tumor-targeting, pH-responsive, and stable unimolecular micelles as drug nanocarriers for targeted cancer therapy. *Bioconjug Chem.*
66. Bae, Y., N. Nishiyama, and K. Kataoka, *In vivo antitumor activity of the folate-conjugated pH-sensitive polymeric micelle selectively releasing adriamycin in the intracellular acidic compartments.* Bioconjug Chem, 2007. **18**(4): p. 1131–1139.
67. Thomas, T.P., et al., *Targeting and inhibition of cell growth by an engineered dendritic nanodevice.* J Med Chem, 2005. **48**(11): p. 3729–3735.
68. Daniels, T.R., et al., *The transferrin receptor part II: targeted delivery of therapeutic agents into cancer cells.* Clin Immunol, 2006. **121**(2): p. 159–176.
69. Gomme, P.T., K.B. McCann, and J. Bertolini, *Transferrin: structure, function and potential therapeutic actions.* Drug Discov Today, 2005. **10**(4): p. 267–273.
70. Tsukagoshi, S., *A new LH-RH agonist for treatment of prostate cancer, 3-month controlled-release formulation of goserelin acetate (Zoladex LA 10.8 mg depot) — outline of pre-clinical and clinical studies.* Gan To Kagaku Ryoho, 2002. **29**(9): p. 1675–1687.
71. Dharap, S.S., et al., *Molecular targeting of drug delivery systems to ovarian cancer by BH3 and LHRH peptides.* J Control Release, 2003. **91**(1–2): p. 61–73.
72. Khandare, J.J., et al., *Novel polymeric prodrug with multivalent components for cancer therapy.* J Pharmacol Exp Ther, 2006. **317**(3): p. 929–937.
73. Heyns, C.F., et al., *Comparative efficacy of triptorelin pamoate and leuprolide acetate in men with advanced prostate cancer.* BJU Int, 2003. **92**(3): p. 226–231.

74. O'Hare, K.B., et al., Polymeric drug-carriers containing doxorubicin and melanocyte-stimulating hormone: *in vitro* and *in vivo* evaluation against murine melanoma. *J Drug Target*, 1993. **1**(3): p. 217–229.
75. Hopewel, J.W., et al., *Preclinical evaluation of the cardiotoxicity of PK2: a novel HPMA copolymer-doxorubicin-galactosamine conjugate antitumour agent.* Hum Exp Toxicol, 2001. **20**(9): p. 461–470.
76. Seymour, L.W., et al., *N*-(2-hydroxypropyl)methacrylamide copolymers targeted to the hepatocyte galactose-receptor: pharmacokinetics in DBA2 mice. *Br J Cancer*, 1991. **63**(6): p. 859–866.
77. Hu, C.-M.J., et al., *Half-antibody functionalized lipid–polymer hybrid nanoparticles for targeted drug delivery to carcinoembryonic antigen presenting pancreatic cancer cells.* Mol Pharm, 2010. **7**(3): p. 914–920.
78. Dhal, P.K., et al., *Functional polymers as therapeutic agents: concept to market place.* Adv Drug Deliv Rev, 2009. **61**(13): p. 1121–1130.
79. Vicent, M.J., H. Ringsdorf, and R. Duncan, *Polymer therapeutics: clinical applications and challenges for development.* Adv Drug Deliv Rev, 2009. **61**(13): p. 1117–1120.
80. Stedronsky, E.R., *Interaction of bile-acids and cholesterol with nonsystemic agents having hypocholesterolemic properties.* Biochim Biophys Acta Lipids Lipid Metab, 1994. **1210**(3): p. 255–287.
81. Mandeville, W.H. and D.I. Goldberg, *The sequestration of bile acids, a non-absorbed method for cholesterol reduction. A review.* Curr Pharm Des, 1997. **3**(1): p. 15–28.
82. Cameron, N.S., A. Eisenberg, and G.R. Brown, Amphiphilic block copolymers as bile acid sorbents: 1. Synthesis of polystyrene-b-poly(*N,N,N*-trimethylammoniumethylene acrylamide chloride). Biomacromolecules, 2002. **3**(1): p. 116–123.
83. Zhang, L., et al., *Enhancing the "stickiness" of bile acids to cross-linked polymers: a bioconjugate approach to the design of bile acid sequestrants.* Bioconjug Chem, 2000. **11**(3): p. 397–400.
84. Huval, C.C., et al., *Ammonium and guanidinium functionalized hydrogels-as bile acid sequestrants: Synthesis, characterization, and biological properties.* J Macromol Sci Pure Appl Chem, 2004. **A41**(3): p. 231–244.
85. Huval, C.C., et al., *Syntheses of hydrophobically modified cationic hydrogels by copolymerization of alkyl substituted diallylamine monomers and their use as bile acid sequestrants.* Eur Polym J, 2004. **40**(4): p. 693–701.
86. Florentin, M., et al., *Colesevelam hydrochloride in clinical practice: a new approach in the treatment of hypercholesterolaemia.* Curr Med Res Op, 2008. **24**(4): p. 995–1009.

87. Staels, B. and F. Kuipers, *Bile acid sequestrants and the treatment of type 2 diabetes mellitus.* Drugs, 2007. **67**(10): p. 1383–1392.

88. Huval, C.C., et al., *Novel cholesterol lowering polymeric drugs obtained by molecular imprinting.* Macromolecules, 2001. **34**(6): p. 1548–1550.

89. Wang, Y.J., et al., *Specific binding of cholic acid by cross-linked polymers prepared by the hybrid imprinting method.* Polymer, 2007. **48**(19): p. 5565–5571.

90. Tamaru, S. and I. Hamachi, *Recent progress of phosphate derivatives recognition utilizing artificial small molecular receptors in aqueous media.* Recognit Anions, 2008. **129**: p. 95–125.

91. Gale, P.A., S.E. Garcia-Garrido, and J. Garric, *Anion receptors based on organic frameworks: highlights from 2005 and 2006.* Chem Soc Rev, 2008. **37**(1): p. 151–190.

92. Holmes-Farley, S.R., et al., *Design and characterization of sevelamer hydrochloride: A novel phosphate-binding pharmaceutical.* J Macromol Sci Pure Appl Chem, 1999. **A36**(7–8): p. 1085–1091.

93. Amin, N., *The impact of improved phosphorus control: use of sevelamer hydrochloride in patients with chronic renal failure.* Nephrol Dial Transplant, 2002. **17**(2): p. 340–345.

94. Goldsmith, D.R., et al., *Sevelamer hydrochloride: a review of its use for hyperphosphataemia in patients with end-stage renal disease on haemodialysis.* Drugs, 2008. **68**(1): p. 85–104.

95. Liu, Z.D. and R.C. Hider, *Design of clinically useful iron(III)-selective chelators.* Med Res Rev, 2002. **22**(1): p. 26–64.

96. Raymond, K.N., *Biomimetic metal encapsulation.* Coordination Chem Rev, 1990. **105**: p. 135–153.

97. Polomoscanik, S.C., et al., *Hydroxamic acid-containing hydrogels for nonabsorbed iron chelation therapy: Synthesis, characterization, and biological evaluation.* Biomacromolecules, 2005. **6**(6): p. 2946–2953.

98. Zhou, T., et al., *Iron binding dendrimers: A novel approach for the treatment of haemochromatosis.* J Med Chem, 2006. **49**(14): p. 4171–4182.

99. Zhou, T., et al., *Synthesis and iron(III)-chelating properties of novel 3-hydroxypyridin-4-one hexadentate ligand-containing copolymers.* Biomacromolecules, 2008. **9**(5): p. 1372–1380.

100. Louie, T.J., et al., *Tolevamer, a novel nonantibiotic polymer, compared with vancomycin in the treatment of mild to moderately severe Clostridium difficile-associated diarrhea.* Clin Infect Dis, 2006. **43**(4): p. 411–420.

101. Vercruysse, K.P. and G.D. Prestwich, *Hyaluronate derivatives in drug delivery.* Crit Rev Ther Drug Carrier Syst, 1998. **15**(5): p. 513–555.

102. Waddell, D.D., *The tolerability of viscosupplementation: low incidence and clinical management of local adverse events.* Curr Med Res Opin, 2003. **19**(7): p. 575–580.

103. Bellamy, N., et al., *Viscosupplementation for the treatment of osteoarthritis of the knee.* Cochrane Database Syst Rev, 2006(2): p. CD005321.

104. Bhardwaj, R. and M.C. Parker, *Impact of adhesions in colorectal surgery.* Colorectal Dis, 2007. **9 Suppl 2**: p. 45–53.

105. Boland, G.M. and R.J. Weigel, *Formation and prevention of postoperative abdominal adhesions.* J Surg Res, 2006. **132**(1): p. 3–12.

106. Zeng, Q., et al., *Efficacy and safety of Seprafilm for preventing postoperative abdominal adhesion: systematic review and meta-analysis.* World J Surg, 2007. **31**(11): p. 2125–2131; discussion 2132.

107. Vasey, P.A., et al., Phase I clinical and pharmacokinetic study of PK1 [*N*-(2-hydroxypropyl)methacrylamide copolymer doxorubicin]: First member of a new class of chemotherapeutic agents — Drug-polymer conjugates. Clin Cancer Res, 1999. **5**(1): p. 83–94.

108. Seymour, L.W., et al., *Hepatic drug targeting: phase I evaluation of polymer-bound doxorubicin.* J Clin Oncol, 2002. **20**(6): p. 1668–1676.

109. Seymour, L.W., et al., *Phase II studies of polymer-doxorubicin (PK1, FCE28068) in the treatment of breast, lung and colorectal cancer.* Int J Oncol, 2009. **34**(6): p. 1629–1636.

110. Vercauteren, R., E. Schacht, and R. Duncan, *Effect of the Chemical Modification of Dextran on the Degradation by Rat Liver Lysosomal Enzymes.* J Bioactive Compatible Polym, 1992. **7**(4): p. 346–357.

111. Auzenne, E., et al., *Superior therapeutic profile of poly-L-glutamic acid-paclitaxel copolymer compared with taxol in xenogeneic compartmental models of human ovarian carcinoma.* Clin Cancer Res, 2002. **8**(2): p. 573–581.

112. *http://www.celltherapeutics.com/pdf/OPAXIO_facts-4pg.pdf.*

113. Paz-Ares, L., et al., *Phase III trial comparing paclitaxel poliglumex vs docetaxel in the second-line treatment of non-small-cell lung cancer.* Br J Cancer, 2008. **98**(10): p. 1608–1613.

114. O'Brien, M.E., et al., *Randomized phase III trial comparing single-agent paclitaxel Poliglumex (CT-2103, PPX) with single-agent gemcitabine or vinorelbine for the treatment of PS 2 patients with chemotherapy-naive advanced non-small cell lung cancer.* J Thorac Oncol, 2008. **3**(7): p. 728–734.

115. Langer, C.J., et al., *Phase III trial comparing paclitaxel poliglumex (CT-2103, PPX) in combination with carboplatin versus standard paclitaxel*

and carboplatin in the treatment of PS 2 patients with chemotherapy-naive advanced non-small cell lung cancer. J Thorac Oncol, 2008. **3**(6): p. 623–630.

116. Wheate, N.J., et al., *The status of platinum anticancer drugs in the clinic and in clinical trials.* Dalton Trans, 2010. **39**(35): p. 8113–8127.

117. Rademaker-Lakhai, J.M., et al., *A phase I and pharmacological study of the platinum polymer AP5280 given as an intravenous infusion once every 3 weeks in patients with solid tumors.* Clin Cancer Res, 2004. **10**(10): p. 3386–3395.

118. Nowotnik, D.P. and E. Cvitkovic, *ProLindac (TM) (AP5346): A review of the development of an HPMA DACH platinum polymer therapeutic.* Adv Drug Deliv Rev, 2009. **61**(13): p. 1214–1219.

119. Yurkovetskiy, A.V. and R.J. Fram, *XMT-1001, a novel polymeric camptothecin pro-drug in clinical development for patients with advanced cancer.* Adv Drug Deliv Rev, 2009. **61**(13): p. 1193–1202.

120. Cheng, J.J., et al., *Synthesis of linear, beta-cyclodextrin-based polymers and their camptothecin conjugates.* Bioconjug Chem, 2003. **14**(5): p. 1007–1017.

121. Davis, M.E., *Design and development of IT-101, a cyclodextrin-containing polymer conjugate of camptothecin.* Adv Drug Deliv Rev, 2009. **61**(13): p. 1189–1192.

122. Folkman, J., *Tumor angiogenesis: therapeutic implications.* N Engl J Med, 1971. **285**(21): p. 1182–1186.

123. Satchi-Fainaro, R., *Targeting tumor vasculature: reality or a dream?* J Drug Target, 2002. **10**(7): p. 529–533.

124. Matsumura, Y. and H. Maeda, *A new concept for macromolecular therapeutics in cancer chemotherapy: mechanism of tumoritropic accumulation of proteins and the antitumor agent smancs.* Cancer Res, 1986. **46**(12 Pt 1): p. 6387–6392.

125. Joralemon, M.J., S. McRae, and T. Emrick, *PEGylated polymers for medicine: from conjugation to self-assembled systems.* Chem Commun (Camb), 2010. **46**(9): p. 1377–1393.

126. Winter, T.A., et al., *Treatment of Crohn's disease with certolizumab pegol.* Expert Rev Clin Immunol, 2007. **3**(5): p. 683–694.

127. Ton, N.C., et al., *Phase I evaluation of CDP791, a PEGylated di-Fab' conjugate that binds vascular endothelial growth factor receptor 2.* Clin Cancer Res, 2007. **13**(23): p. 7113–7118.

128. Einhorn, S. and D. Grander, *Why do so many cancer patients fail to respond to interferon therapy?* J Interferon Cytokine Res, 1996. **16**(4): p. 275–281.

129. Harris, J.M. and R.B. Chess, *Effect of pegylation on pharmaceuticals.* Nat Rev Drug Discov, 2003. **2**(3): p. 214–221.

130. Vogel, C.L., et al., *First and subsequent cycle use of pegfilgrastim prevents febrile neutropenia in patients with breast cancer: a multicenter, double-blind, placebo-controlled phase III study.* J Clin Oncol, 2005. **23**(6): p. 1178–1184.

131. Levy, Y., et al., *Adenosine deaminase deficiency with late onset of recurrent infections: response to treatment with polyethylene glycol-modified adenosine deaminase.* J Pediatr, 1988. **113**(2): p. 312–317.

132. Satchi-Fainaro, R., R. Duncan, and C.M. Barnes, *Polymer therapeutics for cancer: Current status and future challenges.* Polym Ther II Polym Drugs Conjug Gene Deliv Syst, 2006. **193**: p. 1–65.

133. Branco, M.C. and J.P. Schneider, *Self-assembling materials for therapeutic delivery.* Acta Biomater, 2009. **5**(3): p. 817–831.

134. Soussan, E., et al., *Drug delivery by soft matter: matrix and vesicular carriers.* Angew Chem Int Ed, 2009. **48**(2): p. 274–288.

135. Wu, X.L., et al., *Tumor-targeting peptide conjugated pH-responsive micelles as a potential drug carrier for cancer therapy.* Bioconjug Chem. **21**(2): p. 208–213.

136. Kim, S., et al., *Overcoming the barriers in micellar drug delivery: loading efficiency, in vivo stability, and micelle-cell interaction.* Expert Opin Drug Deliv. **7**(1): p. 49–62.

137. Lee, K.S., et al., *Multicenter phase II trial of Genexol-PM, a Cremophor-free, polymeric micelle formulation of paclitaxel, in patients with metastatic breast cancer.* Breast Cancer Res Treat, 2008. **108**(2): p. 241–250.

138. Saif, M.W., et al., *Phase II clinical trial of paclitaxel loaded polymeric micelle in patients with advanced pancreatic cancer.* Cancer Invest. **28**(2): p. 186–194.

139. Kim, D.W., et al., *Multicenter phase II trial of Genexol-PM, a novel Cremophor-free, polymeric micelle formulation of paclitaxel, with cisplatin in patients with advanced non-small-cell lung cancer.* Ann Oncol, 2007. **18**(12): p. 2009–2014.

140. Ahmed, F., et al., *Shrinkage of a rapidly growing tumor by drug-loaded polymersomes: pH-triggered release through copolymer degradation.* Mol Pharm, 2006. **3**(3): p. 340–350.

141. Haag, R. and F. Kratz, *Polymer therapeutics: concepts and applications.* Angew Chem Int Ed Engl, 2006. **45**(8): p. 1198–1215.

142. Jain, K., et al., *Dendrimer toxicity: Let's meet the challenge.* Int J Pharm, 2010. **394**(1–2): p. 122–142.

143. Qiu, L.Y. and Y.H. Bae, *Polymer architecture and drug delivery.* Pharm Res, 2006. **23**(1): p. 1–30.

144. Namazi, H. and M. Adell, *Dendrimers of citric acid and poly (ethylene glycol) as the new drug-delivery agents.* Biomaterials, 2005. **26**(10): p. 1175–1183.

145. Domanski, D.M., M. Bryszewska, and G. Salamonczyk, *Preliminary evaluation of the behavior of fifth-generation thiophosphate dendrimer in biological systems.* Biomacromolecules, 2004. **5**(5): p. 2007–2012.

146. Agrawal, P., U. Gupta, and N.K. Jain, *Glycoconjugated peptide dendrimers-based nanoparticulate system for the delivery of chloroquine phosphate.* Biomaterials, 2007. **28**(22): p. 3349–3359.

147. Gillies, E.R., et al., *Biological evaluation of polyester dendrimer: Poly(ethylene oxide) "Bow-Tie" hybrids with tunable molecular weight and architecture.* Mo Pharm, 2005. **2**(2): p. 129–138.

148. Malik, N., et al., *Dendrimers: Relationship between structure and biocompatibility in vitro, and preliminary studies on the biodistribution of I-125-labelled polyamidoamine dendrimers in vivo.* J Control Release, 2000. **65**(1–2): p. 133–148.

149. Zhang, W., et al., *Triazine dendrimers for drug delivery: Evaluation of solubilization properties, activity in cell culture; and in vivo toxicity of a candidate vehicle.* Supramol Chem, 2003. **15**(7–8): p. 607–617.

150. Singh, P., et al., *Folate and folate-PEG-PAMAM dendrimers: synthesis, characterization, and targeted anticancer drug delivery potential in tumor bearing mice.* Bioconjug Chem, 2008. **19**(11): p. 2239–2252.

151. Zhang, Y.Q., et al., *Synthesis, biodistribution, and microsingle photon emission computed tomography (SPECT) imaging study of technetium-99m labeled PEGylated dendrimer poly(amidoamine) (PAMAM)-folic acid conjugates*, 2010. J Med Chem,. **53**(8): p. 3262–3272.

152. Geng, Y., et al., *Shape effects of filaments versus spherical particles in flow and drug delivery.* Nat Nanotechnol, 2007. **2**(4): p. 249–255.

153. Saad, M., et al., *Receptor targeted polymers, dendrimers, liposomes: Which nanocarrier is the most efficient for tumor-specific treatment and imaging?* J Control Release, 2008. **130**(2): p. 107–114.

154. Gary, D.J., N. Puri, and Y.Y. Won, *Polymer-based siRNA delivery: Perspectives on the fundamental and phenomenological distinctions from polymer-based DNA delivery.* J Control Release, 2007. **121**(1–2): p. 64–73.

155. Sun, X.L. and N. Zhang, *Cationic Polymer Optimization for Efficient Gene Delivery.* Mini Rev Med Chem, 2010. **10**(2): p. 108–125.

156. Akagi, D., et al., *Biocompatible micellar nanovectors achieve efficient gene transfer to vascular lesions without cytotoxicity and thrombus formation.* Gene Ther, 2007. **14**(13): p. 1029–1038.

157. Ofek, P., et al., *In vivo delivery of small interfering RNA to tumors and their vasculature by novel dendritic nanocarriers.* FASEB J. **24**(9): p. 3122–3134.

158. Davis, M.E., et al., *Evidence of RNAi in humans from systemically administered siRNA via targeted nanoparticles.* Nature. **464**(7291): p. 1067–U140.

159. Greco, F. and M.J. Vicent, *Combination therapy: opportunities and challenges for polymer-drug conjugates as anticancer nanomedicines.* Adv Drug Deliv Rev, 2009. **61**(13): p. 1203–1213.

160. Vicent, M.J., et al., *Polymer therapeutics designed for a combination therapy of hormone-dependent cancer.* Angew Chem Int Ed, 2005. **44**(26): p. 4061–4066.

161. Santucci, L., et al., *Nitric oxide modulates proapoptotic and antiapoptotic properties of chemotherapy agents: the case of NO-pegylated epirubicin.* FASEB J., 2006: p. 05-4452fje.

162. Krakovicova, H., T. Etrych, and K. Ulbrich, *HPMA-based polymer conjugates with drug combination.* Eur J Pharm Sci, 2009. **37**(3–4): p. 405–412.

163. Bae, Y., et al., *Mixed polymeric micelles for combination cancer chemotherapy through the concurrent delivery of multiple chemotherapeutic agents.* J Control Release, 2007. **122**(3): p. 324–330.

164. Wang, Y., et al., *Co-delivery of drugs and DNA from cationic core-shell nanoparticles self-assembled from a biodegradable copolymer.* Nat Mater, 2006. **5**(10): p. 791–796.

165. Gaspar, R. and R. Duncan, *Polymeric carriers: preclinical safety and the regulatory implications for design and development of polymer therapeutics.* Adv Drug Deliv Rev, 2009. **61**(13): p. 1220–1231.

166. Maeda, H., *Tumor-selective delivery of macromolecular drugs via the EPR effect: background and future prospects.* Bioconjug Chem, 1992. **21**(5): p. 797–802.

Chapter 5

Polysaccharides as Nanomaterials for Therapeutics

Shoshy Mizrahy[a,b] and Dan Peer[a,b]
[a] *Laboratory of Nanomedicine, Department of Cell Research and Immunology, George S. Wise Faculty of Life Science, Tel Aviv University, Tel Aviv, Israel*
[b] *Center for Nanoscience and Nanotechnology, Tel Aviv University, Tel Aviv, Israel*
peer@post.tau.ac.il

The use of polysaccharides as building blocks in the development of nano-size drug delivery systems is rapidly growing. This can be attributed to the outstanding virtues of polysaccharides such as biocompatibility, biodegradability, low toxicity, and low cost. In addition, the variety of physicochemical properties and the ease of chemical modifications enable the preparation of a wide array of nanoparticles. This chapter describes the properties of common polysaccharides and the main mechanisms for polysaccharide-based nanoparticle preparation and provides examples from the conceptual design toward pre-clinical and clinical applications.

5.1 Introduction

Over the past two decades, nanoparticle-based therapeutics have been introduced for the treatment of cancer, diabetes, allergy,

Handbook of Harnessing Biomaterials in Nanomedicine: Preparation, Toxicity, and Applications
Edited by Dan Peer

ISBN 978-981-4316-46-0 (Hardback), 978-981-4364-27-0 (eBook)
www.panstanford.com

inflammation, and infections [1, 2]. The growing interest in nanoparticles derives from the outstanding advantages they offer, which include protection of the drug from premature degradation, lower therapeutic toxicity, ability to deliver poorly-water-soluble drugs, controlled drug release mechanisms, and improved intracellular penetration [2].

The size and surface characteristics of a nanoparticle are crucial for the control of its biodistribution *in vivo*. The small size, which enables nanoparticles to pass through the smallest capillaries also promotes passive tumor targeting due to the enhanced permeability and retention (EPR) effect of the tumor vasculature. The passive targeting is achieved by extravasation of nanoparticles through increased permeability of the tumor vasculature and ineffective lymphatic drainage [2]. In addition, it has been shown that a combination of nanometric size and hydrophilic surface delays particle uptake by the mononuclear phagocyte system (MPS) and therefore promotes long circulation [3].

As the requirements from the nanoparticle are becoming clear, so are the requirements from the materials used for their preparation. These materials should be biocompatible and preferably biodegradable, well characterized, and easily functionalized [2]. Polysaccharides successfully fulfill all of these requirements and are therefore widely used for the preparation of nanoparticles for drug delivery.

5.2 Polysaccharides

Polysaccharides are polymers of monosaccharides joined by glycosidic bonds. These highly abundant molecules are from various origins, including algal origin (e.g., alginate and carrageenan), plant origin (e.g., cellulose, pectin and guar gum), microbial origin (e.g., dextran and xanthan gum), and animal origin (e.g., chitosan, hyaluronan, chondroitin and heparin) [4]. Naturally occurring polysaccharides are diverse in their physiochemical properties; there are multiple chemical structures (Figure 5.1), the chemical composition greatly varies and so do the molecular weight (Mw) and ionic nature. This versatility also contributes to a wide range of biological activities. From a pharmaceutical standpoint, polysaccharides possess many favorable characteristics such as lack of toxicity, good biocompatibility, stability, low cost, hydrophilic nature, and availability of reactive sites for chemical modification. In addition, many polysaccharides possess bioadhesive properties, especially for mucosal surfaces, which have been used for both targeting and prolonging drug residence time. All of these qualities have led to the growing use of polysaccharides in drug delivery systems.

The properties of common polysaccharides used for the preparation of drug delivery systems are detailed below.

5.2.1 Chitosan

Chitosan is a linear polysaccharide composed of β-(1,4)-linked D-glucosamine and *N*-acetyl-D-glucomasine (Figure 5.1). Chitosan is obtained by deacetylation from chitin, a highly abundant polysaccharide, which is the main component of crustaceans exoskeleton [5]. Chitosan and its derivates are currently the most widely used polysaccharides in newly developed drug delivery systems. Chitosan-based delivery systems have been described for nasal, ocular, oral, parenternal, and transdermal drug delivery [6–9]. Among the many advantages of chitosan are its low cytotoxicity and biocompatibility [10, 11]. In addition, chitosan is positively charged and therefore can interact with negatively charged molecules such as negatively charged polysaccharides, polyanions, nucleic acid and negatively charged proteins. Its positive charge also facilitates adherence to mucosal surfaces, which are mostly negatively charged [12, 13]. In addition, the ability of chitosan to open tight junctions between epithelial cells and therefore increase the permeation of macromolecular drugs across the mucosal epithelia has been demonstrated [14, 15]. In spite of these advantages, chitosan is inherently insoluble in aqueous solutions above pH 6.5 [16, 17]. High degree of deacetylation, low molecular weight, and chemical modification can facilitate water solubility of chitosan. These factors also affect particle properties such as size, surface charge, drug entrapment efficiency, and stability [18].

5.2.2 Alginate

Alginate is a linear anionic polysaccharide composed of alternating blocks of 1,4-linked β-D-mannuronic acid (M) and α-l-guluronic acid (G) residues (Figure 5.1). The monomer composition of alginate is variable and can consist of homopolymeric blocks and alternating M and G residues [19]. The composition, sequence, and molecular weight determine the physical properties of alginate [20]. Alginates are extracted mainly from brown algae and acetylated forms of alginate can be isolated from the bacteria *Pseudomonas* and *Azotobacter* [20].

As a polymer for drug delivery purposes, alginate possesses several attractive properties: It is biocompatible, non-toxic, and water soluble and has the highest mucoadhesive strength compared with other natural polysaccharides such as chitosan and carboxymethylcellulose [21, 22].

5.2.3 Hyaluronan

Hyaluronan (HA) is a linear high-Mw glycosaminoglycan (GAG) composed of alternating disaccharide units of D-glucuronic acid and *N*-acetyl-D-glucosamine with β-(1 , 4) interglycosidic linkage [23] (Figure 5.1). Hyaluronan possesses remarkable hydrodynamic properties, especially related to its viscosity and ability to retain water [24]. It was previously regarded important mostly for joint lubrication or organ structural stability [24]. However, HA was found to be essential for proper cell growth, embryonic development, healing processes, inflammation, and tumor development [24, 25]. As opposed to other GAGs, HA is not sulfated, not linked to a protein and naturally produced by bacteria as a capsule [23]. Commercially available HA is either produced through bacterial fermentation of *Streptococcus* species or extracted from rooster combs, umbilical cords, synovial fluids, or vitreous humor [26]. However, HA obtained from these production methods is usually very polydispersed; therefore, a method to produce HA of a defined size has also been developed [27, 28].

There are several advantages of HA that make it suitable for drug delivery: It is water soluble, biodegradable, biocompatible, non-toxic, and non-immunogenic and can be easily chemically modified [29, 30]. In addition, it is the major ligand for CD44 and RHAMM (CD168) and therefore is suitable for targeting CD44 and RHAMM-expressing cells [25, 31]. CD44 and CD168 are overexpressed by various tumors, for example, squamous cell carcinoma , ovarian, colon, stomach, glioma, and many types of leukemia , lymphoma, and myeloma [32–34], which makes the use of HA as a targeting agent even more attractive.

5.2.4 Dextran

Dextran is a high-Mw branched polysaccharide composed of α-(1,6)-linked glucan with side chains attached to the three positions of the backbone glucose units (Figure 5.1). Dextran is obtained from bacterial cultures of the lactic-acid bacteria such as *Leuconostoc mesenteroides* NRRL B-512 [4]. Dextran is water soluble and is also soluble in a wide range of solvents, among them methyl sulphoxide, ethylene glycol, glycerol, and 4-methylmorpholine-4-oxide. Low-Mw dextran and not the native dextran is usually used for both clinical purposes (mainly due to its antithrombotic effect) and nanoparticle preparation. Low-Mw dextran is usually achieved by acid hydrolysis of the native dextran [35]. The polyanion dextran sulfate is derivate of dextran, which contains approximately two to three sulfate groups per glucosyl residue [36]. Dextran sulfate is a biodegradable polymer that has been widely used in pharmaceutical applications [36]. However, dextran sulfate is not completely inert material. It has inhibitory and stimulatory effects on several enzymes [37], and it possesses the ability to stimulate B-cell proliferation [38] and to increase permeability of lymphocytes [39].

5.2.5 Cyclodextrins

Cyclodextrins are cyclic oligomers of α-(1,4) linked-glucopyranosyl that are produced from starch by enzymatic conversion (Figure 5.1). There are three main members of the cyclodextrin family, composed of six, seven, and eight glucose units and known as α-, β-, and γ-CD, respectively. Cyclodextrins have a hydrophilic exterior and a hydrophobic cavity that enables them to act as hosts to hydrophobic molecules [40]. This ability to form inclusion complexes has been widely studied since its discovery. It is utilized in many industrial products, analytical methods, and technologies [41], including the production of cyclodextrin-based nanoparticles [42]. Cyclodextrins are biocompatible, do not elicit immune responses, and have low toxicities in animals and humans [43]. Therefore, they are used in pharmaceutical applications for numerous purposes, including improving the bioavailability of drugs [43]. Cyclodextrin-based therapeutics have been reviewed elsewhere [43].

5.2.6 Arabinogalactan

Arabinogalactan is a long, highly branched natural polysaccharide composed mostly of galactose and arabinose. Arabinogalactan is extracted mainly from the Larix tree and is available at 99.9% purity with reproducible Mw and physicochemical properties [44]. The unusual water solubility (70% w/w in water), biocompatibility, biodegradability, and ease of drug conjugation in an aqueous medium make arabinogalactan attractive as a potential drug carrier [44].

5.2.7 Pullulan

Pullulan is neutral, homopolysaccharide consisting of α-(1,6)-linked maltotriose residues (Figure 5.1). It is produced from starch primarily by strains of the fungus *Aureobasidium pullulans* [45]. Pullulan's structure unique linkage pattern contributes to exceptional physiochemical properties such as adhesiveness, water solubility, and relatively low viscosity upon dissolving in water. Therefore, pullulan and its derivatives have been used industrially in foods and pharmaceuticals [45].

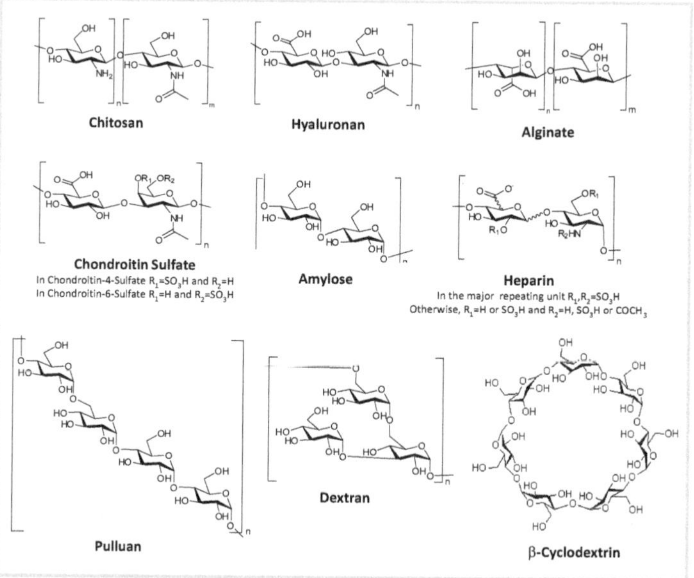

Figure 5.1 Chemical structures of polysaccharides. β-Cyclodextrin structure obtained with permission from http://www.chemblink.com

5.2.8 Heparin

Heparin is a linear glycosaminoglycan (GAG) composed of repeating disaccharide units of 1,4-linked uronic acid (D-glucuronic (GlcAor l-iduronic acid (IdoA) and D-glucosamine (GlcN) (Figure 5.1). The uronic acid usually comprises 90 percent l-idopyranosyluronic acid (l-iduronic acid, IdoA) and 10 percent D-glucopyranosyluronic acid (D-glucuronic acid, GlcA). In addition, there are structural variations at the disaccharide level [46]. Due to high content of sulfo and carboxyl groups, heparin has the highest negative charge density of any known biological molecule [46]. The Mw of heparin varies between 5–40 kDa and it is extracted mainly from mucosal tissues of porcine and bovine [46]. Clinically, heparin has been used as an anticoagulant since the 1930s [46]. The anticoagulant activity of heparin requires direct interaction with the serine protease inhibitor antithrombin III, which causes a conformational change that allows antithrombin III to inhibit thrombin and other serine proteases within the coagulation cascade [47]. Heparin is produced exclusively by mast cells (as opposed to the structurally related GAG heparan sulphate) [23]. Beyond its anticoagulant activity, heparin has been shown to have antiviral activity and ability to inhibit complement activation, tumor growth and angiogenesis [47].

5.3 Main Mechanisms of Nanoparticle Preparation from Polysaccharides

5.3.1 Cross-Linking

In cross-linked nanoparticles, the polymeric chains are interconnected by cross-linkers, leading to the formation of a 3D network (Figure 5.2A,B) [48]. The main factor that determines the properties of a cross-linked nanoparticle such as drug release and mechanical strength is the cross-linking density, which is determined by the molar ratio between the cross-linker and the polymer repeating units [48]. There are two types of cross-linked nanoparticles determined by the nature of the cross-linking agents: covalently cross-linked nanoparticles and ionically cross-linked nanoparticles.

5.3.1.1 Covalent cross-linking

In a covalently cross-linking nanoparticle, the network structure is permanent since irreversible chemical links are formed (Figure 5.2A) [48]. The rigid network allows absorptions of water and bioactive compounds without the dissolution of the nanoparticle even when the pH drastically changes [48]. A covalently cross-linked nanoparticle can contain more than one type of polysaccharide. The covalent bonds are the main interactions that form the 3D network although secondary interactions such as hydrogen bonds and hydrophobic interactions also exist [48]. Covalent cross-linkers are molecules with at least two reactive functional groups that allow the formation of bridges between the polymeric chains [49]. The most common covalent cross-linkers used with polysaccharides are dialdehydes such as glutaraldehyde [50, 51]. However, dialdehydes are highly toxic, and therefore biocompatible alternatives have been tested. For example, natural di- and tricarboxilic acids have been used for intramolecular cross-linking of chitosan, which was facilitated by the condensation agent 1-ethyl-3-[3-dimethylaminopropyl] carbodiimide hydrochloride (EDC) [52]. Genipin, a natural biocompatible cross-linker isolated from the fruits of *Gardenia jasminoides* Ellis, is another option [53].

5.3.1.2 Ionic cross-linking

Ionic cross-linking represents a simple alternative to covalent cross-linking for charged polysaccharides. This method enables the preparation of nanoparticles by the formation of reversible ionic cross-linking and since no harsh preparation or toxic cross-linkers are used these nanoparticles are generally considered biocompatible [48]. Charged polysaccharide can form ionic cross-linked nanoparticles with oppositely charged ions or small ionic molecules (Figure 5.2B). For example, the polyanion tripolyphosphate (TPP) has been widely used to cross-link the chitosan, and divalent cations such as Ca^{2+} have been used to cross-link alginate [54, 55]. The mechanism of nanoparticle formation is based on electrostatic interactions between the polysaccharide and oppositely charged ionic cross-linker [56]. The ionic bonds form bridges between the polysaccharide chains and are the main interactions inside the network, although as with covalent cross-linking, additional interaction such as hydrogen bonds are also present [48]. Several factors influence the cross-linking reaction, most crucial are the size of the cross-linker and the global charge of the cross-linker and the polysaccharide [48, 57]. Unlike covalently cross-linked nanoparticles, ionic cross-linked nanoparticles are generally pH sensitive, a welcome trait for drug delivery purposes. However, this pH sensitivity also contributes to instability of the ionic cross-linked network [48, 58, 59].

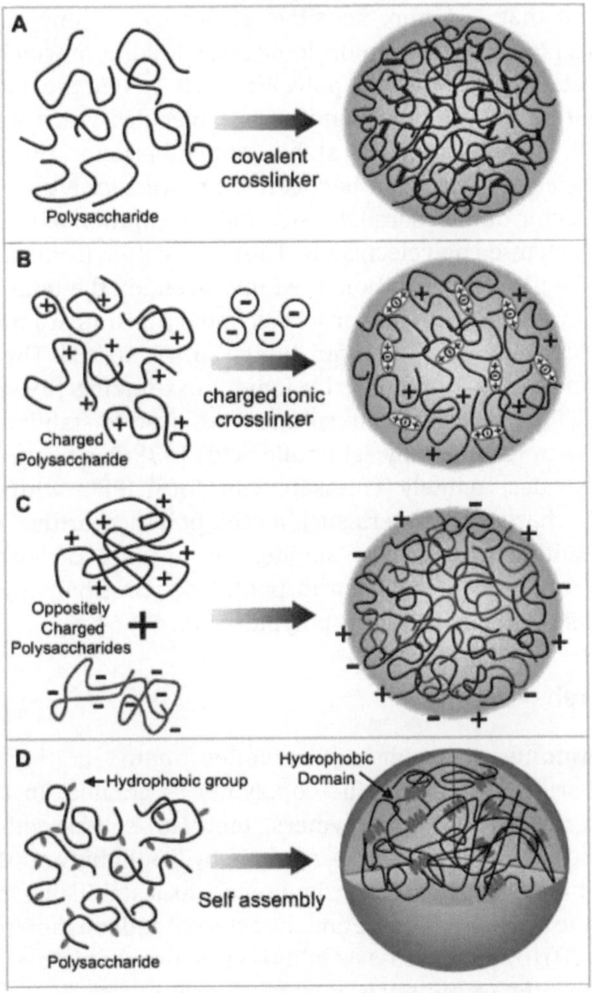

Figure 5.2 Common mechanism for polysaccharide based nanoparticle preparation. (A) Covalent cross-linking. (B) Ionic cross-linking. (C) Polyelectrolyte complexation (PEC). (D) Self-assembly of hydrophobically modified polysaccharides. See also Color Insert.

5.3.2 Polyelectrolyte Complexation (PEC)

Polyelectrolyte complexes (PEC) are formed by direct electrostatic interactions of oppositely charged polyelectrolytes in solution (Figure 5.2C). PEC represents another biocompatible option for drug delivery since no toxic covalent cross-linkers are used. These complexes resemble ionic cross-linking since non-permanent networks are formed that are more sensitive to changes in environmental conditions [26]. However, unlike ionic cross-linking, in which ions or ionic molecules react with the polyelectrolyte, in PEC the interaction is between the polyelecrolyte and larger molecules with a broad MW range [60]. The formation and stability of PEC is determined mainly by the degree of interaction between the polyelectrolytes [49]. The later is a factor of the charge density and distribution of each of the oppositely charged polyelectrolyte. The chemical environment is also crucial: The pH of the solution, the ionic strength, the temperature, and the duration and mixing order. Secondary factors are the Mw of the polyelectrolytes and their flexibility [26, 49, 60, 61]. The formed interaction can be reinforced by ionic cross-linking [49, 62]. For example, TPP and magnesium sulfate were used to stabilize PEC of chitosan with gamma poly (glutamic acid) [63]. Positively charged polysaccharides, namely chitosan, can form PEC with variety negatively charged polymers such as the polysaccharides alginate, dextran sulfate, chondroitin sulfate, hyaluronan, carboxymethyl cellulose, carrageenan and heparin, peptides such as poly-g-glutamic acid ,nucleic acid and synthetic polymers [49, 61, 64–66].

5.3.3 Self-Assembly

Upon grafting hydrophobic moieties onto a hydrophilic polysaccharide an amphiphilic copolymer is created. In aqueous solutions, amphiphilic copolymers tend to self-assemble into nanoparticles in which the inner core is hydrophobic and the shell is hydrophilic. The hydrophilic shell serves as a stabilizing interface between the hydrophobic core and the external aqueous environment (Figure 5.2D) [67]. This self-assembly is via hydrophobic interactions, mainly in order to minimize interfacial free energy [61, 64]. The formed nanoparticles are characterized by prolonged circulation and thermodynamic stability [68]. In addition, since the core is hydrophobic, these nanoparticles have been used for the delivery of hydrophobic drugs. Several properties such as size, surface charge, loading efficiency, stability, and biodistribution can be altered for a particular application. For example, the size of the nanoparticles can be controlled by adjusting the length of the hydrophobic moiety and the length of the polymer [67]. Scaling relations for this purpose have been developed [67]. In addition, the surface charge, which affects particle serum stability and cellular uptake, can be altered by controlling the degree of substitution, the length of the hydrophobic moiety or the nature of the hydrophobic moiety [61, 69]. For example, a cationic derivatization of the hydrophobic moiety has been used to promote cellular uptake [70]: amine bearing cholesterol but not cholesterol without an amine, demonstrated protein cellular delivery when grafted onto pullulan to create self-assembled nanoparticles [70].

Polysaccharides can be modified with a wide range of hydrophobic moieties among them bile acids (e.g., 5β-cholanic acid, cholic acid and deoxycholic acid), fatty acids (e.g., palmitoyl acid, stearic acid, oleic acid) [61], cholesterol, and hydrophobic drugs.

5.4 Polysaccharide-Based Nanoparticles

5.4.1 Chitosan-Based Nanoparticles

Chitosan's nature and the ease of chemical modifications enable multiple nanoparticle preparation schemes among them: covalent cross-linking, ionic cross-linking, polyelectrolyte complexation, desolvation, and self-assembly [71].

Early works describing chitosan nanoparticles for drug delivery were based on covalently crossing chitosan with glutaraldehyde [50]. However, since glutaraldehyde is highly toxic, biocompatible alternatives for covalent cross-linking have been developed, such as condensation reactions with 1-ethyl-3-[3-dimethylaminopropyl]carbodiimide hydrochloride, which was used to facilitate intramolecular cross-linking of chitosan by natural di- and tricarboxylic acids [52]. This method allows the formation of polycations, polyanions, and polyampholyte nanoparticles.

Since chitosan is positively charged, ionic cross-linked nanoparticles can be prepared using polyanions; among them the most widely used is tripolyphosphate (TPP). The wide use of TPP in the preparation of chitosan nanoparticles is a result of both being non-toxic and of the ability to modulate particle size, morphological properties and surface charge mainly by controlling the chitosan to TPP weight ratio [72]. The first TPP cross-linked chitosan nanoparticles for drug delivery were developed by Alonso's group [73]. The method was based on a principle reported previously by Bodmeier et al. [56]. Alonso's group later reported the use of these particles for protein [74, 75], oligonucleotide, and plasmid DNA delivery [76, 77]. The resulting chitosan/TPP nanoparticles for DNA delivery were in the range of 100–300 nm depending on the Mw of the chitosan and showed high physical stability and encapsulation efficiencies both for plasmid DNA and dsDNA oligomers (20-mers), independent of chitosan's Mw. The low-Mw chitosan/TPP nanoparticles gave high gene expression levels in HEK 293 cells and mediated a strong beta-galactosidase expression *in vivo* after intratracheal administration. Chitosan/TPP nanoparticles were also developed for the delivery of double-stranded small interfering RNA (siRNA) [78]. In this study, particle size was shown to be affected by chitosan's Mw, concentration, chitosan-to-TPP weight ratio, and pH. *In vitro* studies of these particles in two types of cells lines, CHO K1 and HEK 293, revealed that chitosan/TPP nanoparticles with entrapped siRNA enhanced gene silencing in comparison with chitosan–siRNA complexes. This was possibly due to their high binding capacity and loading efficiency.

As mentioned, the positive charge of chitosan enables the formation of polyelectrolyte complexes (PEC) with negatively charged polymers such as negatively charged polysaccharides, nucleic acids, negatively charged peptides and poly(acrylic acid). Polyelectrolyte complexation is one of the most frequently used methods to prepare chitosan nanoparticles. PEC of chitosan with gamma-poly-(glutamic acid), a natural, non-toxic, and biodegradable negatively charged polymer have been prepared for oral administration of insulin [63]. These nanoparticles, which were stabilized with TPP and magnesium sulfate were pH sensitive and had an average size of 218 nm in diameter. The particles were shown to be safe, adhere to mucosal surfaces and to induce a significant hypoglycemic action for at least 10 h in diabetic rats when administered orally. The bioavailability of insulin, which was determined from plasma insulin concentration, was of 15%. The same group previously reported transdermal delivery of DNA containing chitosan–gamma-poly-(glutamic acid) nanoparticles

[79]. These nanoparticles shown improved skin penetration and enhanced gene expression in comparison with nanoparticles solely comprised of chitosan and DNA. This can be attributed to a greater density of the gamma-poly-(glutamic acid)-containing nanoparticles, which contributed to a larger penetration momentum into the skin barrier. In a following study [80] the gamma-poly-(glutamic acid)-containing nanoparticles showed a significant increase in cellular uptake and transfection efficiency of HT1080 (human fibrosarcoma) cells in comparison with DNA-chitosan nanoparticles. Another study describing PEC of chitosan and DNA have reported by Krishnendu et al. [81] who have shown that theses PEC can generate immunologic protection in a murine model of peanut allergy. The mice who received nanoparticles containing a dominant peanut allergen gene produced secretory IgA and serum IgG2a and showed a substantial reduction in allergen-induced anaphylaxis associated with reduced levels of IgE, plasma histamine and vascular leakage. More recently, plasmid-chitosan PEC was applied in the delivery of FGF-2 and PDGF-BB [82]. Plasmid-chitosan PEC containing FGF-2/PDGF-BB genes were injected into BALB/C mice. Several formulations were tested, which differed in the degree of chitosan deacetylation and Mw. ELISA assays performed on mice sera showed FGF-2 and PDGF-BB expression. In addition, induction of specific antibodies against these proteins has been shown. PEC containing highly deacetylated low-Mw chitosan, were found to efficiently induce protein expression with minimal production of neutralizing antibodies, which was also confirmed by histological analyses.

Recently, PEC of ultrapure chitosan monomers was used for ocular gene delivery [83]. The nanoparticle preparation which was based on a method developed by Koping-Hoggard et al. [84] had an average size of ~ 100 nm in diameter and a strong positive charge. This formulation demonstrated effective transfection of COS-7 cells *in vitro* and luciferase gene expression 5.4 times greater than polyethylenimine-DNA nanoparticles upon injection to rat corneas. The preparation method of PEC of chitosan and DNA was further improved by Artursson, who optimized the balance between stability and unpacking of PEC containing chitosan oligomers of different sizes [85]. PEC of chitosan oligomers and pDNA have several advantages over PEC of high-Mw chitosan and pDNA: High-Mw chitosan form extremely stable PEC with DNA, which delays the release of DNA and therefore results in a slow onset of action. In addition, these PEC are of aggregated shapes, their viscosity at concentration used for *in vivo* delivery is very high and their solubility at a physiological pH is low [84].

Chemical modification, usually by utilizing the primary amino groups of chitosan, is another way to improve its physiochemical properties. For example, conjugation of hydrophobic moieties such as deoxycholic acid and cholesterol to chitosan allows solvent induced self-assembly into nanoparticles [86, 87]. This principle was used for preparation of 5β-cholanic acid (HGC)-modified glycol chitosan nanoparticles for the delivery of the antiangiogenic peptide RGD [88]. The RGD (Arg–Gly–Asp) peptides can specifically target $\alpha_v\beta_3$ integrins on angiogenic endothelial cells and therefore inhibit angiogenesis and tumor growth [89]; however, these peptides have short half-life *in vivo*, and thus a delivery system is required. The self-assembled polymeric nanoparticles of glycol chitosan nanoparticles modified with hydrophobic bile acid analogs have hydrophilic shells of glycol chitosan and hydrophobic cores of bile acid derivatives. The hydrophobically modified glycol chitosan was prepared by covalently attaching 5β-cholanic acid through amide formation. The nanoparticles have a diameter of 230 nm and loading efficiency >85%. The nanoparticles demonstrated prolonged and sustained release and inhibition of HUVEC adhesion *in vitro*. In the *in vivo* study, the RGD containing nanoparticles inhibited bFGF-induced angiogenesis and significantly decreased tumor growth and microvessel density in comparison with native RGD peptide. These particles were previously used by the same group for gene delivery and for the chemotherapeutic agents doxorubicin and paclitaxel [90, 91]. Other modifications of chitosan such as addition of thiol groups and trimethylation can improve the mucoadhesive and permeation-enhancing properties of chitosan [92]. Trimethylated chitosan (TMC) is also characterized by increased solubility in neutral pH [93]. Finally, targeted delivery of chitosan nanoparticles has been achieved simply by conjugation of targeting ligand to chitosan for example; nanoparticles containing galactosylated chitosan were used for hepatic gene delivery [94]. In addition, folate-conjugated chitosan nanoparticles were used for the delivery of interleukin-1 receptor antagonist (IL-1Ra) gene in rats with adjuvant induced arthritis [95]. IL-1Ra is a natural blocker of the inflammatory cytokine IL-1. When administered *in vivo*, the folate modified chitosan-DNA nanoparticles offered improved protection against inflammation and abnormal bone metabolism in comparison with naked DNA and chitosan–DNA complexes.

5.4.2 Alginate-Based Nanoparticles

The early preparations of alginate-based nanoparticles were based on the ability of alginate to form 3D network upon ionic inter- and intramolecular cross-linking with divalent ions [56]. Ever since, several preparation mechanisms have been utilized and alginate-based nanoparticles have been developed for the delivery of proteins, genes, antitubercular and antifungal drugs [96].

Calcium cross-linked alginate nanoparticles containing econazole and antitubercular drugs were utilized for the treatment of murine tuberculosis [54]. The encapsulated drugs were detectable above minimum inhibitory concentration for 15 days after administration in lung, liver and spleen of the treated mice in comparison with 12–24 h of the free drugs. In addition, the alginate nanoparticles managed to reduce bacterial burden in the lung and spleen of mice infected with *Mycobacterium tuberculosis* by more than 90% at 15 fold lower dosages in comparison with free drugs.

Chitosan alginate nanoparticles were used for the transmucosal delivery of insulin [97]. The nanoparticles were prepared by ionic cross-linking of chitosan and TPP, which was followed by complexation with alginate. Insulin was associated to the CS-TPP-AL nanoparticles with loading efficiency of 41–52%. The CS-TPP-AL nanoparticles were administered nasally and exhibited a capacity to enhance systemic absorption of insulin. The duration of the hypoglycemic response was dependent on the Mw of alginate.

Recently, surfactant–alginate hybrid nanoparticles have been employed for dual chemotherapy and photodynamic therapy on a murine drug-resistant tumor model [98]. The obtained nanoparticles had an average size of 73 nm measured by dynamic light scattering (DLS) and contained doxorubicin and methylene blue with encapsulation efficiencies of 78% and 82%, respectively. Following administration to Balb/c mice bearing syngeneic JC tumors (mammary adenocarcinoma), the dual therapy managed to significantly inhibit tumor growth and improved animal survival. The treatment resulted in enhanced tumor accumulation of both doxorubicin and methylene blue, significant inhibition of tumor cell proliferation, and increased induction of apoptosis.

Chemically modified alginate has also been used for the preparation of nanoparticles. As with chitosan, chemical modifications improve the physiochemical characteristics of alginate. For example, thiolated alginate achieved by covalent attachment of cysteine improves the mucoadhesive properties of alginate and provides improved stability of the drug delivery system [99]. Hydrophobically modified alginate have also been produced [100].

5.4.3 Hyaluronan-Based Nanoparticles

HA-based nanocarriers were developed using several approaches such as HA–drug conjugates, which restore their cytotoxicity upon cell internalization by receptor-mediated endocytosis [32], PEC with polycations and ionically cross-linked nanoparticles. Chemically modified HA have also been widely used for the delivery of proteins, peptides, and nucleotides [101]. Chemical modifications assist in prolonging HA half-life; however, beyond a certain level of modification, HA loses the ability to bind its receptors [101].

HA–drug conjugates utilize several chemical groups on hyaluronan: the carboxylate on the glucuronic acid, the *N*-acetylglucosamine hydroxyl, the reducing end, and the acetyl group, which can be enzymatically removed from the *N*-acetylglucosamine [25]. In addition to targeting, HA conjugation has been used to increase drug solubility. This quality was used for the delivery of the hydrophobic antimitotic chemotherapeutic agent paclitaxel [102–104]. HA–paclitaxel conjugates exhibited greater cytotoxicity to CD44 overexpressing cells (HCT-116 and MCF-7) and reduced cytotoxicity to CD44-deficient cells (NIH-3T3) in comparison with free paclitaxel [103]. HA–drug conjugates are internalized via CD44 receptor-mediated endocytosis and drug is released mainly by intracellular enzymatic hydrolysis [25]. Recently, HA conjugation was used for the delivery and improved serum stability of exendin 4 [105]. Exendin 4 (exenatide) is a 39-amino acid peptide incretin mimetic that exhibits gluco-regulatory activities [106]. Exendin 4 has been shown to induce glucose-dependent enhancement of insulin secretion, glucose-dependent suppression of inappropriately high glucagon secretion, slowing of gastric emptying, reduction of food intake and body weight, and an increase in β-cell mass [105]. However, exendin 4 has a significantly short half-life, which limits its clinical applications [105]. Conjugation to vinyl sulfone-modified HA resulted in 20 times improved *in vitro* serum stability without loss of bioactivity. The size of these HA–exendin 4 conjugates was not reported. HA–exendin 4 conjugates lowered glucose levels in type 2 db/db mice and the hypoglycemic effect lasted up to 3 days after injection. In addition, insulin immunohistochemical analysis of islets in db/db mice confirmed the improved insulinotropic activity of the HA–exendin 4 conjugates. HA conjugates have also been suggested for the treatment of acute promyelocytic leukemia (APL) [107]. APL patients often relapse due to resistance to the therapy, all-trans retinoic acid. Because of the molecular basis of APL alteration and previous success with treating tumors with HA conjugated to the histone deacetylase inhibitor butyric acid [108, 109], conjugation of HA to both all-trans retinoic acid and butyric acid has been tested. The size of these HA conjugates was not reported. *In vitro*, the HA conjugates induced growth arrest and terminal differentiation in retinoic acid sensitive cells and apoptosis in retinoic acid resistant cells. *In vivo*, HA conjugates led to a significant increase in survival time of a retinoic acid sensitive APL murine model in comparison with that induced by a maximum tolerated dose of retinoic acid alone. In addition, in a retinoic acid resistant murine model, the HA conjugates were active in contrast to retinoic acid that was completely ineffective [107].

As described above, PEC have been used to prepare HA-based nanoparticles. HA-chitosan nanoparticles have demonstrated the ability to transport genes across the ocular mucosa and transfect ocular tissue [110]. The nanoparticles were prepared by ionically cross-linking of chitosan with TPP, which was followed by PEC with HA. The HA-low-Mw chitosan nanoparticles led to high expression levels of the transfected alkaline phosphatase in a human corneal epithelium model. Upon topical administration to rabbits, the nanoparticles managed to overcome cellular barriers and were located inside the corneal and conjunctival cells, suggesting that they penetrate the epithelia by a transcellular pathway. In addition, the *in vivo* transfection levels reached were significant.

As with other polysaccharides, self-assembly of hydrophobically modified HA has been used for nanoparticle preparation. Poly(lactic-co-(glycolic acid)) (PLGA)-modified HA copolymers were shown to self-assemble in aqueous solution into micelle nanoparticles [111]. The sizes of doxorubicin loaded HA micelle nanoparticles were ranging from 120–285 nm in diameter depending on the Mw of HA and the percent of grafted PLGA. *In vitro*, the micelles exhibited higher cellular uptake and greater cytotoxicity in comparison with free doxorubicin for CD44 over-expressing cells (HCT-116) suggesting that they were taken up by the cells via HA receptor-mediated endocytosis [111]. The same group has recently prepared self-assembled HA nanoparticles for the delivery of paclitaxel by grafting an amine-terminated hydrotropic oligomer onto HA [112]. Active tumor targeting by self-assembled HA-5β-cholanic acid nanoparticles has also been shown [113]. Particle size could be controlled in the range of 240–430 nm by varying the degree of substitution of the hydrophobic moiety. *In vitro*, fluorescently labeled Cy5.5-HA-nanoparticles were detected in the cytosol of CD44 overexpressing cells (SCC7) to a much greater extent than cells with low CD44 expression (CV-1). When administered systemically to tumor-bearing mice, the nanoparticles were shown to selectively accumulate in tumor sites. Smaller HA-NPs were able to reach the tumor site more effectively than larger HA-NPs. In addition, the concentration of the nanoparticles in the tumor site was dramatically reduced when mice were pretreated with free HA. This suggests an additional active targeting mechanism, beyond the passive targeting of the EPR effect.

5.4.4 Dextran-Based Nanoparticles

Several strategies have been reported for dextran-based nanoparticles among them dextran–drug conjugates and self-assembly of hydrophobically modified dextran [114, 115]. The cardiotoxicity of doxorubicin can be significantly reduced by conjugation to dextran and followed by encapsulation in chitosan nanoparticle [116]. Upon conjugation of poorly water-soluble drugs to dextran, hydrophobic derivatives that self-assemble into nanoparticles are formed [117]. The self-assembled nanoparticles were shown to have high loading efficiency. Particle size was strongly influenced by the degree of dextran modification and preparation technique.

Dextran sulfate-based nanoparticles have been mostly prepared by PEC, exploiting the anionic nature of dextran sulfate for electrostatic interaction with positively charged polycations (for example, chitosan and polyethylenimine.) Huang et al. [118] prepared chitosan–dextran sulfate PEC for the controlled release of vascular endothelial growth factor (VEGF). VEGF, a growth factor that stimulates angiogenesis and therefore desired as a therapeutic approach for ischemic conditions was shown to generate new blood vessels *in vivo*. However, intravenously injected VEGF was not clinically successful and implantable controlled release devices have shown that localized and sustained release of VEGF is required for its favorable action. Nanoparticles of ~250 nm were prepared in which the heparin-binding domain of VEGF was utilized to bind the polyanion dextran sulfate. The encapsulation efficiency of VEGF was high (85%) and controlled release (near linear) of active VEGF was persisted was persistent for more than 10 days. The activity of VEGF was determined by ELISA and by the ability to stimulate endothelial cell proliferation (mitogenic assay). PEC containing different polycations (polyethylenimine and poly-L-lysine) were also tested; however, chitosan–dextran sulfate complexes were preferred because of their biodegradability, desirable particle size, higher entrapment efficiency, controlled release, and mitogenic activity. In a following study by the same group [119], Repifermin®-containing nanoparticles were prepared in the same manner. Repifermin® is a truncated form of fibroblast growth factor-10 that exhibits promise in wound-healing applications. The challenge of the delivery lies in the instability of this protein. The resulting 250 nm nanoparticles showed high encapsulation efficiency and the release of active Repifermin® was controlled for more than 10 days. In addition, the mitogenic activity of Repifermin® on human umbilical cord vascular endothelial cells was only demonstrated for encapsulated and not free Repifermin®.

Zinc-stabilized complexes of dextran sulfate and polyethylenimine have been used for the delivery of proteins [62], DNA, and the poorly water-soluble antifungal agent amphotericin B [120]. The preparation method of these nanoparticles was complex coacervation, a method that was usually used for microencapsulation [120]. The effects of preparation conditions and composition on the physicochemical properties of the particles have been determined [120]. The sizes of the amphotericin B-containing nanoparticles were 100–600 nm, a zeta potential of 30 mV and drug recovery efficiency of up to 85%. Particle size was shown to be controlled by processing parameters such as the pH of the PEI solutions, the ratio of the two polymers and the concentrations of dextran sulfate and zinc sulfate. The amphotericin B-containing nanoparticles displayed no toxicity in tissue culture in contrast to free drug and were almost as efficacious as free drug in killing *Candida albicans*.

5.4.5 Cyclodextrin-Based Nanoparticles

Amphiphilic cyclodextrins have been widely used for the preparation of nanoparticles for drug delivery. This can be attributed to the outstanding drug-loading efficiencies of amphiphilic cyclodextrin-based nanoparticles that do not require the presence of surfactant in the preparation [121]. In addition, nanoparticles can be prepared directly from pre-formed inclusion complexes of drug with amphiphilic cyclodextrins, which ensures both high drug loading and delayed burst effect [121]. Interestingly, the first experimental therapeutic to provide targeted delivery of siRNA in humans utilized a cyclodextrin-based nanoparticle [122].

Choisnard et al. prepared self-assembled nanoparticles of decanoate β-cyclodextrin esters and hexanoate β-cyclodextrin esters [123]. The mean size and polydispersity were significantly affected by the nature of solvent used in the nano-precipitation technique. In addition, the globular shape of nanoparticle was determined by the hydrophobic moiety used for modification [123].

Cyclodextrin-containing polymers have demonstrated unique capabilities for nucleic acid delivery: They have demonstrated low *in vitro* and *in vivo* toxicities when compared with other non-cyclodextrin-containing polycations such as poly-L-lysine and polyethylenimine. In addition, these polycations form self-assembled nanoparticles with oligonucleotides [124]. These advantages have been utilized for the preparation of the first clinically tested nanoparticle for siRNA delivery, which is composed of cyclodextrin-containing polycation, a polythethylene glycol (PEG) steric stabilization agent, and human transferrin as a targeting ligand [122]. Structurally, the cyclodextrin-containing polycation assembles with the siRNA primarily via electrostatic interactions. It condenses siRNA and protects it from nuclease degradation. The cyclodextrins within the polymer chains that reside on the surface of the nanoparticles are used for assembling PEG, which is conjugated to adamantine. The assembly of PEG-adamantine is due to inclusion complex formation between the adamantine and cyclodextrin. The same principle is applied for the assembly of the targeting ligand transferrin, which was chosen since its receptor is upregulated on cancer cells. Primary results from phase I clinical trials using RRM2 siRNA-containing nanoparticles have been recently published [125]. Following systemic administration to patients with solid cancers, tumor biopsies revealed intracellular and dose dependent localization of the nanoparticles. In addition, specific reductions of both RRM2 mRNA and protein levels were observed. 5-RLM-RACE analyses have shown that this reduction was mediated by an RNAi mechanism [125]. The paper describing results from the clinical studies did not contain data regarding the effects on human metabolism and immune response. However, following long-term administration to mice, no abnormalities in interleukin-12 and IFN-alpha, liver and kidney function tests, complete blood counts, or pathology of major organs were observed [42]. The administered nanoparticles used for delivery of *EWS-FLI1* siRNA, demonstrated a significant and ligand specific inhibition of tumor growth in a murine model of metastatic Ewing's sarcoma [42].

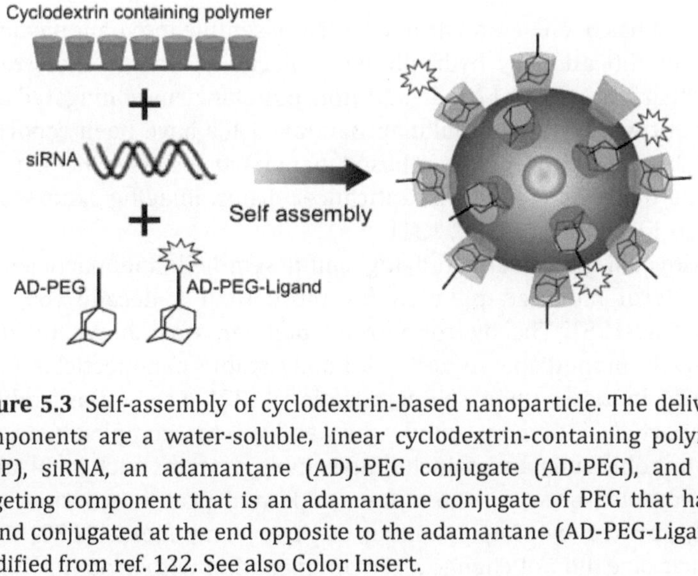

Figure 5.3 Self-assembly of cyclodextrin-based nanoparticle. The delivery components are a water-soluble, linear cyclodextrin-containing polymer (CDP), siRNA, an adamantane (AD)-PEG conjugate (AD-PEG), and the targeting component that is an adamantane conjugate of PEG that has a ligand conjugated at the end opposite to the adamantane (AD-PEG-Ligand). Modified from ref. 122. See also Color Insert.

5.4.6 Arabinogalactan-Based Nanoparticles

Arabinogalactan has been used as a carrier for drug conjugates [44,126]. Recently, Arabinogalactan–folic acid–drug conjugates for targeted delivery and activated drug release were prepared [127]. The targeted nanovehicle was formed by conjugation of folic acid and the anticancer drug methotrexate to arabinogalactan. The use of folic acid as a targeting ligand derives from fact that cancer cells overexpress receptors for nutrients in order to maintain their fast-growing metabolism [2] one of these receptor is folate receptor, which is overexpressed in malignant cells including ovary, brain, kidney, breast, colon, and lung [127]. Another advantage of using nutrient receptors as targets is that they enable internalization of the nanocarrier via receptor-mediated endocytosis. The activated drug release was achieved by linking methotrexate to arabinogalactan by an endosomally cleavable peptide Gly-Phe-Leu-Gly (GFLG). The nanocarrier displayed significant cytotoxic activity to folate receptor overexpressing cells in comparison with folate receptor-deficient cells.

5.4.7 Pullulan-Based Nanoparticles

Pullulan has been demonstrated to self-assemble into nanoparticles after modification by hydrophobic molecules, such as cholesterol and stearic acid [128,129]. In addition, pullulan drug conjugated and covalently cross-linked pullulan nanoparticles have been reported [130,131]. Overall, pullulan-based nanoparticles have been used for the delivery of proteins, anticancer drugs, imaging agents, and nucleotides [69, 129, 130, 131].

Akiyoshi has been studying self-assembled nanoparticles of cholesterol modified pullulan for more than a decade [69, 70, 129, 132–135]. The hydrophobized pullulan was shown to form relatively monodisperse and colloidally stable nanoparticles (20–30 nm) in water upon self-aggregation [132]. The self-assembled nanoparticles demonstrated the ability to complex various hydrophobic substances, including soluble proteins such as Insulin. The complex between the nanoparticle and protein solution was easily formed by simply mixing the two components [129]. The particle size did not change after complexation with proteins [136]. The complexation with insulin occurred faster than with larger proteins such as α-chymotrypsin or BSA. The nanoparticles showed high colloidal stability and no dissociation of insulin or precipitation were observed. The complexation contributed greatly to the thermal stability of insulin (even after heating for 6 h at 90°C) and protected insulin from enzymatic degradation. *In vivo* experiments demonstrated preservation insulin's bioavailability [129]. The ability of these nanoparticles to thermally stabilize proteins was investigated further [133]. The molecular chaperon-like activity was demonstrated on proteins using a system consisting of the cholesterol–pullulan nanoparticles and β-cyclodextrin. Capture of heat-denatured unfolded protein and the release of the refolded form were achieved and the irreversible protein aggregation upon heating was completely prevented, recovering almost 100% of protein activity. Intracellular protein delivery by self-assembled nanoparticles of cationic cholesteryl group-bearing pullulans was also demonstrated [69]. While particle size did not change significantly upon replacing the cholesterol with the cationic cholesteryl group, the zeta potential became positive (+7.7 ± 0.1 mV in comparison with −1.3 ± 0.4). In addition, the binding constant to the model protein, BSA, significantly grew. The cholesteryl–pullulan nanoparticles demonstrated a more effective internalization of protein to into HeLa cells in comparison with cationic liposomes and a protein transduction domain (PTD)-based carrier. Upon cell internalization, the protein-containing nanoparticle dissociated and the protein was released. Recently, cholesteryl–pullulan nanoparticles were used as an antigenic protein delivery system for adjuvant-free intranasal vaccines [70]. Intranasal delivery of a non-toxic subunit fragment of Clostridium botulinum type-A neurotoxin using these nanoparticles induced vigorous botulinum-neurotoxin-A-neutralizing serum IgG and secretory IgA antibody responses. In addition, intranasally immunization of tetanus toxoid with the nanoparticles induced strong tetanus-toxoid-specific systemic and mucosal immune responses.

5.5 Polysaccharide-Coated Nanoparticles

Surface modification of nanoparticles with polysaccharides, an outcome of the cell surface polysaccharide discovery, has remarkable advantages for drug delivery systems: It endows the nanoparticle with long-term circulation and increased stability. In addition, it provides targeting abilities: pullulan coating have been used for hepatic delivery [137], alginate and chitosan coating have been used for mucosal delivery [138], mannan coating facilitated uptake by macrophages [139] and HA-coated nanoparticles have been used to target CD44 overexpressing cells [3, 140, 141]. Another advantage is cryoprotection, which has been reported for several polysaccharides

[18,142]. Polysaccharide-decorated liposomes demonstrated reduced permeability to water-soluble encapsulated materials and protection from degradation by lipases [143].

Coating nanoparticles with polysaccharide can be achieved by adsorption, incorporation, copolymerization, or covalent grafting [144] and has been reported for many polysaccharides, including pectin, pullulan, mannan, HA, heparin, chitosan, and dextran [144, 145].

5.5.1 Chitosan-Coated Nanoparticles

The cationic nature of chitosan enables its adherence to mucosal surfaces. In addition, the ability of chitosan to open tight junctions between epithelial cells has also been demonstrated [14]. These characteristics make chitosan appealing as a coating agent of nanocarriers designed for mucosal delivery. For example, chitosan-coated poly-ε-caprolactone (PECL) nanoparticles allowed the bioavailability of the anti-inflammatory drug indomethacin in the cornea and aqueous humor following topical ocular instillation [144]. In addition, chitosan coating of liposomes enhanced mucosal adhesion in rat intestine [146]. The degree of adhesion showed strong correlation to the amount of chitosan on the surface of the liposomes. When the chitosan-coated liposomes were used for the delivery of insulin, the effect determined by blood glucose levels was more significant and longer lasting in comparison with uncoated liposomes possibly due to mucoadhesion facilitated by the chitosan coat.

Chitosan coating can be used to replace the cationic polymers and lipids currently used for nucleic acid delivery thus overcoming the toxicity, which is the major obstacle in using these compounds. Chitosan-coated nanoparticles can interact with nucleic acids, improving the nanoparticle loading efficiency and transfection properties [144].

Structural benefits of coating nanoparticles with chitosan have also been demonstrated: Chitosan-coated liposomes were more stable in stimulated gastric fluids in comparison with uncoated liposomes [147]. Chitosan-coated PECL nanoparticles also demonstrated enhanced physical stability [18]. In addition, the chitosan coating also facilitated the redispersion of lyophilized PECL nanoparticles.

5.5.2 Hyaluronan-Coated Nanoparticles

The HA capsule of group A streptococci enables it to escape the host immune response [148] and therefore provides long-term circulation. This trait has been successfully adopted for the delivery of mitomycin C using HA-coated liposomes (tHA-LIP) (Figure 5.4A) [141]. tHA-LIP were 7-fold and 70-fold longer circulating in comparison with uncoated liposomes and free mitomycin C in three murine tumor models: BALB/c-bearing C-26 solid tumors; C57BL/6-bearing B16F10.9, or D122 lung metastasis [141]. The HA on the tHA-LIP was covalently attached using EDC via the glucuronic carboxylate to phosphatidylethanolamine in the pre-formed liposomes. The tHA-LIP demonstrated slower drug efflux and higher encapsulation efficiency. In addition, since the effect of tHA-LIP is CD44 dependent, these nanoparticles demonstrated significantly higher cytotoxicity *in vitro* on CD44 overexpressing cells and increased drug accumulation in tumors *in vivo*. The later resulted in decreased metastasis, inhibition of tumor growth, and prolonged survival. These effects were later demonstrated with doxorubicin-loaded tHA-LIP [3]. This study also compared tHA-LIP with poly(ethylenglycol) (PEG)-coated liposomes ("stealth" liposomes). This was done since PEGylation, a common hydrophilic surface modification of drug delivery systems, has demonstrated prevention of recognition by the immune system. The tHA-LIP were long circulating more than all tested controls, including uncoated and PEGylated liposomes in healthy and tumor-bearing mice.

Recently, HA-coated paclitaxel-clusters (PTX-GAGs) have been prepared for selective tumor targeting (Figure 5.4B) [149] (see also Chapter 1 in this book). The aqueous insolubility of PTX was utilized in this preparation by mixing it with lipids that self-assembled into nano-size clusters. The clusters were then coated with HA to facilitate targeting of CD44. When tested *in vivo*, these nanoparticles managed to induce tumor arrest in a murine model of colon adenocarcinoma and were significantly more potent than free PTX .

Targeting of CD44 was also demonstrated for liposomes decorated with HA oligomers [140, 150]. Unlike in the preparation of the previously described tHA-LIP, the HA oligosaccharides were conjugated by reductive amination to phosphatidylethanolamine prior to liposome preparation. The oligosaccharide-decorated liposomes demonstrated CD44-dependent uptake, that could be blocked by both free HA and anti-CD44 antibodies. Liposome uptake was dependent on ligand density; however, as little as 0.1 HA molar percent managed to facilitate targeting. In addition, doxorubicin encapsulated in the oligosaccharide-decorated liposomes was significantly more cytotoxic to CD44 overexpression cells in comparison with free drug.

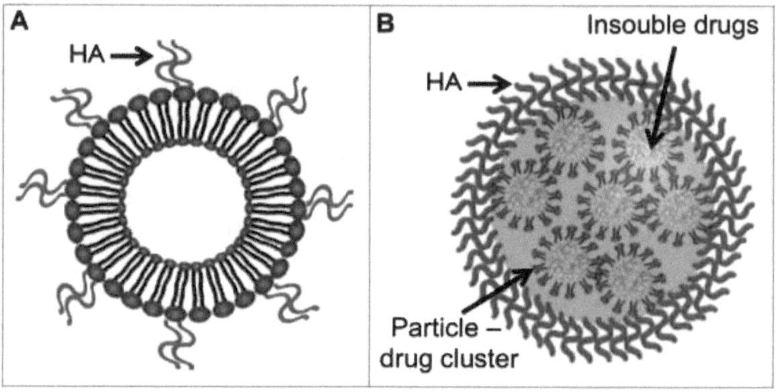

Figure 5.4 Hyaluronan-coated nanoparticles: (A) Hyaluronan-coated liposome (tHA-LIP). (B) Paclitaxel-clusters coated with hyaluronan (PTX-GAGs). See also Color Insert.

Another clinically relevant advantage of the liposomal HA coat is cryoprotection [142]. Cryoprotection provides the liposomes with a longer shelf life since it prevents the reversion of lyophilized unilamellar liposomes to multilamellar liposomes upon rehydration. The tested lyophilized tHA-LIP demonstrated the ability to retain the same dimensions, zeta potentials, encapsulation efficiencies and half-life of drug release of the original systems upon redispersion. HA cryoprotects possibly by providing substitute structure-stabilizing H-bonds.

5.5.3 Heparin- and Dextran-Coated Nanoparticles

Heparin has been shown to inhibit complement activation at different stages by increasing the activity of protein H [151]. Since the activation of the complement system plays an important role in opsonization and uptake of particles by the mononuclear phagocyte system (MPS), surface modification of nanoparticles with heparin seemed promising [151]. And indeed, a heparin coat significantly promoted long-term circulation of nanoparticle [151]. The heparin-modified poly(methyl methacrylate) (PMMA) nanoparticles elongated the *in vivo* half-life from only a few minutes to 5 h [151]. Dextran-coated nanoparticles also demonstrated longer *in vivo* half-life but to a lesser extent in comparison with heparin, probably since dextran has been shown to activate the complement system [152]. *In vitro*, the heparin- or dextran-coated nanoparticles were also demonstrated to be less taken up by a macrophagic cell line in comparison with uncoated nanoparticles [151]. The steric barrier formed by dense brush-like arrangement of the attached polysaccharide chains could contribute to the long-circulating properties of the heparin (or dextran)-coated PMMA nanoparticles.

Recently, an artificial oxygen carrier based on a polysaccharide-decorated nanoparticle was demonstrated [153]. The core-shell nanoparticles, developed as red blood cell substitutes, were covered with a long brush of polysaccharides (heparin, dextran, or dextran sulfate) and demonstrated very low complement activation. The nanoparticles were obtained by using a redox radical polymerization mechanism in aqueous medium, which was followed by adsorption or coupling of hemoglobin. Interestingly, a former heparin-coated oxygen carrier developed by the same group demonstrated a highly improved cell line tolerance in the presence of hemoglobin [154]. In addition, the anticoagulant properties of heparin were preserved upon coating the nanoparticles with heparin. When benzene tetracarboxylic acid (BTCA) was used as a coupling agent for hemoglobin to dextran-coated nanoparticles, the loading capacity showed a 9.3-fold increase. The modification of nanoparticles by BTCA slightly increased complement activation; however, this activation was reverted by the further addition of hemoglobin. The bound hemoglobin preserved its ability for exchanging oxygen [153].

5.6 Summary

The variety of naturally occurring polysaccharide properties has been successfully utilized to create multiple nano-size drug delivery systems. The advantages of polysaccharides enable the preparation of nanocarriers for the delivery of proteins, peptides, antibiotics and nucleic acids using several administration routes. In addition, preliminary results from the first phase I clinical trial using a polysaccharide nanocarrier for siRNA delivery have been presented.

Further understanding of the mechanisms involved in drug delivery will result in improved drug delivery systems tailor-made for a particular application.

Acknowledgments

The authors wish to thank Dr. Micha Fridman from the TAU School of Chemistry for his help in the presentation of the polysaccharide chemical structures.

References

1. Petros RA, DeSimone JM (2010) Strategies in the design of nanoparticles for therapeutic applications. *Nat Rev Drug Discov* 9: 615–627.
2. Peer D, Karp JM, Hong S, Farokhzad OC, Margalit R, et al. (2007) Nanocarriers as an emerging platform for cancer therapy. *Nat Nanotechnol* 2: 751–760.
3. Peer D, Margalit R (2004) Tumor-targeted hyaluronan nanoliposomes increase the antitumor activity of liposomal doxorubicin in syngeneic and human xenograft mouse tumor models. *Neoplasia* 6: 343–353.
4. Sinha VR, Kumria R (2001) Polysaccharides in colon-specific drug delivery. *Int J Pharm* 224: 19–38.
5. Muzzarelli R (1973) Chitosan. In: Muzzarelli, editor. *Natural Chelating Polymers*: Pergamon Press, Oxford pp. 144–176.
6. Alpar HO, Somavarapu S, Atuah KN, Bramwell VW (2005) Biodegradable mucoadhesive particulates for nasal and pulmonary antigen and DNA delivery. *Adv Drug Deliv Rev* 57: 411–430.
7. Paolicelli P, de la Fuente M, Sanchez A, Seijo B, Alonso MJ (2009) Chitosan nanoparticles for drug delivery to the eye. *Expert Opin Drug Deliv* 6: 239–253.
8. Takeuchi H, Yamamoto H, Kawashima Y (2001) Mucoadhesive nanoparticulate systems for peptide drug delivery. *Adv Drug Deliv Rev* 47: 39–54.
9. Valenta C, Auner BG (2004) The use of polymers for dermal and transdermal delivery. *Eur J Pharm Biopharm* 58: 279–289.
10. Sashiwa H, Saimoto H, Shigemasa Y, Ogawa R, Tokura S (1990) Lysozyme susceptibility of partially deacetylated chitin. *Int J Biol Macromol* 12: 295–296.
11. Muzzarelli R, Baldassarre V, Conti F, Ferrara P, Biagini G, et al. (1988) Biological activity of chitosan: ultrastructural study. *Biomaterials* 9: 247–252.

12. Illum L, Farraj NF, Davis SS (1994) Chitosan as a novel nasal delivery system for peptide drugs. *Pharm Res* 11: 1186–1189.

13. Lehr CM, Bouwstra JA, Schacht EH, Junginger HE (1992) *In vitro* evaluation of mucoadhesive properties of chitosan and some other natural polymers. *Int J Pharm* 78: 43–48.

14. Artursson P, Lindmark T, Davis SS, Illum L (1994) Effect of chitosan on the permeability of monolayers of intestinal epithelial cells (Caco-2). *Pharm Res* 11: 1358–1361.

15. Thanou M, Verhoef JC, Marbach P, Junginger HE (2000) Intestinal absorption of octreotide: *N*-trimethyl chitosan chloride (TMC) ameliorates the permeability and absorption properties of the somatostatin analogue *in vitro* and *in vivo*. *J Pharm Sci* 89: 951–957.

16. Kubota N, Eguchi Y (1997) Facile preparation of water-soluble *N*-acetylated chitosan and molecular weight dependence of its water-solubility. *Polym J* 29: 123–127.

17. Varum KM, Ottoy MH, Smidsrod O (1994) Water-solubility of partially *N*-acetylated chitosans as a function of Ph — effect of chemical-composition and depolymerization. *Carbohydr Polym* 25: 65–70.

18. Calvo P, RemunanLopez C, VilaJato JL, Alonso MJ (1997) Development of positively charged colloidal drug carriers: chitosan coated polyester nanocapsules and submicron-emulsions. *Colloid Polym Sci* 275: 46–53.

19. Bhattarai N, Zhang MQ (2007) Controlled synthesis and structural stability of alginate-based nanofibers. *Nanotechnology* 18: 455601.

20. George M, Abraham TE (2006) Polyionic hydrocolloids for the intestinal delivery of protein drugs: alginate and chitosan — a review. *J Control Release* 114: 1–14.

21. Shilpa A, Agrawal SS, Ray AR (2003) Controlled delivery of drugs from alginate matrix. *J Macromol Sci Polym Rev* C43: 187–221.

22. Ch'ng HS, Park H, Kelly P, Robinson JR (1985) Bioadhesive polymers as platforms for oral controlled drug delivery II: synthesis and evaluation of some swelling, water-insoluble bioadhesive polymers. *J Pharm Sci* 74: 399–405.

23. Varki A (2009) *Essentials of Glycobiology*. Cold Spring Harbor, N.Y.: Cold Spring Harbor Laboratory Press. xxix, 784 p.

24. Toole BP (2004) Hyaluronan: from extracellular glue to pericellular cue. *Nat Rev Cancer* 4: 528–539.

25. Platt VM, Szoka FC, Jr. (2008) Anticancer therapeutics: targeting macromolecules and nanocarriers to hyaluronan or CD44, a hyaluronan receptor. *Mol Pharm* 5: 474–486.

26. Hamman JH (2010) Chitosan based polyelectrolyte complexes as potential carrier materials in drug delivery systems. *Mar Drugs* 8: 1305–1322.
27. Jing W, DeAngelis PL (2004) Synchronized chemoenzymatic synthesis of monodisperse hyaluronan polymers. *J Biol Chem* 279: 42345–42349.
28. DeAngelis PL, Oatman LC, Gay DF (2003) Rapid chemoenzymatic synthesis of monodisperse hyaluronan oligosaccharides with immobilized enzyme reactors. *J Biol Chem* 278: 35199–35203.
29. Pouyani T, Prestwich GD (1994) Functionalized derivatives of hyaluronic acid oligosaccharides: drug carriers and novel biomaterials. *Bioconjug Chem* 5: 339–347.
30. Prestwich GD, Marecak DM, Marecek JF, Vercruysse KP, Ziebell MR (1998) Controlled chemical modification of hyaluronic acid: synthesis, applications, and biodegradation of hydrazide derivatives. *J Control Release* 53: 93–103.
31. Mohapatra S, Yang X, Wright JA, Turley EA, Greenberg AH (1996) Soluble hyaluronan receptor RHAMM induces mitotic arrest by suppressing Cdc2 and cyclin B1 expression. *J Exp Med* 183: 1663–1668.
32. Day AJ, Prestwich GD (2002) Hyaluronan-binding proteins: tying up the giant. J Biol Chem 277: 4585–4588.
33. Shigeishi H, Fujimoto S, Hiraoka M, Ono S, Taki M, et al. (2009) Overexpression of the receptor for hyaluronan-mediated motility, correlates with expression of microtubule-associated protein in human oral squamous cell carcinomas. *Int J Oncol* 34: 1565–1571.
34. Krause DS, Spitzer TR, Stowell CP (2010) The concentration of CD44 is increased in hematopoietic stem cell grafts of patients with acute myeloid leukemia, plasma cell myeloma, and non-Hodgkin lymphoma. *Arch Pathol Lab Med* 134: 1033–1038.
35. Borgstrom S, Gelin LE, Zederfeldt B (1959) The formation of vein thrombi following tissue injury: an experimental study in rabbits. *Acta Chir Scand Suppl* 247: 1–36.
36. Nimesh S, Kumar R, Chandra R (2006) Novel polyallylamine-dextran sulfate-DNA nanoplexes: highly efficient non-viral vector for gene delivery. *Int J Pharm* 320: 143–149.
37. Zimmermann K, Preinl G, Ludwig H, Greulich KO (1983) Inhibition of hyaluronidase by dextran sulfate and its possible application in anticancer treatment. *J Cancer Res Clin Oncol* 105: 189–190.
38. Wetzel GD, Kettman JR (1981) Activation of murine B cells. II. Dextran sulfate removes the requirement for cellular interaction during lipopolysaccharide-induced mitogenesis. *Cell Immunol* 61: 176–189.

39. Ataullakhanov RI, Ataullakhanov FI, Abdullaev DM (1984) Increase in the permeability of the lymphocyte plasma membrane for uni- and bivalent cations and low-molecular metabolites following exposure to mitogenic polyanions. *Biull Eksp Biol Med* 98: 81–84.
40. Sallas F, Darcy R (2008) Amphiphilic cyclodextrins — advances in synthesis and supramolecular chemistry. *Eur J Org Chem* 6: 957–969.
41. Szejtli J (1998) Introduction and general overview of cyclodextrin chemistry. *Chem Rev* 98: 1743–1754.
42. Hu-Lieskovan S, Heidel JD, Bartlett DW, Davis ME, Triche TJ (2005) Sequence-specific knockdown of EWS-FLI1 by targeted, nonviral delivery of small interfering RNA inhibits tumor growth in a murine model of metastatic Ewing's sarcoma. *Cancer Res* 65: 8984–8992.
43. Davis ME, Brewster ME (2004) Cyclodextrin-based pharmaceutics: past, present and future. *Nat Rev Drug Discov* 3: 1023–1035.
44. Falk R, Domb AJ, Polacheck I (1999) A novel injectable water-soluble amphotericin B-arabinogalactan conjugate. *Antimicrob Agents Chemother* 43: 1975–1981.
45. Leathers TD (2003) Biotechnological production and applications of pullulan. *Appl Microbiol Biotechnol* 62: 468–473.
46. Linhardt RJ (2003) 2003 Claude S. Hudson Award address in carbohydrate chemistry. Heparin: structure and activity. *J Med Chem* 46: 2551–2564.
47. Kemp MM, Linhardt RJ (2010) Heparin-based nanoparticles. *Wiley Interdiscip Rev Nanomed Nanobiotechnol* 2: 77–87.
48. Berger J, Reist M, Mayer JM, Felt O, Peppas NA, et al. (2004) Structure and interactions in covalently and ionically crosslinked chitosan hydrogels for biomedical applications. *Eur J Pharm Biopharm* 57: 19–34.
49. Berger J, Reist M, Mayer JM, Felt O, Gurny R (2004) Structure and interactions in chitosan hydrogels formed by complexation or aggregation for biomedical applications. *Eur J Pharm Biopharm* 57: 35–52.
50. Ohya Y, Shiratani M, Kobayashi H, Ouchi T (1994) Release behavior of 5-fluorouracil from chitosan-gel nanospheres immobilizing 5-fluorouracil coated with polysaccharides and their cell-specific cytotoxicity. *J Macromol Sci Pure Appl Chem* A31: 629–642.
51. Banerjee T, Mitra S, Kumar Singh A, Kumar Sharma R, Maitra A (2002) Preparation, characterization and biodistribution of ultrafine chitosan nanoparticles. *Int J Pharm* 243: 93–105.
52. Bodnar M, Hartmann JF, Borbely J (2005) Preparation and characterization of chitosan-based nanoparticles. *Biomacromolecules* 6: 2521–2527.

53. Chen KY, Liao WJ, Kuo SM, Tsai FJ, Chen YS, et al. (2009) Asymmetric chitosan membrane containing collagen I nanospheres for skin tissue engineering. *Biomacromolecules* 10: 1642–1649.
54. Ahmad Z, Sharma S, Khuller GK (2007) Chemotherapeutic evaluation of alginate nanoparticle-encapsulated azole antifungal and antitubercular drugs against murine tuberculosis. *Nanomedicine* 3: 239–243.
55. Ahmad Z, Sharma S, Khuller GK (2005) Inhalable alginate nanoparticles as antitubercular drug carriers against experimental tuberculosis. *Int J Antimicrob Agents* 26: 298–303.
56. Bodmeier R, Chen HG, Paeratakul O (1989) A novel approach to the oral delivery of micro- or nanoparticles. *Pharm Res* 6: 413–417.
57. Mi FL, Shyu SS, Lee ST, Wong TB (1999) Kinetic study of chitosan-tripolyphosphate complex reaction and acid-resistive properties of the chitosan-tripolyphosphate gel beads prepared by in-liquid curing method. *J Polym Sci Part B Poly Phys* 37: 1551–1564.
58. Draget KI, Varum KM, Moen E, Gynnild H, Smidsrod O (1992) Chitosan cross-linked with Mo(VI) polyoxyanions: a new gelling system. *Biomaterials* 13: 635–638.
59. Mi FL, Chen CT, Tseng YC, Kuan CY, Shyu SS (1997) Iron(III)-carboxymethylchitin microsphere for the pH-sensitive release of 6-mercaptopurine. *J Control Rel* 44: 19–32.
60. Bhattarai N, Gunn J, Zhang M (2010) Chitosan-based hydrogels for controlled, localized drug delivery. *Adv Drug Deliv Rev* 62: 83–99.
61. Park JH, Saravanakumar G, Kim K, Kwon IC (2010) Targeted delivery of low molecular drugs using chitosan and its derivatives. *Adv Drug Deliv Rev* 62: 28–41.
62. Tiyaboonchai W, Woiszwillo J, Sims RC, Middaugh CR (2003) Insulin containing polyethylenimine-dextran sulfate nanoparticles. *Int J Pharm* 255: 139–151.
63. Sonaje K, Lin YH, Juang JH, Wey SP, Chen CT, et al. (2009) *In vivo* evaluation of safety and efficacy of self-assembled nanoparticles for oral insulin delivery. *Biomaterials* 30: 2329–2339.
64. Liu Z, Jiao Y, Wang Y, Zhou C, Zhang Z (2008) Polysaccharides-based nanoparticles as drug delivery systems. *Adv Drug Deliv Rev* 60: 1650–1662.
65. Howard KA, Paludan SR, Behlke MA, Besenbacher F, Deleuran B, et al. (2009) Chitosan/siRNA nanoparticle-mediated TNF-alpha knockdown in peritoneal macrophages for anti-inflammatory treatment in a murine arthritis model. *Mol Ther* 17: 162–168.

66. Oyarzun-Ampuero FA, Brea J, Loza MI, Torres D, Alonso MJ (2009) Chitosan-hyaluronic acid nanoparticles loaded with heparin for the treatment of asthma. *Int J Pharm* 381: 122–129.

67. Allen C, Maysinger D, Eisenberg A (1999) Nano-engineering block copolymer aggregates for drug delivery. *Colloids Surf B Biointerfaces* 16: 3–27.

68. Letchford K, Burt H (2007) A review of the formation and classification of amphiphilic block copolymer nanoparticulate structures: micelles, nanospheres, nanocapsules and polymersomes. *Eur J Pharm Biopharm* 65: 259–269.

69. Ayame H, Morimoto N, Akiyoshi K (2008) Self-assembled cationic nanogels for intracellular protein delivery. *Bioconjug Chem* 19: 882–890.

70. Nochi T, Yuki Y, Takahashi H, Sawada S, Mejima M, et al. (2010) Nanogel antigenic protein-delivery system for adjuvant-free intranasal vaccines. *Nat Mater* 9: 572–578.

71. Janes KA, Calvo P, Alonso MJ (2001) Polysaccharide colloidal particles as delivery systems for macromolecules. *Adv Drug Deliv Rev* 47: 83–97.

72. Gan Q, Wang T, Cochrane C, McCarron P (2005) Modulation of surface charge, particle size and morphological properties of chitosan-TPP nanoparticles intended for gene delivery. *Colloids Surf B Biointerfaces* 44: 65–73.

73. Calvo P, RemunanLopez C, VilaJato JL, Alonso MJ (1997) Novel hydrophilic chitosan-polyethylene oxide nanoparticles as protein carriers. *J Appl Polym Sci* 63: 125–132.

74. Fernandez-Urrusuno R, Calvo P, Remunan-Lopez C, Vila-Jato JL, Alonso MJ (1999) Enhancement of nasal absorption of insulin using chitosan nanoparticles. *Pharm Res* 16: 1576–1581.

75. De Campos AM, Sanchez A, Alonso MJ (2001) Chitosan nanoparticles: a new vehicle for the improvement of the delivery of drugs to the ocular surface. Application to cyclosporin A. *Int J Pharm* 224: 159–168.

76. Csaba N, Koping-Hoggard M, Alonso MJ (2009) Ionically crosslinked chitosan/tripolyphosphate nanoparticles for oligonucleotide and plasmid DNA delivery. *Int J Pharm* 382: 205–214.

77. Csaba N, Koping-Hoggard M, Fernandez-Megia E, Novoa-Carballal R, Riguera R, et al. (2009) Ionically crosslinked chitosan nanoparticles as gene delivery systems: effect of PEGylation degree on *in vitro* and *in vivo* gene transfer. *J Biomed Nanotechnol* 5: 162–171.

78. Katas H, Alpar HO (2006) Development and characterisation of chitosan nanoparticles for siRNA delivery. *J Control Release* 115: 216–225.

79. Lee PW, Peng SF, Su CJ, Mi FL, Chen HL, et al. (2008) The use of biodegradable polymeric nanoparticles in combination with a low-pressure gene gun for transdermal DNA delivery. *Biomaterials* 29: 742–751.

80. Peng SF, Yang MJ, Su CJ, Chen HL, Lee PW, et al. (2009) Effects of incorporation of poly(gamma-glutamic acid) in chitosan/DNA complex nanoparticles on cellular uptake and transfection efficiency. *Biomaterials* 30: 1797–1808.

81. Roy K, Mao HQ, Huang SK, Leong KW (1999) Oral gene delivery with chitosan–DNA nanoparticles generates immunologic protection in a murine model of peanut allergy. *Nat Med* 5: 387–391.

82. Jean M, Smaoui F, Lavertu M, Methot S, Bouhdoud L, et al. (2009) Chitosan-plasmid nanoparticle formulations for IM and SC delivery of recombinant FGF-2 and PDGF-BB or generation of antibodies. *Gene Ther* 16: 1097–1110.

83. Klausner EA, Zhang Z, Chapman RL, Multack RF, Volin MV (2010) Ultrapure chitosan oligomers as carriers for corneal gene transfer. *Biomaterials* 31: 1814–1820.

84. Koping-Hoggard M, Varum KM, Issa M, Danielsen S, Christensen BE, et al. (2004) Improved chitosan-mediated gene delivery based on easily dissociated chitosan polyplexes of highly defined chitosan oligomers. *Gene Ther* 11: 1441–1452.

85. Strand SP, Lelu S, Reitan NK, de Lange Davies C, Artursson P, et al. (2010) Molecular design of chitosan gene delivery systems with an optimized balance between polyplex stability and polyplex unpacking. *Biomaterials* 31: 975–987.

86. Zahr AS, Davis CA, Pishko MV (2006) Macrophage uptake of core-shell nanoparticles surface modified with poly(ethylene glycol). *Langmuir* 22: 8178–8185.

87. Zhang J, Chen XG, Li YY, Liu CS (2007) Self-assembled nanoparticles based on hydrophobically modified chitosan as carriers for doxorubicin. *Nanomedicine* 3: 258–265.

88. Kim JH, Kim YS, Park K, Kang E, Lee S, et al. (2008) Self-assembled glycol chitosan nanoparticles for the sustained and prolonged delivery of antiangiogenic small peptide drugs in cancer therapy. *Biomaterials* 29: 1920–1930.

89. Pasqualini R, Koivunen E, Ruoslahti E (1997) Alpha v integrins as receptors for tumor targeting by circulating ligands. *Nat Biotechnol* 15: 542–546.

90. Son YJ, Jang JS, Cho YW, Chung H, Park RW, et al. (2003) Biodistribution and anti-tumor efficacy of doxorubicin loaded glycol-chitosan nanoaggregates by EPR effect. *J Control Release* 91: 135–145.

91. Kim JH, Kim YS, Kim S, Park JH, Kim K, et al. (2006) Hydrophobically modified glycol chitosan nanoparticles as carriers for paclitaxel. *J Control Release* 111: 228–234.

92. Kast CE, Bernkop-Schnurch A (2001) Thiolated polymers--thiomers: development and *in vitro* evaluation of chitosan-thioglycolic acid conjugates. *Biomaterials* 22: 2345–2352.

93. Florea BI, Thanou M, Junginger HE, Borchard G (2006) Enhancement of bronchial octreotide absorption by chitosan and *N*-trimethyl chitosan shows linear *in vitro/in vivo* correlation. *J Control Release* 110: 353–361.

94. Jiang HL, Kwon JT, Kim YK, Kim EM, Arote R, et al. (2007) Galactosylated chitosan-graft-polyethylenimine as a gene carrier for hepatocyte targeting. *Gene Ther* 14: 1389–1398.

95. Fernandes JC, Wang H, Jreyssaty C, Benderdour M, Lavigne P, et al. (2008) Bone-protective effects of nonviral gene therapy with folate-chitosan DNA nanoparticle containing interleukin-1 receptor antagonist gene in rats with adjuvant-induced arthritis. *Mol Ther* 16: 1243–1251.

96. Hamidi M, Azadi A, Rafiei P (2008) Hydrogel nanoparticles in drug delivery. *Adv Drug Deliv Rev* 60: 1638–1649.

97. Goycoolea FM, Lollo G, Remunan-Lopez C, Quaglia F, Alonso MJ (2009) Chitosan-alginate blended nanoparticles as carriers for the transmucosal delivery of macromolecules. *Biomacromolecules* 10(7): 1736–1743.

98. Khdair A, Chen D, Patil Y, Ma L, Dou QP, et al. (2010) Nanoparticle-mediated combination chemotherapy and photodynamic therapy overcomes tumor drug resistance. *J Control Release* 141: 137–144.

99. Bernkop-Schnurch A, Kast CE, Richter MF (2001) Improvement in the mucoadhesive properties of alginate by the covalent attachment of cysteine. *J Control Release* 71: 277–285.

100. Leonard M, De Boisseson MR, Hubert P, Dalencon F, Dellacherie E (2004) Hydrophobically modified alginate hydrogels as protein carriers with specific controlled release properties. *J Control Release* 98: 395–405.

101. Oh EJ, Park K, Kim KS, Kim J, Yang JA, et al. (2010) Target specific and long-acting delivery of protein, peptide, and nucleotide therapeutics using hyaluronic acid derivatives. *J Control Release* 141: 2–12.

102. Luo Y, Prestwich GD (1999) Synthesis and selective cytotoxicity of a hyaluronic acid-antitumor bioconjugate. *Bioconjug Chem* 10: 755–763.

103. Lee H, Lee K, Park TG (2008) Hyaluronic acid-paclitaxel conjugate micelles: synthesis, characterization, and antitumor activity. *Bioconjug Chem* 19: 1319–1325.

104. Xin D, Wang Y, Xiang J (2010) The use of amino acid linkers in the conjugation of paclitaxel with hyaluronic acid as drug delivery system: synthesis, self-assembled property, drug release, and *in vitro* efficiency. *Pharm Res* 27: 380–389.

105. Kong JH, Oh EJ, Chae SY, Lee KC, Hahn SK (2010) Long acting hyaluronate–exendin 4 conjugate for the treatment of type 2 diabetes. *Biomaterials* 31: 4121–4128.

106. Buse JB, Henry RR, Han J, Kim DD, Fineman MS, et al. (2004) Effects of exenatide (exendin-4) on glycemic control over 30 weeks in sulfonylurea-treated patients with type 2 diabetes. *Diabetes Care* 27: 2628–2635.

107. Coradini D, Pellizzaro C, Scarlata I, Zorzet S, Garrovo C, et al. (2006) A novel retinoic/butyric hyaluronan ester for the treatment of acute promyelocytic leukemia: preliminary preclinical results. *Leukemia* 20: 785–792.

108. Coradini D, Pellizzaro C, Miglierini G, Daidone MG, Perbellini A (1999) Hyaluronic acid as drug delivery for sodium butyrate: improvement of the anti-proliferative activity on a breast-cancer cell line. *Int J Cancer* 81: 411–416.

109. Coradini D, Zorzet S, Rossin R, Scarlata I, Pellizzaro C, et al. (2004) Inhibition of hepatocellular carcinomas *in vitro* and hepatic metastases *in vivo* in mice by the histone deacetylase inhibitor HA-But. *Clin Cancer Res* 10: 4822–4830.

110. de la Fuente M, Seijo B, Alonso MJ (2008) Bioadhesive hyaluronan-chitosan nanoparticles can transport genes across the ocular mucosa and transfect ocular tissue. *Gene Ther* 15: 668–676.

111. Lee H, Ahn CH, Park TG (2009) Poly[lactic-co-(glycolic acid)]-grafted hyaluronic acid copolymer micelle nanoparticles for target-specific delivery of doxorubicin. *Macromol Biosci* 9: 336–342.

112. Saravanakumar G, Choi KY, Yoon HY, Kim K, Park JH, et al. (2010) Hydrotropic hyaluronic acid conjugates: Synthesis, characterization, and implications as a carrier of paclitaxel. *Int J Pharm* 394: 154–161.

113. Choi KY, Chung H, Min KH, Yoon HY, Kim K, et al. (2010) Self-assembled hyaluronic acid nanoparticles for active tumor targeting. *Biomaterials* 31: 106–114.

114. Lemarchand C, Couvreur P, Besnard M, Costantini D, Gref R (2003) Novel polyester-polysaccharide nanoparticles. *Pharm Res* 20: 1284–1292.

115. Choi KC, Bang JY, Kim C, Kim PI, Lee SR, et al. (2009) Antitumor effect of adriamycin-encapsulated nanoparticles of poly(DL-lactide-co-glycolide)-grafted dextran. *J Pharm Sci* 98: 2104–2112.

116. Bisht S, Maitra A (2009) Dextran-doxorubicin/chitosan nanoparticles for solid tumor therapy. *Wiley Interdiscip Rev Nanomed Nanobiotechnol* 1: 415–425.

117. Hornig S, Bunjes H, Heinze T (2009) Preparation and characterization of nanoparticles based on dextran-drug conjugates. *J Colloid Interface Sci* 338: 56–62.

118. Huang M, Vitharana SN, Peek LJ, Coop T, Berkland C (2007) Polyelectrolyte complexes stabilize and controllably release vascular endothelial growth factor. *Biomacromolecules* 8: 1607–1614.

119. Huang M, Berkland C (2009) Controlled release of repifermin from polyelectrolyte complexes stimulates endothelial cell proliferation. *J Pharm Sci* 98: 268–280.

120. Tiyaboonchai W, Woiszwillo J, Middaugh CR (2001) Formulation and characterization of amphotericin B-polyethylenimine-dextran sulfate nanoparticles. *J Pharm Sci* 90: 902–914.

121. Memisoglu-Bilensoy E, Vural I, Bochot A, Renoir JM, Duchene D, et al. (2005) Tamoxifen citrate loaded amphiphilic beta-cyclodextrin nanoparticles: *in vitro* characterization and cytotoxicity. *J Control Release* 104: 489–496.

122. Davis ME (2009) The first targeted delivery of siRNA in humans via a self-assembling, cyclodextrin polymer-based nanoparticle: from concept to clinic. *Mol Pharm* 6: 659–668.

123. Choisnard L, Geze A, Putaux JL, Wong YS, Wouessidjewe D (2006) Nanoparticles of beta-cyclodextrin esters obtained by self-assembling of biotransesterified beta-cyclodextrins. *Biomacromolecules* 7: 515–520.

124. Spinner NB, Gibas Z, Kline R, Berger B, Jackson L (1992) Placental mosaicism in a case of 46,XY,-22,+t(22;22)(p11;q11) or i(22q) diagnosed at amniocentesis. *Prenat Diagn* 12: 47–51.

125. Davis ME, Zuckerman JE, Choi CH, Seligson D, Tolcher A, et al. (2010) Evidence of RNAi in humans from systemically administered siRNA via targeted nanoparticles. *Nature* 464: 1067–1070.

126. Elgart A, Farber S, Domb AJ, Polacheck I, Hoffman A (2010) Polysaccharide pharmacokinetics: amphotericin B arabinogalactan conjugate — a drug delivery system or a new pharmaceutical entity? *Biomacromolecules* 11: 1972–1977.

127. Pinhassi RI, Assaraf YG, Farber S, Stark M, Ickowicz D, et al. (2010) Arabinogalactan-folic acid–drug conjugate for targeted delivery and target-activated release of anticancer drugs to folate receptor-overexpressing cells. *Biomacromolecules* 11: 294–303.

128. Akiyama E, Morimoto N, Kujawa P, Ozawa Y, Winnik FM, et al. (2007) Self-assembled nanogels of cholesteryl-modified polysaccharides: effect of the polysaccharide structure on their association characteristics in the dilute and semidilute regimes. *Biomacromolecules* 8: 2366–2373.

129. Akiyoshi K, Kobayashi S, Shichibe S, Mix D, Baudys M, et al. (1998) Self-assembled hydrogel nanoparticle of cholesterol-bearing pullulan as a carrier of protein drugs: complexation and stabilization of insulin. *J Control Release* 54: 313–320.

130. Lu D, Wen X, Liang J, Gu Z, Zhang X, et al. (2009) A pH-sensitive nano drug delivery system derived from pullulan/doxorubicin conjugate. *J Biomed Mater Res B Appl Biomater* 89: 177–183.

131. Gupta M, Gupta AK (2004) Hydrogel pullulan nanoparticles encapsulating pBUDLacZ plasmid as an efficient gene delivery carrier. *J Control Release* 99: 157–166.

132. Akiyoshi K, Deguchi S, Moriguchi N, Yamaguchi S, Sunamoto J (1993) Self-aggregates of hydrophobized polysaccharides in water — formation and characteristics of nanoparticles. *Macromolecules* 26: 3062–3068.

133. Akiyoshi K, Sasaki Y, Sunamoto J (1999) Molecular chaperone-like activity of hydrogel nanoparticles of hydrophobized pullulan: thermal stabilization with refolding of carbonic anhydrase B. *Bioconjug Chem* 10: 321–324.

134. Hasegawa U, Sawada S, Shimizu T, Kishida T, Otsuji E, et al. (2009) Raspberry-like assembly of cross-linked nanogels for protein delivery. *J Control Release* 140: 312–317.

135. Sawada S, Akiyoshi K (2010) Nano-encapsulation of lipase by self-assembled nanogels: induction of high enzyme activity and thermal stabilization. *Macromol Biosci* 10: 353–358.

136. Nishikawa T, Akiyoshi K, Sunamoto J (1994) Supramolecular assembly between nanoparticles of hydrophobized polysaccharide and soluble-protein complexation between the self-aggregate of cholesterol-bearing pullulan and alpha-chymotrypsin. *Macromolecules* 27: 7654–7659.

137. Cui Z, Mumper RJ (2002) Plasmid DNA-entrapped nanoparticles engineered from microemulsion precursors: *in vitro* and *in vivo* evaluation. *Bioconjug Chem* 13: 1319–1327.

138. Borges O, Cordeiro-da-Silva A, Romeijn SG, Amidi M, de Sousa A, et al. (2006) Uptake studies in rat Peyer's patches, cytotoxicity and release studies of alginate coated chitosan nanoparticles for mucosal vaccination. *J Control Release* 114: 348–358.

139. Cui Z, Hsu CH, Mumper RJ (2003) Physical characterization and macrophage cell uptake of mannan-coated nanoparticles. *Drug Dev Ind Pharm* 29: 689–700.

140. Eliaz RE, Szoka FC, Jr. (2001) Liposome-encapsulated doxorubicin targeted to CD44: a strategy to kill CD44-overexpressing tumor cells. *Cancer Res* 61: 2592–2601.

141. Peer D, Margalit R (2004) Loading mitomycin C inside long circulating hyaluronan targeted nano-liposomes increases its antitumor activity in three mice tumor models. *Int J Cancer* 108: 780–789.

142. Peer D, Florentin A, Margalit R (2003) Hyaluronan is a key component in cryoprotection and formulation of targeted unilamellar liposomes. *Biochim Biophys Acta* 1612: 76–82.

143. Sunamoto J, Iwamoto K (1986) Protein-coated and polysaccharide-coated liposomes as drug carriers. *Crit Rev Ther Drug Carrier Syst* 2: 117–136.

144. Lemarchand C, Gref R, Couvreur P (2004) Polysaccharide-decorated nanoparticles. *Eur J Pharm Biopharm* 58: 327–341.

145. Jones MN (1994) Carbohydrate-mediated liposomal targeting and drug-delivery. *Adv Drug Delivery Rev* 13: 215–249.

146. Takeuchi H, Yamamoto H, Niwa T, Hino T, Kawashima Y (1996) Enteral absorption of insulin in rats from mucoadhesive chitosan-coated liposomes. *Pharm Res* 13: 896–901.

147. Filipovic-Grcic J, Skalko-Basnet N, Jalsenjak I (2001) Mucoadhesive chitosan-coated liposomes: characteristics and stability. *J Microencapsul* 18: 3–12.

148. Ouskova G, Spellerberg B, Prehm P (2004) Hyaluronan release from *Streptococcus* pyogenes: export by an ABC transporter. *Glycobiology* 14: 931–938.

149. Rivkin I, Cohen K, Koffler J, Melikhov D, Peer D, et al. (2010) Paclitaxel-clusters coated with hyaluronan as selective tumor-targeted nanovectors. *Biomaterials* 31: 7106–7114.

150. Eliaz RE, Nir S, Szoka FC, Jr. (2004) Interactions of hyaluronan-targeted liposomes with cultured cells: modeling of binding and endocytosis. *Methods Enzymol* 387: 16–33.

151. Passirani C, Barratt G, Devissaguet JP, Labarre D (1998) Long-circulating nanoparticles bearing heparin or dextran covalently bound to poly(methyl methacrylate). *Pharm Res* 15: 1046–1050.

152. Passirani C, Barratt G, Devissaguet JP, Labarre D (1998) Interactions of nanoparticles bearing heparin or dextran covalently bound to poly(methyl methacrylate) with the complement system. *Life Sci* 62: 775–785.

153. Chauvierre C, Manchanda R, Labarre D, Vauthier C, Marden MC, et al. (2010) Artificial oxygen carrier based on polysaccharides-poly(alkylcyanoacrylates) nanoparticle templates. *Biomaterials* 31: 6069–6074.

154. Chauvierre C, Leclerc L, Labarre D, Appel M, Marden MC, et al. (2007) Enhancing the tolerance of poly(isobutylcyanoacrylate) nanoparticles with a modular surface design. *Int J Pharm* 338: 327–332.

Chapter 6

RNAi as New Class of Nanomedicines

Monika Dominska and Derek M. Dykxhoorn
John T. Macdonald Foundation Department of Human Genetics and the Department of Microbiology and Immunology, University of Miami Miller School of Medicine, 1501 NW 10th Ave, Miami, FL 33136, USA
DDykxhoorn@med.miami.edu

RNA interference (RNAi)-based gene-silencing technologies provide a novel approach for the treatment of a variety of diseases through the sequence-specific silencing of gene expression. The application of small interfering RNA (siRNA) as potential therapeutic agents requires the development of clinically feasible delivery strategies that enhance their pharmacological properties. To be effective, siRNAs must be delivered to and taken up by specific target cells and tissues, enter the cytoplasm, and associate with the RNA-induced silencing complex (RISC) to guide the sequence-specific cleavage of appropriate messenger RNA (mRNA). This chapter will focus on recent progress made in the development of safe and effective therapeutic strategies for the siRNA-based silencing of gene expression.

6.1 Introduction

RNA interference (RNAi) is a highly conserved regulatory mechanism of post-transcriptional gene silencing that uses small double-

Handbook of Harnessing Biomaterials in Nanomedicine: Preparation, Toxicity, and Applications
Edited by Dan Peer

ISBN 978-981-4316-46-0 (Hardback), 978-981-4364-27-0 (eBook)
www.panstanford.com

stranded RNA (dsRNA) molecules to control gene expression [3, 12, 45, 95, 161]. The two major classes of small regulatory RNAs are small interfering RNAs (siRNAs) and microRNAs (miRNAs) [52]. miRNAs are expressed as long, hairpin structured primary transcripts, primary miRNAs (pri-miRNAs), that are processed in the nucleus through the concerted actions of the RNase III family member Drosha and its dsRNA binding partner Pasha [94, 99, 100, 107, 158]. This processing results in the production of an ~70-nt stem loop precursor miRNA (pre-miRNA), which is exported to the cytoplasm and cleaved by the enzyme Dicer to generate the mature ~22-nt miRNA [86, 87] (Figure 6.1).

One strand of the miRNA (guide strand) is incorporated into the RNA-induced silencing complex (RISC), where it guides the silencing complex to target mRNAs containing imperfectly complementary binding sites (usually present in the 3′ untranslated regions (UTR)), to inhibit translation and/or promote mRNA degradation [9, 51, 52, 56].

Originally, siRNAs were thought to be derived from either exogenously added dsRNAs, such as intermediate products of viral replication, or experimentally introduced long dsRNAs [38, 40, 41, 142, 161]. However, recent studies have identified siRNAs derived from endogenously expressed hairpin RNAs or bidirectional transcription, termed endo-siRNAs [24, 50, 81, 114–116]. Processing of these long dsRNAs by the RNase III family member Dicer results in the production of ~21-nt duplexed siRNAs bearing 2-nt 3′ overhangs and 5′ terminal phosphate groups [60, 82, 114, 116]. One of the two strands of the duplexed siRNA is loaded onto Argonaute 2 (Ago2), the key catalytic component of the RISC. The thermodynamic stability of the 5′ termini determines the degree to which each strand of the siRNA participates in RNAi [83, 130]. The strand with a lower stability at the 5′ end is preferentially taken up into the RISC, and this strand provides the specificity determinant to guide RISC to the appropriate target mRNA. Attachment of the siRNA guide strand to the complementary binding site on the target mRNA positions the mRNA into the RNase H domain of Ago2, which results in the cleavage of the mRNA and the suppression of gene expression [38, 39, 103]. The discovery by Tuschl and colleagues that the introduction of chemically synthesized siRNAs into mammalian cells suppressed gene expression in a sequence-specific manner raised the prospect of harnessing this potent and specific gene-silencing mechanism for biomedical research and therapy [20, 30, 31, 38, 106, 141].

Pioneering preclinical studies have shown that potent silencing responses could be produced in mammalian cells through the introduction of specific siRNAs, which have been designed to target genes involved in a variety of pathogenic processes, including viral infections, tumor and metastases formation, and neurodegeneration [35, 48, 49, 121, 143, 147, 146]. Two basic strategies are employed to trigger the RNAi pathway for targeted gene knockdown: (1) delivery of synthetic siRNAs to the cytoplasm of cells and (2) expression from DNA-based vectors of short hairpin RNAs (shRNAs) that are recognized and processed by Dicer into active siRNAs [32, 33]. shRNAs are highly effective and frequently used experimentally for gene function analysis where permanent knockdown of a gene is desirable. However, stable over-expression of shRNAs *in vivo* has, in some cases, been associated with cytotoxic effects resulting from outcompeting endogenous molecules for limiting amounts of RNAi pathway components [6, 55]. In addition, toxicities associated with the integration of retroviral-based vectors, a commonly used approach for the stable delivery of shRNAs to many cell types, into the host cell genome have raised concerns about the safety of these delivery systems [113]. Once integrated, these vectors are maintained for the life span of the target cells and, presumably, retain siRNA expression even after their therapeutic utility has been exhausted. In contrast, the delivery of chemically synthesized siRNAs can efficiently silence gene expression without altering the host genetic material. The transient nature of the silencing response mediated by synthetic siRNAs means that repeated doses of the siRNA may be needed to maintain robust silencing [98, 135]. As a result of this transient silencing phenotype, the use of synthetic siRNAs allows for the gene-silencing treatment to be tailored to the specific clinical needs, thereby, providing a greater range of therapeutic options. This can be helpful if the target sequence needs to be altered (for example, siRNAs targeting sequences that are subject to mutation and selection like that seen during the replication of HIV), as well as if changing the dosage or discontinuing the treatment is desired due to untoward side effects or the achievement of a clinical end point. This chapter will focus on the delivery of synthetic siRNAs as mediators of the therapeutic gene silencing.

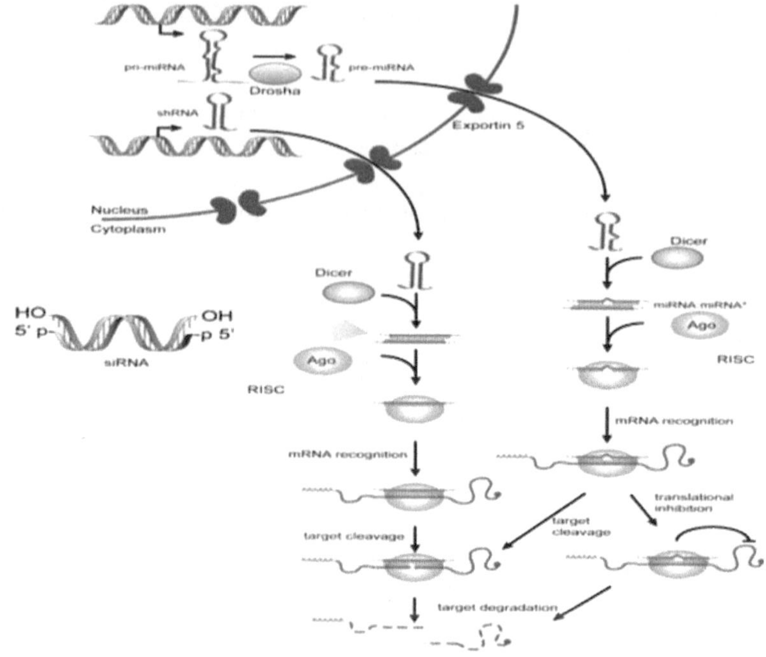

Figure. 6.1 RNAi-mediated gene silencing. RNA interference (RNAi) is a highly conserved regulatory mechanism of post-transcriptional gene silencing that uses small double-stranded RNA (dsRNA) molecules, principally siRNAs and miRNAs, to control gene expression. Micro RNAs (miRNAs) are encoded from highly structured, RNA polymerase II-derived transcripts, which are processed through the sequential cleavages by the RNase III-family members, Drosha and Dicer. In the nucleus, Drosha recognizes and cleaves specific structural elements of the miRNA-containing hairpin releasing an ~70-nt stem loop, the precursor (pre)-miRNA. The pre-miRNA is translocated to the cytoplasm by Exportin 5 where upon it is cleaved into the transiently double stranded miRNA:miRNA* duplex. The mature miRNA strand associates with Argonaute (Ago), the key component of the RNA-induced silencing complex (RISC), to direct the translational inhibition and/or degradation of the target mRNAs to which they bear partial complementarity. SiRNAs can be either directly transfected into the target cells or can be derived from short hairpin RNAs expressed from DNA-based vectors and cleaved by Dicer into the active siRNA. The guide strand of the siRNA is taken up by Ago2 into RISC. The siRNA guides RISC to the complementary site on the target mRNA, which engages the endonucleolytic activity of Ago2, resulting in mRNA cleavage.

One of the biggest challenges facing the *in vivo* application of RNAi-based silencing technologies is the delivery of siRNAs to the cytoplasm of appropriate target cell type(s). Broadly speaking, delivery approaches can be divided into two routes of administration: localized and systemic delivery. The route of administration can affect several parameters associated with effective silencing, including the delivery vehicle used, the dose of the siRNA needed to achieve effective silencing, the tissue distribution, and the potential for off-target effects in bystander tissues. To date, localized delivery of siRNAs to readily accessible tissues and organs has moved the most rapidly into the clinic. Preclinical studies in experimental animals using localized delivery to the eye, lung, muscle, subcutaneous tissues (e.g., tumors), vagina, and skin have shown effective *in vivo* silencing and protection in disease models [8, 14, 42, 59, 66, 118, 137, 140, 156]. Several RNAi methods have already entered clinical trials, including the treatment of respiratory syncytial virus (RSV) infection by intranasal or intratracheal installation of siRNAs, the treatment of Age-related macular degeneration (AMD) and diabetic macular edema through intraocular injection, and the treatment of pachyonychia congenita via transdermal siRNA application [4, 14, 27, 96, 97, 145]. Although localized delivery of siRNAs works for a handful of disorders, the majority of diseases require systemic delivery approaches.

Systemic siRNA delivery for therapeutic applications offers both the greatest opportunities and the greatest challenges. The physicochemical properties of siRNAs, including their net negative charge, relatively small size, and susceptibility to nucleases, present several challenges to their efficient delivery into the cytoplasm of target cells. To be effective, the systemic delivery methods need to protect siRNAs from degradation by serum nucleases as well as clearance from the circulatory system by renal filtration while facilitate effective biodistribution and accumulation at the appropriate tissues, and promote efficient siRNA uptake and intracellular trafficking into the cytoplasm of the target cells [30].

To stabilize siRNA in serum, chemical modifications of the 2′-OH of the ribose, the phosphate linkage, or the base have been employed [10]. As some of these modifications inhibit knockdown efficacy, a balance must be maintained between the incorporation of chemical modifications and the functional activity of the siRNAs [153].

Since siRNAs fall below the size threshold for renal filtration and are rapidly cleared from the circulatory system, a variety of approaches have been developed to promote their systemic delivery *in vivo*. Direct conjugation of one or both of the siRNA strands with lipid or cholesterol molecules improves both circulation time and cellular uptake of these bioconjugates, and consequently gene silencing [104, 138]. The improved cellular uptake of siRNAs is a result of cell membrane permeability to these hydrophobic bioconjugates. Cell penetrating peptides (CPPs) have also been conjugated to siRNAs to enhance their cellular delivery. Short extensions with positively charged amino acids of CPPS help their translocation across the cell membrane and delivery of siRNAs directly to the cytoplasm. This highly efficient cellular uptake of CPP-siRNA conjugates takes place in a receptor-independent fashion [111].

Mixing the siRNAs with various delivery agents can increase their circulation time either by exceeding the upper limit of the particle size for renal clearance or by promoting their association with serum proteins (e.g., serum albumin). A number of delivery carriers have been developed for improved *in vivo* delivery of siRNA, which are based on cationic nanoparticles [110], lipids, and liposomes [2, 155]. Negatively charged siRNA molecules spontaneously interact electrostatically with cationic liposomes or cationic polymers. The positively charged core of the delivery nanoparticle also allows enhanced interactions with cellular membrane leading to internalization via adsorptive pinocytosis [160].

Most of the approaches developed to date can be divided into two major categories: non-specific accumulation and targeted delivery. Non-specific delivery utilizes the bias of macromolecules to accumulate in cancerous or inflamed tissues due to the increased permeability of the blood vessels, and retention associated with dysfunctional lymphatic drainage, an effect commonly known as enhanced permeability and retention (EPR) [72, 105]. This EPR effect has been employed to successfully deliver siRNAs against KLF5 (a transcription factor that is known to play a role in tumor angiogenesis) to solid tumors. siRNAs mixed with neutral lipids and coated with polyethylene glycol (PEG) for increased retention time, resulted in the knockdown of KLF5 and subsequent suppression of both angiogenesis within tumors and tumor growth [157]. However, if the cells do not efficiently internalize the siRNAs, accumulation of delivery nanoparticles within the tumor microenvironment by the EPR effect may not correlate well with the therapeutic outcome.

One of the first approaches used to systemically deliver siRNAs involved rapid injection of siRNAs in a large volume of physiological buffer, termed hydrodynamic injection [11, 101, 108, 136, 163]. The rapid injection of large fluid volumes leads to right-sided heart failure resulting in an elevated venous pressure and the transient disruption of the plasma membrane of cells in highly vascular tissues, including lung, liver, spleen, and pancreas. This transient disruption of the plasma membrane facilitates the uptake of the siRNAs and the concomitant targeted silencing of gene expression. The ease of delivery to the liver and the susceptibility of the liver to variety of agents that induce acute or chronic liver injury (for example, viral infections, autoimmune hepatitis, toxins, and liver transplantation) has made the liver an attractive target for siRNA-mediated therapeutic gene silencing [15, 127, 136, 162]. The targeted silencing of Fas by hydrodynamic delivery of siRNAs protected mice from fulminant hepatitis induced by the intraperitoneal injection of a fas agonist antibody [136]. Although effective, this approach requires a high dose of siRNAs to achieve effective silencing with only a relatively small fraction of the siRNAs actually entering the target tissue. In addition, systemic hydrodynamic injection is too risky for human therapeutic applications.

6.2 Cell-Type Specific Delivery

Effective systemic delivery requires agents that facilitate the transport of siRNAs to specific cell type(s) (Figure 6.3). Cell type-specific delivery approaches reduce potential toxicities to neighboring bystander cells, promote the accumulation of the siRNA at the target tissue, and lower the therapeutic dose necessary to achieve effective silencing in the cells of interest. Typically, these approaches take advantage of molecules that recognize specific surface antigens expressed on distinct cells or tissues. These antigens can define a very narrow or broad spectrum of cell types depending on the breadth of their distribution. Several different types of molecules, including antibodies, ligands, and aptamers, have been successfully used for cell type-specific siRNA delivery [30, 31].

6.2.1 Antibody-Mediated siRNA Delivery

Antibodies are proteins expressed by B cells that recognize and bind specific antigens with high affinity and selectivity. Under normal circumstances, the immune system produces antibodies to defend against foreign pathogens, but antibodies can also be produced against non-pathogen-associated molecules when a specific protein or peptide is introduced into a foreign species. The use of antibodies for therapeutic purposes is limited by their large and complex molecular structure, the cost of production and purification, and the potential for binding to complement or Fc receptors inducing cell lysis, opsonization and degranulation of mast cells, eosinophils and basophils [1, 149, 154]. To circumvent some of these limitations, antibody fragments have been used that retain the antigen recognition domain, but have lost the heavy chain Fc domain. This reduces the overall size of the molecule and reduces many of the negative side effects of antibody treatments. To facilitate siRNA delivery, the antigen recognition domain of an antibody can be fused to a cationic polymer to which siRNAs bind. Using a fragment antibody (FAb) that specifically recognizes the HIV-1 envelope glycoprotein (gp160) fused to protamine, Song and colleagues were able to deliver anti-HIV siRNAs exclusively to hard-to-transfect, HIV-1 infected CD4+ T lymphocytes resulting in the suppression of the viral infection [137]. In addition, the growth of subcutaneously implanted tumors that transgenically expressed the HIV-1 envelope, but not of envelope negative control tumors, was inhibited following the intratumoral or intravenous injection of a cocktail of siRNAs (c-MYC, VEGF, and MDM2 siRNAs), bound to the antibody-protamine fusion protein. In a similar manner, a single-chain antibody specific for the pan T cell marker CD7 fused to a polyarginine tract (scFvCD7-9R) was able to deliver anti-HIV siRNAs to T lymphocytes in a humanized mouse model of HIV-1 [91]. This treatment resulted in the suppression of viral replication and prevention of the disease-associated loss of CD4+ T cells. Since antibodies can be generated to very specific epitopes, it is possible to target distinct isoforms or conformations of a protein. Peer and colleagues demonstrated this exquisite specificity using an antibody that recognized a conformationally distinct, activated form of the lymphocyte function-associated antigen-1 (LFA-1) [123]. This reagent facilitated siRNA delivery to cells that bore the activated, but not the latent form of the receptor. Although these studies demonstrated the feasibility of using antibodies to direct siRNAs to specific cell populations, the cationic proteins or peptides have a limited siRNA binding capacity (approximately 6 siRNAs/fusion molecule).

To improve the efficiency of antibody mediated siRNA delivery, antibodies can be attached to the surface of liposome-based nanoparticles. The encapsulation of cyclin D1 siRNAs in lipid nanoparticles coated on their outer surface with an anti-β_7 integrin antibody effectively silenced cyclin D1 expression in gut mononuclear leukocytes following intravenous injection [122]. The knockdown of cyclin D1 in these cells reversed the lymphocyte proliferation and inflammatory cytokine expression patterns associated with dextran sodium sulfate (DSS)-induced colitis in mice. A single-chain antibody (scAb) to the transferrin receptor, whose expression is elevated in a wide variety of tumor types, including breast and pancreatic tumors, facilitated the delivery of Her2 siRNAs to subcutaneously implanted tumor cells [17]. The siRNA-mediated silencing of Her2 sensitized the tumor cells to treatment with chemotherapeutic agents leading to a reduction in tumor size. Zheng et al. also achieved effective siRNA-mediated silencing of CD40 in dendritic cells treated with immunoliposomes coated with anti-DEC-205 antibodies *in vitro* and *in vivo* [164].

6.2.2 Ligand-Mediated siRNA Delivery

As an alternative to antibodies, cell type-specific delivery could be achieved by taking advantage of the specificity of ligands, including peptides, hormones, chemokines, sugars, and lipids, which recognize and bind specific cell surface molecules. The conjugation of a cholesterol molecule to the 3′ terminus of the passenger strand of a siRNA targeting ApoB led to uptake of the siRNA by cells of the liver and jujenum bearing lipoprotein receptors [138]. This treatment resulted in decreased ApoB mRNA and protein levels and a concomitant decrease in serum cholesterol in ApoB siRNA treated mice compared with control siRNA treatment. In a similar manner, cholesterol-conjugated siRNAs were used to deliver an siRNA targeting a mutant version of the huntingtin gene to neuronal cells. The intrastriatal injection of the cholesterol-conjugated siRNA was able to attenuate the abnormal behavior associated with a rapid onset model of Huntington's disease in mice [29]. The conjugation of α-Tocopherol (Vitamin E) to the 5′ terminus of the guide strand of a Dicer substrate siRNA (an elongated double-stranded RNA molecule (~27-mer) that is processed by Dicer into an active siRNA) facilitated the delivery of an ApoB siRNA into mice hepatocytes [112]. The transferrin receptor, which is overexpressed on the surface of many tumor types, has been the target for a variety of delivery strategies including antibody-mediated (see above) and ligand mediated delivery. In one iteration, systemic administration of nanoparticles composed of cyclodextrin coated with transferrin (Tf) and containing siRNAs targeting the EWS-FLI1 fusion gene, effectively inhibited tumor growth in a mouse model of Ewing's sarcoma [69]. Similarly, lipoplexes coated with Tf facilitated siRNA delivery to primary cortical neuron *in vitro* and *in vivo* after injection into the striatum of mice [17, 18]. Clinical studies have begun to test the safety and efficacy of targeted nanoparticles for the treatment of therapy-refractory solid tumors. Davis and colleagues used nanoparticles composed of a linear, cyclodextrin-based polymer and a hydrophilic polymer, PEG, and coated with Tf to deliver siRNAs to transferrin receptor bearing tumors [26]. This formulation had been shown previously to be well tolerated in non-human primates [63]. Transmission electron microscopy analysis of tumor biopsies showed accumulation of the nanoparticles in the tumor tissue. In addition, quantitative real-time PCR and western blot analysis demonstrated a significant reduction in the M2 subunit of ribonucleotide reductase (RRM2) (the target of the siRNA) mRNA and protein, respectively, in treated tumors compared with the pretreatment biopsy samples. Delivered siRNAs have been shown to engage the RNAi machinery since the siRNA cleavage site on the RRM2 mRNA could be identified using 5′ RLM-RACE analysis in the treated tumor samples [26]. Other ligands that have been used for siRNA delivery, include *N*-acetyl galactosamine and galactose, which bind asialoglycoprotein receptors, and apolipoprotein A-1, which binds the scavenger receptor class B type 1 [84, 128].

Most viruses take advantage of endogenous cell surface molecules to infect target cells. The rabies virus glycoprotein (RVG) binds to the nicotine acetylcholine receptor present on the surface of neuronal cells. The fusion of a peptide derived from the RVG to a polyarginine tract (nona-arginine peptide, 9dR) capable of non-covalently binding siRNAs specifically targeted neuronal cells for siRNA uptake [92]. Treatment with an siRNA targeting Japanese encephalitis virus (JEV) bound to the RVG-polyarginine fusion molecule protected mice from a subsequent lethal challenge with infectious JEV. Recently, the RVG-polyarginine fusion molecule was used to deliver siRNAs targeting tumor necrosis factor α (TNFα) to macrophage/microglial cells expressing the nicotine acetylcholine receptor [85]. The systemic administration of the TNFα siRNA complexed with the RVG-9dR fusion molecule inhibited neuroinflammation in lipopolysaccharide (LPS)-treated mice. In a similar manner, a 12-amino acid peptide (DC3) identified from a phage display peptide library that specifically binds to a cell surface antigen on dendritic cells was fused to the nona-D-arginine peptide (DC3-9dR) [139]. This fusion molecule was used to deliver siRNAs targeting the Dengue virus envelope to monocyte-derived dendritic cells, CD34+ hematopoietic stem cell-derived Langerhan DCs, and peripheral blood DCs resulting in the efficient inhibition of Dengue virus replication. The delivery of siRNAs targeting TNFα to DCs inhibited Dengue virus-induced TNFα in cultured cells and poly(I:C)-induced TNFα expression in humanized mice.

6.2.3 Aptamer-Mediated siRNA Delivery

Aptamers are structured nucleic acid molecules (RNA or DNA aptamers) *in vitro* selected through multiple rounds to bind with high affinity to specific target molecules in a process termed the systematic evolution of ligands by exponential enrichment or SELEX. RNA aptamers can be produced by *in vitro* transcription and readily purified in high yield. This ease of production gives aptamers an advantage over ligands and antibodies, which need to be purified from cultured mammalian cells, insect cells, yeast or bacteria and require extensive purification before they are amenable for therapeutic applications. An aptamer, which efficiently binds to the prostate-specific membrane antigen (PSMA), effectively delivered anti-tumor siRNAs (for example, siRNAs targeting PLK1 or BCL2) to PSMA-expressing tumor cells resulting in a regression in tumor size in a mouse prostate cancer model [109]. Modification of the siRNA structure and the appending of a PEG moiety helped to increase the silencing activity and improve the bioavailability of these molecules [25]. In a variation of these experiments, a streptavidin-biotin bridge was employed to connect the PSMA aptamer to siRNAs [22]. Aptamers targeting the HIV-1 envelope glycoprotein (gp120) have been shown to specifically deliver siRNAs to HIV-1 infected cells and suppress HIV-1 replication [19, 165, 166]. This inhibition of HIV-1 occurred through the synergistic action of the aptamer, which itself had anti-viral properties and the attached anti-HIV siRNA.

6.3 Intracellular Trafficking of siRNAs

Whether cationic lipids, nanoparticles or cell-type-specific delivery reagents deliver them, the intracellular trafficking of siRNAs begins in early endosomal vesicles [30]. The contents of the early endosomes are transferred to sorting endosomes and subsequently to the late endosomes that are acidified (pH 5–6) by membrane-bound proton-pump ATPases. The contents of the late endosomes are transported to the lysosomes, which are further acidified (pH ~4.5) and which contain various nucleases that promote degradation of the siRNAs. To avoid lysosomal degradation, siRNAs (free or complexed with the delivery vehicle) must escape from the endosome into the cytosol, where they can associate with the RNAi machinery. This endosomal escape is one of the major barriers for efficient siRNA delivery. In the following sections, we focus on strategies that have been developed to promote endosomal release of siRNA, including the use of fusogenic lipids, polymers with high buffering capacity and membrane-interacting peptides.

6.4 Strategies for Endosomal Escape

6.4.1 Cationic Lipids

There is a class of cationic lipids (e.g., phosphatidylethanolamines, PE) that assembles in the inversed hexagonal phase — wherein the lipid molecules adopt micelle-like structures to form non-bilayer assemblies under physiological conditions [90, 102]. Complexes composed of these cationic lipids and nucleic acids (lipoplexes) have been shown to attach themselves to anionic membranes such as endosomal membranes and rapidly fuse with them, resulting in the release of their contents into the cell interior [90]. The incorporation of cationic lipids, such as dioleoylphosphatidylethanolamine (DOPE), into other lipoplexes improves the release of endosomal content by increasing the net positive charge on the lipoplex surface and consequently amplifying the rate of electrostatic interactions between the lipoplexes and endosomal membranes [44, 65, 102]. The efficacy of siRNA delivery by a commercially available lipid-based transfection reagent JetSI™ was also enhanced after mixing it with fusogenic lipids [61].

6.4.2 pH-Sensitive Lipoplexes

A variety of modifications to lipid-based delivery carriers have been designed to protect positively charged fusogenic lipoplexes from interactions with serum proteins and macrophages while maintaining the fusogenic character necessary for efficient endosomal escape and intracellular trafficking of the siRNAs. One of the approaches used to protect these carriers and their cargo is a modification of the outer surface of the lipoplex with hydrophilic, pH-sensitive polymers [57, 58, 131]. These polymer-liposome conjugates are stable in the circulatory system. However, upon endocytosis and lowering the pH inside the endosomal vesicle, the polymer molecules are rapidly hydrolyzed exposing the underlying lipoplexes and promoting their fusion with endosomal membranes and the release of their contents into the cytosol. Coating the liposomal surface with PEG-polycation block copolymers has been shown to be much more efficient at targeted silencing when compared with a commercially available transfection reagent (Oligofectamine™) [7].

In a similar manner, Carmona et al. developed liposomes composed of DOPE lipid and an aminoxy cholesteryl lipid, which enables covalent attachment of biocompatible polymers, such as PEG [19]. This bioconjugation produces oxime bonds, which are stable at neutral pH, but readily hydrolyze at pH 5.5 and lower. This pH sensitivity of the siRNA carrier allows the PEG desorption that leads to nanoparticle destabilization and, consequently, escape from the early endosome.

6.4.3 pH-Sensitive Polyplexes

A number of pH-sensitive, endosomal buffering polymers have been developed to improve gene knockdowns through more effective siRNA delivery. The high efficiency of nucleic acid delivery by protonable cationic polymers has been primarily attributed to their high buffering capacity that is thought to act as a 'proton sponge' and mediate endosomal release. In this approach, proton absorbance by buffering polymers prevents acidification of endosomal vesicles, thereby increasing the ATPase-mediated influx of protons as well as counterions (which enter the vesicles to balance the proton flux). Increased concentration of the counterions inside the endosome leads to osmotic swelling, followed by endosomal membrane rupture, and eventually to the leakage of the polyplex and its contents into the cytosol [134]. Polyethyleneimine (PEI) is one of the most widely investigated cationic polymers for nucleic acid delivery [124, 125, 144]. Positively charged amine groups of PEI both facilitate their interaction with negatively charged nucleic acid molecules and enable endosomal release through their action as proton sponges. However, treatment with PEI has toxic side effects that directly correlate to the size of the polymer and this has impeded its application for therapeutic drug delivery.

Polyethyleneimine and polyamidoamine dendrimers (symmetrically and repeatedly branched polymers) have also been utilized for siRNA delivery owing to their excellent proton-absorbing properties [119, 120]. This excellent buffering capacity of dendrimers is attributed to the high density of readily protonable tertiary amine groups. However, maintaining the neutral character of the outer surface of these cationic dendrimers is important for controlling morphology of the polyplexes and protection of the concentrated siRNA molecules inside. In addition, the presence of dense modifiable peripheral groups facilitates attachment of target recognition elements for cell specific delivery [120].

More sophisticated polymeric siRNA carriers with tunable pH sensitivities have been developed by Wang and colleagues [150]. They have developed a multifunctional polymeric siRNA carriers composed of a proton-sponge domain, a hydrophobic domain, and a domain of polymerizable cysteine residues. The presence of various protonable amino groups with differing pK_a values increases the buffering capacity of the complex. The hydrophobic portion of the particle improves the overall stability of the carrier allowing the formation of a compact structure enclosing the siRNA molecules. The presence of disulfide bonds formed between the cysteine residues stabilizes the nanoparticles even further. After endosomal release, disulfide bonds are reduced by cytosolic glutathione resulting in dissociation of the nanoparticles and release of siRNA into the cytoplasm. In addition, the presence of disulfides on the nanoparticle surface permits chemical modifications for targeted delivery [151, 152].

6.4.4 Fusogenic Proteins

As an alternative strategy to improve endosomal escape of siRNAs, lipid- or polymer-based nanoparticles can be supplemented with fusogenic or cell penetrating peptides (CPPs) — short peptides that are capable of penetrating biological membranes and entering the cell [43]. Because cargo molecules covalently attached to CPPs can translocate into the cell in concert with CPPs, these peptides have been utilized in manufacturing nanoparticles of improved efficiency of cytoplasmic delivery of nucleic acids [62, 88, 89]. A rough sketch of this kind of nanoparticle depicts a nucleic acid cargo enclosed inside the liposome, which is further wrapped in a mixture of "masking" polymers, cell-specific ligands, and CPPs. A polymeric coat helps to maintain nanoparticle stability in serum, while cell-recognition elements direct the nanoparticle to target cells or tissues, and CPPs allow ultimate penetration of endosomal membranes and delivery of the cargo directly to the cell cytoplasm. Even commercially available transfection reagents such as Lipofectamine™ supplemented with influenza-derived fusogenic peptides have shown enhanced silencing properties due to more efficient endosomal release of siRNA [117].

Finally, membrane-destabilization mechanism of viroporins has also been utilized for gene delivery purposes [93]. The main action of these highly hydrophobic proteins is to create channels in cell membranes, which facilitate ion flow across them and eventually to osmolytic membrane rupture [53]. The membrane disruption mechanism of viroporins, unlike fusogenic polymers, is pH-insensitive and is therefore not limited to delivery through endosomes.

6.4.5 Dynamic Polyconjugates

In vivo delivery systems are becoming increasingly sophisticated incorporating multiple components to optimize each stage of the delivery process from the initial administration, transportation through the circulatory system to the appropriate tissue, recognition of the target cells and deposition of the siRNAs into the cytoplasm where they can associate with the RISC. To that end, Rozema and colleagues developed a multifunctional polymer-based 'device' designed to maximize each step in the delivery process — from target cell recognition (by using the targeting ligand *N*-acetylgalactosamine) to endosomal escape (by using the amphipatic poly(vinyl ether), PBAVE, which acts as an endosomolytic agent) and silencing (by using appropriate siRNAs) (Figure 6.2) [127]. They referred to this system as a dynamic polyconjugate because each component is revealed in a systematic manner. *N*-acetylgalactosamine is present for delivery of the siRNA to hepatocytes, but it is released from the polymer in the acidic environment of the endosome. At the same time, the endosomolytic agent (PBAVE) is revealed through the dissociation of a PEG shielding group, facilitating the translocation of the siRNA from the endosomal compartment to the cytoplasm. The siRNA molecules are attached to PBAVE through a disulfide linkage that is cleaved in the reducing environment of the cytosol, releasing the siRNA, which is free to interact with RISC and direct target mRNA cleavage. These multifunctional delivery reagents will become more important as RNAi-based gene-silencing technologies make their way into the clinic.

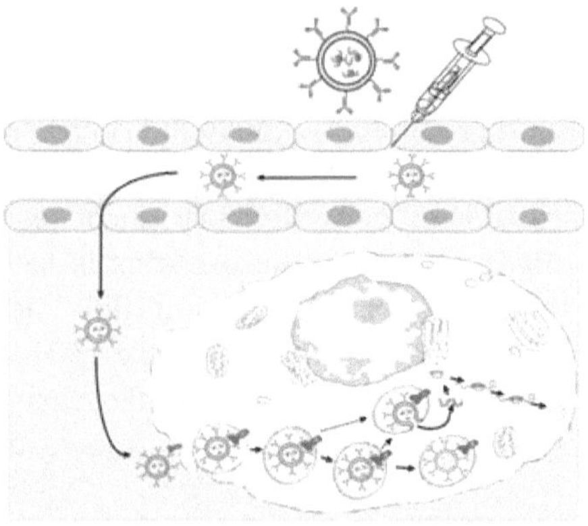

Figure 6.2 Barriers to siRNA delivery *in vivo*. To be effective, systemic delivery approaches need to protect siRNAs from degradation by serum nucleases, avoid clearance from the circulatory system by renal filtration, transport across the vascular endothelial barrier, facilitate effective biodistribution and accumulation at the appropriate tissue, and promote efficient siRNA uptake and endosomal escape into the cytoplasm of the target cells where they can associated with RISC and guide the cleavage of target mRNA.

6.5 Off-Target Effects of siRNAs

Early RNAi-based gene-silencing experiments suggested that the treatment of mammalian cells with synthetic siRNAs led to the highly specific silencing of target gene expression without the induction of non-specific interferon (IFN) responses [5, 16, 41, 67, 71]. In fact, siRNAs could be identified that discriminated between transcripts that varied by a single nucleotide polymorphism (SNP) attesting to their high degree of specificity [5, 34, 41, 67, 129]. However, it has become apparent that, under some conditions, the treatment with siRNAs can have toxic effects. These toxicities can result from several potential sources, including off-target silencing of genes that bear partial complementarity to the siRNA, the engagement of innate immune responses, and competition with endogenous RNAi effector molecules, such as, miRNAs, for limited RNAi pathway components [55, 73, 76, 126]. Recent microarray-based experiments have shown that siRNA treatments can alter the expression levels of a large number of transcripts. Informatic analysis has shown that these alterations in transcript levels are sequence-dependent and largely the result of the pairing of the 'seed region' (corresponding to nucleotides 2 to 8) of the siRNA to sites on off target mRNAs, particularly in the 3' UTR, and therefore operating in much the same manner as miRNAs [13, 75]. These "miRNA-like" off-target effects could be generated from either strand of the siRNA duplex. The impact that these off-target effects have on cellular functionality needs to be determined experimentally and could potentially confound the interpretation of experimental results. Since these effects are sequence-specific, testing of multiple siRNAs against a given target mRNA can help to delineate specific targeting from off-target effects. Alteration of the thermodynamic properties of the siRNA ends to favor incorporation of the guide strand could help to reduce off-target effects by reducing the probability of incorporation of the passenger strand into the RISC. Testing of multiple siRNAs targeting the gene of interest, each with a unique seed sequence, is one approach that can be used to ensure that the observed phenotype results from the knockdown of the intended target and is not a result of the off-target silencing [23]. In addition, rescue experiments can be performed by over-expressing an siRNA-resistant, functional version of the target gene to rescue the observed phenotype [36, 37].

Innate immune responses function as a mechanism to recognize and eliminate pathogens, while aiding in the establishment of adaptive immunity. This recognition requires a diverse family of pattern recognition receptors to detect a variety of bacterial and viral-associated molecules, such as, lipopolysaccharides, bacterial DNA, and viral RNAs [77, 78]. Originally, siRNAs were believed to be unable to engage the RNA-dependent protein kinase (PKR) pathway due to their small size (<30bp) [38]. However, more recent studies have shown that, in some cases, synthetic siRNAs could stimulate aspects of the innate immune response through the engagement of Toll-like receptors (TLRs), in particular, TLR7 and TLR8 [68, 79, 132]. It has been suggested that the sequence-independent engagement of TLR3 on dendritic cells and endothelial cells could be a source of additional toxicity [80, 133]. However, TLR3 signaling does not appear to be a major determinant of innate immune activation by siRNAs. On the other hand, the sequence-specific engagement of TLR7 and TLR8 seems to be the primary mechanism for the induction of innate immune activation by synthetic siRNAs [28, 46, 64]. Both TLR7 and TLR8 are expressed in the endosomes and their signaling requires endosomal acidification. Although similar in function and intracellular localization, they are expressed in different subsets of cells, with TLR7 predominating in plasmacytoid dendritic cells and B cells, while TLR8 expression is restricted to dendritic cells, monocytes and macrophages. Although the immunostimulatory effects of siRNAs have not been fully characterized, it appears that these receptors recognize GU-rich RNA sequences [28, 64, 68, 79]. Selecting siRNAs that avoid these GU-rich motifs can help to reduce the immunostimulatory nature of certain siRNAs [79]. However, GU-rich sequences alone can't account for the full range of siRNA immunogenicity. While GU-rich sequences have been shown to engage TLR7 and TLR8, AU-rich sequences were found to preferentially activate TLR8 [46]. Additional factors, including the position of immunostimulatory motifs within the siRNA, sequence context, and the length of the siRNA molecule, have been suggested to influence the immunostimulatory nature of siRNAs [54, 68].

The incorporation of chemical modifications into the siRNA has been used to improve several aspects of the pharmacokinetic properties of siRNAs including serum nuclease stability and reduction of off-target gene silencing [5]. Several different modifications have been incorporated into siRNAs including the substitution of phosphorothioate bonds for the phosphodiester bonds and 2′ sugar modifications (e.g., a fluorine substitution) [21, 47, 148]. However, the selective incorporation of 2′ O-methyl groups on the sugar backbone has been the most common substitution used for the protection of siRNAs from serum nucleases and the reduction of off-target effects, including the inhibition of the proinflammatory effects of some siRNAs and the targeting of partially complementary mRNAs. The incorporation of 2′ *O*-methyl modifications within the seed region of the guide strand of the siRNA reduced both the number and the magnitude of off-target silencing without adversely affecting the on-target silencing efficacy [74].

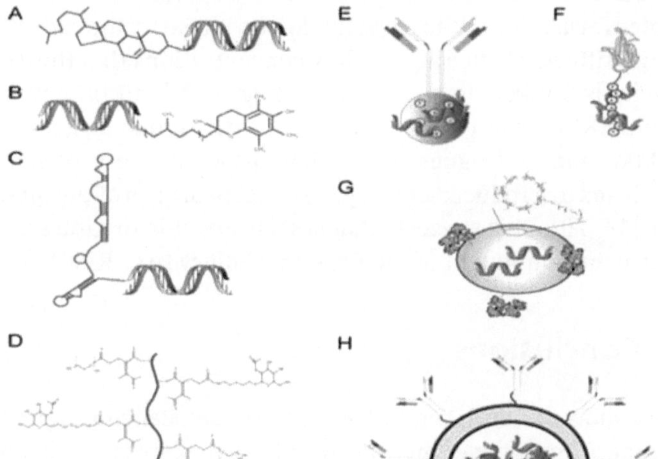

Figure 6.3 Strategies for cell type-specific siRNA delivery *in vivo*. A variety of approach have been used for the cell type-specific delivery of siRNAs, including the direct conjugation of targeting molecules, such as, ligands (cholesterol (A) and a-tocopherol (B)), aptamers (C), or polymers (Dynamic polyconjugates (D). In addition, the negatively charged siRNA will spontaneous bind to positively charged proteins or peptides fused to an antibody (E) or a ligand (eg., a portion of the rabies virus glycoprotein (RVG)). SiRNAs can be encapsulated into polymeric (eg. cyclodextrin (G) coated with the ligand transferring) or lipid nanoparticles (eg., immunoliposomes (H), lipid nanoparticles coated with an antibody).

An additional source of potential toxicity is the saturation of the RNAi machinery by excessive exogenously introduced silencing RNA molecules [6, 55]. This has been shown to be the case for highly expressed shRNAs. Similar to miRNA, shRNAs are expressed in the nucleus and exported to the cytoplasm where they are processed into active siRNAs. Cell culture experiments demonstrated that high-level expression of shRNAs inhibited the maturation of endogenous miRNAs but saturating the activity of Exportin 5 [159]. Similarly, the sustained over-expression of shRNAs in the liver of adult mice resulted in dose-dependent liver injury and death [55]. These toxic side effects were correlated with decreased expression of liver-derived miRNAs. The reduction of shRNA expression using weaker promoters was found to greatly lower these cytotoxic effects. Although siRNAs silence at such low concentrations that this source of toxicity is unlikely in most cells, it may set a limit on how many different siRNAs can be used simultaneously in one target cell. In fact, Bitko and colleagues found that the co-delivery of multiple siRNAs leads to a reduced efficacy of silencing of each of the intended targets [14, 70]. This suggests that siRNAs are able to saturate some downstream component of the RNAi machinery (e.g., RISC).

6.6 Conclusions

In a very short period of time, RNAi-based gene-silencing approaches have gone from a novel mechanism of gene expression regulation in *C. elegans* to a potential therapeutic approach for the treatment of a variety of intractable human diseases. This has necessitated the development of a variety of novel delivery strategies that seek to improve the pharmacokinetic properties of siRNAs. To be effective, these delivery approaches need to optimize each step in the delivery process from the initial administration of the siRNA to the uptake into RISC and the cleavage of the target mRNA. This will minimize the therapeutic dose required for effective silencing and, as a consequence, reduce some the potential off-target toxicities. These advances have included the incorporation of chemical modifications into the siRNA to improve their stability, the use of targeting agents to facilitate siRNA delivery to specific cell types and tissues, the development of novel lipid formulations to maximize intracellular trafficking and endosomal escape, and improvement in siRNA design to optimize RISC uptake and gene silencing. In spite of these advances, there are still a number of concerns that need to be addressed as these technologies begin to make their way into the clinic. Foremost among these concerns is the need for a more comprehensive understanding of the potential toxicities associated with siRNAs and the delivery vehicles. Improvements in design and the selective incorporation of chemical modifications have served to reduce these off-target effects, but further improvements are warranted to ensure the safety of these gene-silencing reagents. Due to the inherent differences between humans and rodents, the use of non-human primates in the drug development process may provide a better model for understanding potential toxicities. In addition, many of the current delivery approaches incorporate multiple components, which increase both the complexity of their manufacture and, as a result, the cost of their production. Although there are still many challenges that need to be overcome, there is hope that siRNA-based therapeutics will soon become a reality and provide novel tools to combat a variety of diseases, particularly for those diseases for which therapeutic options are limited or non-existent.

References

1. Adams, G.P., and L.M. Weiner (2005). Monoclonal antibody therapy of cancer, *Nat Biotechnol.* **23**: pp. 1147–1157.
2. Akinc, A., A. Zumbuehl, M. Goldberg, E.S. Leshchiner, V. Busini, N. Hossain, S.A. Bacallado, D.N. Nguyen, J. Fuller, R. Alvarez, A. Borodovsky, T. Borland, R. Constien, A. de Fougerolles, J.R. Dorkin, K. Narayanannair Jayaprakash, M. Jayaraman, M. John, V. Koteliansky, M. Manoharan, L. Nechev, J. Qin, T. Racie, D. Raitcheva, K.G. Rajeev, D.W. Sah, J. Soutschek, I. Toudjarska, H.P. Vornlocher, T.S. Zimmermann, R. Langer, and D.G. Anderson (2008). A combinatorial library of lipid-like materials for delivery of RNAi therapeutics, *Nat Biotechnol.* **26**: pp. 561–569.
3. Almeida, R., and R.C. Allshire (2005). RNA silencing and genome regulation, *Trends Cell Biol.* **15**: pp. 251–258.
4. Alvarez, R., S. Elbashir, T. Borland, I. Toudjarska, P. Hadwiger, M. John, I. Roehl, S.S. Morskaya, R. Martinello, J. Kahn, M. Van Ranst, R.A. Tripp, J.P. DeVincenzo, R. Pandey, M. Maier, L. Nechev, M. Manoharan, V. Kotelianski, and R. Meyers (2009). RNA interference-mediated silencing of the respiratory syncytial virus nucleocapsid defines a potent antiviral strategy, *Antimicrob Agents Chemother.* **53**: pp. 3952–3962.

5. Amarzguioui, M., T. Holen, E. Babaie, and H. Prydz (2003). Tolerance for mutations and chemical modifications in a siRNA, *Nucleic Acids Res.* **31**: pp. 589–595.
6. An, D.S., F.X. Qin, V.C. Auyeung, S.H. Mao, S.K. Kung, D. Baltimore, and I.S. Chen (2006). Optimization and functional effects of stable short hairpin RNA expression in primary human lymphocytes via lentiviral vectors, *Mol Ther.* **14**: pp. 494–504.
7. Auguste, D.T., K. Furman, A. Wong, J. Fuller, S.P. Armes, T.J. Deming, and R. Langer (2008). Triggered release of siRNA from poly(ethylene glycol)-protected, pH-dependent liposomes, *J Control Release.* **130**: pp. 266–274.
8. Azuma, M., P. Ritprajak, and M. Hashiguchi Topical application of siRNA targeting cutaneous dendritic cells in allergic skin disease, *Methods Mol Biol.* **623**: pp. 373–381.
9. Bartel, D.P. (2009). MicroRNAs: target recognition and regulatory functions, *Cell.* **136**: pp. 215–233.
10. Behlke, M.A. (2008). Chemical modification of siRNAs for *in vivo* use, *Oligonucleotides.* **18**: pp. 305–319.
11. Beider, K., A. Nagler, O. Wald, S. Franitza, M. Dagan-Berger, H. Wald, H. Giladi, S. Brocke, J. Hanna, O. Mandelboim, M. Darash-Yahana, E. Galun, and A. Peled (2003). Involvement of CXCR4 and IL-2 in the homing and retention of human NK and NK T cells to the bone marrow and spleen of NOD/SCID mice, *Blood.* **102**: pp. 1951–1958.
12. Bernstein, E., A.A. Caudy, S.M. Hammond, and G.J. Hannon (2001). Role for a bidentate ribonuclease in the initiation step of RNA interference, *Nature.* **409**: pp. 363–366.
13. Birmingham, A., E.M. Anderson, A. Reynolds, D. Ilsley-Tyree, D. Leake, Y. Fedorov, S. Baskerville, E. Maksimova, K. Robinson, J. Karpilow, W.S. Marshall, and A. Khvorova (2006). 3′ UTR seed matches, but not overall identity, are associated with RNAi off-targets, *Nat Methods.* **3**: pp. 199–204.
14. Bitko, V., A. Musiyenko, O. Shulyayeva, and S. Barik (2005). Inhibition of respiratory viruses by nasally administered siRNA, *Nat Med.* **11**: pp. 50–55.
15. Bradley, S.P., C. Rastellini, M.A. da Costa, T.F. Kowalik, A.B. Bloomenthal, M. Brown, L. Cicalese, G.P. Basadonna, and M.E. Uknis (2005). Gene silencing in the endocrine pancreas mediated by short-interfering RNA, *Pancreas.* **31**: pp. 373–379.
16. Caplen, N.J., S. Parrish, F. Imani, A. Fire, and R.A. Morgan (2001). Specific inhibition of gene expression by small double-stranded RNAs

in invertebrate and vertebrate systems, *Proc Natl Acad Sci USA*. **98**: pp. 9742–9747.

17. Cardoso, A.L., S. Simoes, L.P. de Almeida, J. Pelisek, C. Culmsee, E. Wagner, and M.C. Pedroso de Lima (2007). siRNA delivery by a transferrin-associated lipid-based vector: a non-viral strategy to mediate gene silencing, *J Gene Med*. **9**: pp. 170–183.
18. Cardoso, A.L., S. Simoes, L.P. de Almeida, N. Plesnila, M.C. Pedroso de Lima, E. Wagner, and C. Culmsee (2008). Tf-lipoplexes for neuronal siRNA delivery: a promising system to mediate gene silencing in the CNS, *J Control Release*. **132**: pp. 113–123.
19. Carmona, S., M. Keller, M.R. Jorgensen, S. Kolli, C. Crowther, F.H. Salazar, P.L. Marion, M. Fujino, Y. Natori, M. Thanou, P. Arbuthnot, and A.D. Miller (2009). Controlling HBV replication *in vivo* by intravenous administration of triggered PEGylated siRNA-nanoparticles, *Mol Pharm*. **6**: pp. 706–717.
20. Castanotto, D., and J.J. Rossi (2009). The promises and pitfalls of RNA-interference-based therapeutics, *Nature*. **457**: pp. 426–433.
21. Chernolovskaya, E.L., and M.A. Zenkova Chemical modification of siRNA, *Curr Opin Mol Ther*. **12**: pp. 158–167.
22. Chu, T.C., K.Y. Twu, A.D. Ellington, and M. Levy (2006). Aptamer mediated siRNA delivery, *Nucleic Acids Res*. **34**: pp. e73.
23. Cullen, B.R. (2006). Enhancing and confirming the specificity of RNAi experiments, *Nat Methods*. **3**: pp. 677–681.
24. Czech, B., C.D. Malone, R. Zhou, A. Stark, C. Schlingeheyde, M. Dus, N. Perrimon, M. Kellis, J.A. Wohlschlegel, R. Sachidanandam, G.J. Hannon, and J. Brennecke (2008). An endogenous small interfering RNA pathway in Drosophila, *Nature*. **453**: pp. 798–802.
25. Dassie, J.P., X.Y. Liu, G.S. Thomas, R.M. Whitaker, K.W. Thiel, K.R. Stockdale, D.K. Meyerholz, A.P. McCaffrey, J.O. McNamara, 2nd, and P.H. Giangrande (2009). Systemic administration of optimized aptamer-siRNA chimeras promotes regression of PSMA-expressing tumors, *Nat Biotechnol*. **27**: pp. 839–849.
26. Davis, M.E., J.E. Zuckerman, C.H. Choi, D. Seligson, A. Tolcher, C.A. Alabi, Y. Yen, J.D. Heidel, and A. Ribas Evidence of RNAi in humans from systemically administered siRNA via targeted nanoparticles, *Nature*. **464**: pp. 1067–1070.
27. DeVincenzo, J., J.E. Cehelsky, R. Alvarez, S. Elbashir, J. Harborth, I. Toudjarska, L. Nechev, V. Murugaiah, A. Van Vliet, A.K. Vaishnaw, and R. Meyers (2008). Evaluation of the safety, tolerability and pharmacokinetics of ALN-RSV01, a novel RNAi antiviral therapeutic

directed against respiratory syncytial virus (RSV), *Antiviral Res.* **77**: pp. 225–231.

28. Diebold, S.S., T. Kaisho, H. Hemmi, S. Akira, and C. Reis e Sousa (2004). Innate antiviral responses by means of TLR7-mediated recognition of single-stranded RNA, *Science.* **303**: pp. 1529–1531.
29. DiFiglia, M., M. Sena-Esteves, K. Chase, E. Sapp, E. Pfister, M. Sass, J. Yoder, P. Reeves, R.K. Pandey, K.G. Rajeev, M. Manoharan, D.W. Sah, P.D. Zamore, and N. Aronin (2007). Therapeutic silencing of mutant huntingtin with siRNA attenuates striatal and cortical neuropathology and behavioral deficits, *Proc Natl Acad Sci USA.* **104**: pp. 17204–17209.
30. Dominska, M., and D.M. Dykxhoorn Breaking down the barriers: siRNA delivery and endosome escape, *J Cell Sci.* **123**: pp. 1183–1189.
31. Dykxhoorn, D.M. Advances in cell-type specific delivery of RNAi-based therapeutics, *IDrugs.* **13**: pp. 325–331.
32. Dykxhoorn, D.M., and J. Lieberman (2005). The silent revolution: RNA interference as basic biology, research tool, and therapeutic, *Annu Rev Med.* **56**: pp. 401–423.
33. Dykxhoorn, D.M., and J. Lieberman (2006). Running interference: prospects and obstacles to using small interfering RNAs as small molecule drugs, *Annu Rev Biomed Eng.* **8**: pp. 377–402.
34. Dykxhoorn, D.M., L.D. Schlehuber, I.M. London, and J. Lieberman (2006). Determinants of specific RNA interference-mediated silencing of human beta-globin alleles differing by a single nucleotide polymorphism, *Proc Natl Acad Sci USA.* **103**: pp. 5953–5958.
35. Eacker, S.M., Dawson, T.M., Dawson, V.L. (2009). Understanding microRNAs in neurodegeneration, *Nat Rev Neurosci.* **10**: pp. 837–841.
36. Echeverri, C.J., P.A. Beachy, B. Baum, M. Boutros, F. Buchholz, S.K. Chanda, J. Downward, J. Ellenberg, A.G. Fraser, N. Hacohen, W.C. Hahn, A.L. Jackson, A. Kiger, P.S. Linsley, L. Lum, Y. Ma, B. Mathey-Prevot, D.E. Root, D.M. Sabatini, J. Taipale, N. Perrimon, and R. Bernards (2006). Minimizing the risk of reporting false positives in large-scale RNAi screens, *Nat Methods.* **3**: pp. 777–779.
37. Echeverri, C.J., and N. Perrimon (2006). High-throughput RNAi screening in cultured cells: a user's guide, *Nat Rev Genet.* **7**: pp. 373–384.
38. Elbashir, S.M., J. Harborth, W. Lendeckel, A. Yalcin, K. Weber, and T. Tuschl (2001). Duplexes of 21-nucleotide RNAs mediate RNA interference in cultured mammalian cells, *Nature.* **411**: pp. 494–498.
39. Elbashir, S.M., J. Harborth, K. Weber, and T. Tuschl (2002). Analysis of gene function in somatic mammalian cells using small interfering RNAs, *Methods.* **26**: pp. 199–213.

40. Elbashir, S.M., W. Lendeckel, and T. Tuschl (2001). RNA interference is mediated by 21- and 22-nucleotide RNAs, *Genes Dev.* **15**: pp. 188–200.

41. Elbashir, S.M., J. Martinez, A. Patkaniowska, W. Lendeckel, and T. Tuschl (2001). Functional anatomy of siRNAs for mediating efficient RNAi in Drosophila melanogaster embryo lysate, *EMBO J.* **20**: pp. 6877–6888.

42. Emerson, M.V., and A.K. Lauer (2007). Emerging therapies for the treatment of neovascular age-related macular degeneration and diabetic macular edema, *BioDrugs.* **21**: pp. 245–257.

43. Endoh, T., and T. Ohtsuki (2009). Cellular siRNA delivery using cell-penetrating peptides modified for endosomal escape, *Adv Drug Delivery Rev.* **61**: pp. 704–709.

44. Farhood, H., N. Serbina, and L. Huang (1995). The role of dioleoyl phosphatidylethanolamine in cationic liposome mediated gene transfer, *Biochim Biophys Acta Biomembr.* **1235**: pp. 289–295.

45. Fire, A., S. Xu, M.K. Montgomery, S.A. Kostas, S.E. Driver, and C.C. Mello (1998). Potent and specific genetic interference by double-stranded RNA in *Caenorhabditis elegans, Nature.* **391**: pp. 806–811.

46. Forsbach, A., J.G. Nemorin, C. Montino, C. Muller, U. Samulowitz, A.P. Vicari, M. Jurk, G.K. Mutwiri, A.M. Krieg, G.B. Lipford, and J. Vollmer (2008). Identification of RNA sequence motifs stimulating sequence-specific TLR8-dependent immune responses, *J Immunol.* **180**: pp. 3729–3738.

47. Gaglione, M., and A. Messere Recent progress in chemically modified siRNAs, *Mini Rev Med Chem.* **10**: pp. 578–595.

48. Garzon, R., G.A. Calin, and C.M. Croce (2009). MicroRNAs in cancer, *Annu Rev Med.* **60**: pp. 167–179.

49. Garzon, R., M. Fabbri, A. Cimmino, G.A. Calin, and C.M. Croce (2006). MicroRNA expression and function in cancer, *Trends Mol Med.* **12**: pp. 580–587.

50. Ghildiyal, M., H. Seitz, M.D. Horwich, C. Li, T. Du, S. Lee, J. Xu, E.L. Kittler, M.L. Zapp, Z. Weng, and P.D. Zamore (2008). Endogenous siRNAs derived from transposons and mRNAs in Drosophila somatic cells, *Science.* **320**: pp. 1077–1081.

51. Ghildiyal, M., J. Xu, H. Seitz, Z. Weng, and P.D. Zamore Sorting of Drosophila small silencing RNAs partitions microRNA* strands into the RNA interference pathway, *RNA.* **16**: pp. 43–56.

52. Ghildiyal, M., and P.D. Zamore (2009). Small silencing RNAs: an expanding universe, *Nat Rev Genet.* **10**: pp. 94–108.

53. Gonzalez, M.E., and L. Carrasco (2003). Viroporins, *FEBS Lett.* **552**: pp. 28–34.

54. Goodchild, A., N. Nopper, A. King, T. Doan, M. Tanudji, G.M. Arndt, M. Poidinger, L.P. Rivory, and T. Passioura (2009). Sequence determinants of innate immune activation by short interfering RNAs, *BMC Immunol.* **10**: pp. 40.

55. Grimm, D., K.L. Streetz, C.L. Jopling, T.A. Storm, K. Pandey, C.R. Davis, P. Marion, F. Salazar, and M.A. Kay (2006). Fatality in mice due to oversaturation of cellular microRNA/short hairpin RNA pathways, *Nature.* **441**: pp. 537–541.

56. Guo, H., N.T. Ingolia, J.S. Weissman, and D.P. Bartel Mammalian microRNAs predominantly act to decrease target mRNA levels, *Nature.* **466**: pp. 835–840.

57. Guo, X., J.A. MacKay, and F.C. Szoka, Jr. (2003). Mechanism of pH-triggered collapse of phosphatidylethanolamine liposomes stabilized by an ortho ester polyethyleneglycol lipid, *Biophys. J.* **84**: pp. 1784–1795.

58. Guo, X., and F.C. Szoka, Jr. (2001). Steric stabilization of fusogenic liposomes by a low-pH sensitive PEG-diortho ester–lipid conjugate, *Bioconjugate Chem.* **12**: pp. 291–300.

59. Hagstrom, J.E., J. Hegge, G. Zhang, M. Noble, V. Budker, D.L. Lewis, H. Herweijer, and J.A. Wolff (2004). A facile nonviral method for delivering genes and siRNAs to skeletal muscle of mammalian limbs, *Mol Ther.* **10**: pp. 386–398.

60. Hammond, S.M., E. Bernstein, D. Beach, and G.J. Hannon (2000). An RNA-directed nuclease mediates post-transcriptional gene silencing in Drosophila cells, *Nature.* **404**: pp. 293–296.

61. Hassani, Z., G.F. Lemkine, P. Erbacher, K. Palmier, G. Alfama, C. Giovannangeli, J.-P. Behr, and B.A. Demeneix (2005). Lipid-mediated siRNA delivery down-regulates exogenous gene expression in the mouse brain at picomolar levels, *J. Gene Med.* **7**: pp. 198–207.

62. Hatakeyama, H., H. Akita, K. Kogure, M. Oishi, Y. Nagasaki, Y. Kihira, M. Ueno, H. Kobayashi, H. Kikuchi, and H. Harashima (2007). Development of a novel systemic gene delivery system for cancer therapy with a tumor-specific cleavable PEG-lipid, *Gene Ther.* **14**: pp. 68–77.

63. Heidel, J.D., Z. Yu, J.Y. Liu, S.M. Rele, Y. Liang, R.K. Zeidan, D.J. Kornbrust, and M.E. Davis (2007). Administration in non-human primates of escalating intravenous doses of targeted nanoparticles containing ribonucleotide reductase subunit M2 siRNA, *Proc Natl Acad Sci USA.* **104**: pp. 5715–5721.

64. Heil, F., H. Hemmi, H. Hochrein, F. Ampenberger, C. Kirschning, S. Akira, G. Lipford, H. Wagner, and S. Bauer (2004). Species-specific recognition of single-stranded RNA via toll-like receptor 7 and 8, *Science.* **303**: pp. 1526–1529.

65. Heyes, J., L. Palmer, K. Bremner, and I. MacLachlan (2005). Cationic lipid saturation influences intracellular delivery of encapsulated nucleic acids, *J Control. Release.* **107**: pp. 276–287.

66. Hickerson, R.P., F.J. Smith, R.E. Reeves, C.H. Contag, D. Leake, S.A. Leachman, L.M. Milstone, W.H. McLean, and R.L. Kaspar (2008). Single-nucleotide-specific siRNA targeting in a dominant-negative skin model, *J Invest Dermatol.* **128**: pp. 594–605.

67. Holen, T., M. Amarzguioui, M.T. Wiiger, E. Babaie, and H. Prydz (2002). Positional effects of short interfering RNAs targeting the human coagulation trigger Tissue Factor, *Nucleic Acids Res.* **30**: pp. 1757–1766.

68. Hornung, V., M. Guenthner-Biller, C. Bourquin, A. Ablasser, M. Schlee, S. Uematsu, A. Noronha, M. Manoharan, S. Akira, A. de Fougerolles, S. Endres, and G. Hartmann (2005). Sequence-specific potent induction of IFN-alpha by short interfering RNA in plasmacytoid dendritic cells through TLR7, *Nat Med.* **11**: pp. 263–270.

69. Hu-Lieskovan, S., J.D. Heidel, D.W. Bartlett, M.E. Davis, and T.J. Triche (2005). Sequence-specific knockdown of EWS-FLI1 by targeted, nonviral delivery of small interfering RNA inhibits tumor growth in a murine model of metastatic Ewing's sarcoma, *Cancer Res.* **65**: pp. 8984–8992.

70. Hutvagner, G., M.J. Simard, C.C. Mello, and P.D. Zamore (2004). Sequence-specific inhibition of small RNA function, *PLoS Biol.* **2**: pp. E98.

71. Hutvagner, G., and P.D. Zamore (2002). A microRNA in a multiple-turnover RNAi enzyme complex, *Science.* **297**: pp. 2056–2060.

72. Iyer, A.K., G. Khaled, J. Fang, and H. Maeda (2006). Exploiting the enhanced permeability and retention effect for tumor targeting, *Drug Discov Today.* **11**: pp. 812–818.

73. Jackson, A.L., S.R. Bartz, J. Schelter, S.V. Kobayashi, J. Burchard, M. Mao, B. Li, G. Cavet, and P.S. Linsley (2003). Expression profiling reveals off-target gene regulation by RNAi, *Nat Biotechnol.* **21**: pp. 635–637.

74. Jackson, A.L., J. Burchard, D. Leake, A. Reynolds, J. Schelter, J. Guo, J.M. Johnson, L. Lim, J. Karpilow, K. Nichols, W. Marshall, A. Khvorova, and P.S. Linsley (2006). Position-specific chemical modification of siRNAs reduces "off-target" transcript silencing, *RNA.* **12**: pp. 1197–1205.

75. Jackson, A.L., J. Burchard, J. Schelter, B.N. Chau, M. Cleary, L. Lim, and P.S. Linsley (2006). Widespread siRNA "off-target" transcript silencing mediated by seed region sequence complementarity, *RNA.* **12**: pp. 1179–1187.

76. Jackson, A.L., and P.S. Linsley Recognizing and avoiding siRNA off-target effects for target identification and therapeutic application, *Nat Rev Drug Discov.* **9**: pp. 57–67.
77. Judge, A., and I. MacLachlan (2008). Overcoming the innate immune response to small interfering RNA, *Hum Gene Ther.* **19**: pp. 111–124.
78. Judge, A.D., G. Bola, A.C. Lee, and I. MacLachlan (2006). Design of noninflammatory synthetic siRNA mediating potent gene silencing *in vivo*, *Mol Ther.* **13**: pp. 494–505.
79. Judge, A.D., V. Sood, J.R. Shaw, D. Fang, K. McClintock, and I. MacLachlan (2005). Sequence-dependent stimulation of the mammalian innate immune response by synthetic siRNA, *Nat Biotechnol.* **23**: pp. 457–462.
80. Kariko, K., P. Bhuyan, J. Capodici, and D. Weissman (2004). Small interfering RNAs mediate sequence-independent gene suppression and induce immune activation by signaling through toll-like receptor 3, *J Immunol.* **172**: pp. 6545–6549.
81. Kawamura, Y., K. Saito, T. Kin, Y. Ono, K. Asai, T. Sunohara, T.N. Okada, M.C. Siomi, and H. Siomi (2008). Drosophila endogenous small RNAs bind to Argonaute 2 in somatic cells, *Nature.* **453**: pp. 793–797.
82. Ketting, R.F., S.E. Fischer, E. Bernstein, T. Sijen, G.J. Hannon, and R.H. Plasterk (2001). Dicer functions in RNA interference and in synthesis of small RNA involved in developmental timing in *C. elegans*, *Genes Dev.* **15**: pp. 2654–2659.
83. Khvorova, A., A. Reynolds, and S.D. Jayasena (2003). Functional siRNAs and miRNAs exhibit strand bias, *Cell.* **115**: pp. 209–216.
84. Kim, S.I., D. Shin, T.H. Choi, J.C. Lee, G.J. Cheon, K.Y. Kim, M. Park, and M. Kim (2007). Systemic and specific delivery of small interfering RNAs to the liver mediated by apolipoprotein A-I, *Mol Ther.* **15**: pp. 1145–1152.
85. Kim, S.S., C. Ye, P. Kumar, I. Chiu, S. Subramanya, H. Wu, P. Shankar, and N. Manjunath (2010). Targeted delivery of siRNA to macrophages for anti-inflammatory treatment, *Mol Ther.* **18**: pp. 993–1001.
86. Kim, V.N. (2005). MicroRNA biogenesis: coordinated cropping and dicing, *Nat Rev Mol Cell Biol.* **6**: pp. 376–385.
87. Kim, V.N., J. Han, and M.C. Siomi (2009). Biogenesis of small RNAs in animals, *Nat Rev Mol Cell Biol.* **10**: pp. 126–139.
88. Kogure, K., H. Akita, and H. Harashima (2007). Multifunctional envelope-type nano device for non-viral gene delivery: Concept and application of Programmed Packaging, *J Control Release* **122**: pp. 246–251.

89. Kogure, K., R. Moriguchi, K. Sasaki, M. Ueno, S. Futaki, and H. Harashima (2004). Development of a non-viral multifunctional envelope-type nano device by a novel lipid film hydration method, *J Control Release* **98**: pp. 317–323.

90. Koltover, I., T. Salditt, J.O. Radler, and C.R. Safinya (1998). An inverted hexagonal phase of cationic liposome-DNA complexes related to DNA release and delivery, *Science (Washington, D. C.)* **281**: pp. 78–81.

91. Kumar, P., H.S. Ban, S.S. Kim, H. Wu, T. Pearson, D.L. Greiner, A. Laouar, J. Yao, V. Haridas, K. Habiro, Y.G. Yang, J.H. Jeong, K.Y. Lee, Y.H. Kim, S.W. Kim, M. Peipp, G.H. Fey, N. Manjunath, L.D. Shultz, S.K. Lee, and P. Shankar (2008). T cell-specific siRNA delivery suppresses HIV-1 infection in humanized mice, *Cell.* **134**: pp. 577–586.

92. Kumar, P., H. Wu, J.L. McBride, K.E. Jung, M.H. Kim, B.L. Davidson, S.K. Lee, P. Shankar, and N. Manjunath (2007). Transvascular delivery of small interfering RNA to the central nervous system, *Nature.* **448**: pp. 39–43.

93. Kwon, E.J., J.M. Bergen, and S.H. Pun (2008). Application of an HIV gp41-derived peptide for enhanced intracellular trafficking of synthetic gene and siRNA delivery vehicles, *Bioconjugate Chem.* **19**: pp. 920–927.

94. Lagos-Quintana, M., R. Rauhut, W. Lendeckel, and T. Tuschl (2001). Identification of novel genes coding for small expressed RNAs, *Science.* **294**: pp. 853–858.

95. Latchman, Y., C.R. Wood, T. Chernova, D. Chaudhary, M. Borde, I. Chernova, Y. Iwai, A.J. Long, J.A. Brown, R. Nunes, E.A. Greenfield, K. Bourque, V.A. Boussiotis, L.L. Carter, B.M. Carreno, N. Malenkovich, H. Nishimura, T. Okazaki, T. Honjo, A.H. Sharpe, and G.J. Freeman (2001). PD-L2 is a second ligand for PD-1 and inhibits T cell activation, *Nat Immunol.* **2**: pp. 261–268.

96. Leachman, S.A., R.P. Hickerson, P.R. Hull, F.J. Smith, L.M. Milstone, E.B. Lane, S.J. Bale, D.R. Roop, W.H. McLean, and R.L. Kaspar (2008). Therapeutic siRNAs for dominant genetic skin disorders including pachyonychia congenita, *J Dermatol Sci.* **51**: pp. 151–157.

97. Leachman, S.A., R.P. Hickerson, M.E. Schwartz, E.E. Bullough, S.L. Hutcherson, K.M. Boucher, C.D. Hansen, M.J. Eliason, G.S. Srivatsa, D.J. Kornbrust, F.J. Smith, W.I. McLean, L.M. Milstone, and R.L. Kaspar (2009). First-in-human mutation-targeted siRNA phase Ib trial of an inherited skin disorder, *Mol Ther.* **18**: pp. 442–446.

98. Lee, S.K., D.M. Dykxhoorn, P. Kumar, S. Ranjbar, E. Song, L.E. Maliszewski, V. Francois-Bongarcon, A. Goldfeld, N.M. Swamy, J. Lieberman, and P. Shankar (2005). Lentiviral delivery of short hairpin RNAs protects CD4 T cells from multiple clades and primary isolates of HIV, *Blood.* **106**: pp. 818–826.

99. Lee, Y., K. Jeon, J.T. Lee, S. Kim, and V.N. Kim (2002). MicroRNA maturation: stepwise processing and subcellular localization, *EMBO J.* **21**: pp. 4663–4670.

100. Lee, Y., M. Kim, J. Han, K.H. Yeom, S. Lee, S.H. Baek, and V.N. Kim (2004). MicroRNA genes are transcribed by RNA polymerase II, *EMBO J.* **23**: pp. 4051–4060.

101. Lewis, D.L., J.E. Hagstrom, A.G. Loomis, J.A. Wolff, and H. Herweijer (2002). Efficient delivery of siRNA for inhibition of gene expression in postnatal mice, *Nat Genet.* **32**: pp. 107–108.

102. Litzinger, D.C., and L. Huang (1992). Phosphatidylethanolamine liposomes: drug delivery, gene transfer and immunodiagnostic applications, *Biochim Biophys Acta Rev Biomembr.* **1113**: pp. 201–227.

103. Liu, J., M.A. Carmell, F.V. Rivas, C.G. Marsden, J.M. Thomson, J.J. Song, S.M. Hammond, L. Joshua-Tor, and G.J. Hannon (2004). Argonaute2 is the catalytic engine of mammalian RNAi, *Science.* **305**: pp. 1437–1441.

104. Lorenz, C., P. Hadwiger, M. John, H.P. Vornlocher, and C. Unverzagt (2004). Steroid and lipid conjugates of siRNAs to enhance cellular uptake and gene silencing in liver cells, *Bioorg Med Chem Lett.* **14**: pp. 4975–4977.

105. Maeda, H., J. Wu, T. Sawa, Y. Matsumura, and K. Hori (2000). Tumor vascular permeability and the EPR effect in macromolecular therapeutics: a review, *J Control Release.* **65**: pp. 271–284.

106. Manjunath, N., and D.M. Dykxhoorn (2010) Advances in synthetic siRNA delivery, *Discov Med.* **9**: pp. 418–430.

107. Martin, R., P. Smibert, A. Yalcin, D.M. Tyler, U. Schafer, T. Tuschl, and E.C. Lai (2009). A Drosophila pasha mutant distinguishes the canonical microRNA and mirtron pathways, *Mol Cell Biol.* **29**: pp. 861–870.

108. McCaffrey, A.P., H. Nakai, K. Pandey, Z. Huang, F.H. Salazar, H. Xu, S.F. Wieland, P.L. Marion, and M.A. Kay (2003). Inhibition of hepatitis B virus in mice by RNA interference, *Nat Biotechnol.* **21**: pp. 639–644.

109. McNamara, J.O., 2nd, E.R. Andrechek, Y. Wang, K.D. Viles, R.E. Rempel, E. Gilboa, B.A. Sullenger, and P.H. Giangrande (2006). Cell type-specific delivery of siRNAs with aptamer-siRNA chimeras, *Nat Biotechnol.* **24**: pp. 1005–1015.

110. Morrissey, D.V., J.A. Lockridge, L. Shaw, K. Blanchard, K. Jensen, W. Breen, K. Hartsough, L. Machemer, S. Radka, V. Jadhav, N. Vaish, S. Zinnen, C. Vargeese, K. Bowman, C.S. Shaffer, L.B. Jeffs, A. Judge, I. MacLachlan, and B. Polisky (2005). Potent and persistent *in vivo* anti-HBV activity of chemically modified siRNAs, *Nat Biotechnol.* **23**: pp. 1002–1007.

111. Muratovska, A., and M.R. Eccles (2004). Conjugate for efficient delivery of short interfering RNA (siRNA) into mammalian cells, *FEBS Lett.* **558**: pp. 63–68.

112. Nishina, K., T. Unno, Y. Uno, T. Kubodera, T. Kanouchi, H. Mizusawa, and T. Yokota (2008). Efficient *in vivo* delivery of siRNA to the liver by conjugation of alpha-tocopherol, *Mol Ther.* **16**: pp. 734–740.

113. Noguchi, P. (2003). Risks and benefits of gene therapy, *N Engl J Med.* **348**: pp. 193–194.

114. Okamura, K., S. Balla, R. Martin, N. Liu, and E.C. Lai (2008). Two distinct mechanisms generate endogenous siRNAs from bidirectional transcription in Drosophila melanogaster, *Nat Struct Mol Biol.* **15**: pp. 581–590.

115. Okamura, K., W.J. Chung, and E.C. Lai (2008). The long and short of inverted repeat genes in animals: microRNAs, mirtrons and hairpin RNAs, *Cell Cycle.* **7**: pp. 2840–2845.

116. Okamura, K., W.J. Chung, J.G. Ruby, H. Guo, D.P. Bartel, and E.C. Lai (2008). The Drosophila hairpin RNA pathway generates endogenous short interfering RNAs, *Nature.* **453**: pp. 803–806.

117. Oliveira, S., I. van Rooy, O. Kranenburg, G. Storm, and R.M. Schiffelers (2007). Fusogenic peptides enhance endosomal escape improving siRNA-induced silencing of oncogenes, *Int. J. Pharm.* **331**: pp. 211–214.

118. Palliser, D., D. Chowdhury, Q.Y. Wang, S.J. Lee, R.T. Bronson, D.M. Knipe, and J. Lieberman (2006). An siRNA-based microbicide protects mice from lethal herpes simplex virus 2 infection, *Nature.* **439**: pp. 89–94.

119. Patil, M.L., M. Zhang, S. Betigeri, O. Taratula, H. He, and T. Minko (2008). Surface-modified and internally cationic polyamidoamine dendrimers for efficient siRNA delivery, *Bioconjugate Chem.* **19**: pp. 1396–1403.

120. Patil, M.L., M. Zhang, O. Taratula, O.B. Garbuzenko, H. He, and T. Minko (2009). Internally cationic polyamidoamine PAMAM-OH dendrimers for siRNA delivery: effect of the degree of quaternization and cancer targeting, *Biomacromolecules* **10**: pp. 258–266.

121. Pauley, K.M., S. Cha, and E.K. Chan (2009). MicroRNA in autoimmunity and autoimmune diseases, *J Autoimmun.* **32**: pp. 189–194.

122. Peer, D., E.J. Park, Y. Morishita, C.V. Carman, and M. Shimaoka (2008). Systemic leukocyte-directed siRNA delivery revealing cyclin D1 as an anti-inflammatory target, *Science.* **319**: pp. 627–630.

123. Peer, D., P. Zhu, C.V. Carman, J. Lieberman, and M. Shimaoka (2007). Selective gene silencing in activated leukocytes by targeting siRNAs to the integrin lymphocyte function-associated antigen-1, *Proc Natl Acad Sci USA.* **104**: pp. 4095–4100.

124. Read, M.L., S. Singh, Z. Ahmed, M. Stevenson, S.S. Briggs, D. Oupicky, L.B. Barrett, R. Spice, M. Kendall, M. Berry, J.A. Preece, A. Logan, and L.W. Seymour (2005). A versatile reducible polycation-based system for efficient delivery of a broad range of nucleic acids, *Nucleic Acids Res.* **33**: pp. e86/81–e86/16.

125. Richards Grayson, A.C., A.M. Doody, and D. Putnam (2006). Biophysical and structural characterization of polyethylenimine-mediated siRNA delivery *in vitro*, *Pharm. Res.* **23**: pp. 1868–1876.

126. Robbins, M., A. Judge, and I. MacLachlan (2009). siRNA and innate immunity, *Oligonucleotides*. **19**: pp. 89–102.

127. Rozema, D.B., D.L. Lewis, D.H. Wakefield, S.C. Wong, J.J. Klein, P.L. Roesch, S.L. Bertin, T.W. Reppen, Q. Chu, A.V. Blokhin, J.E. Hagstrom, and J.A. Wolff (2007). Dynamic polyconjugates for targeted *in vivo* delivery of siRNA to hepatocytes, *Proc Natl Acad Sci USA*. **104**: pp. 12982–12987.

128. Sato, A., M. Takagi, A. Shimamoto, S. Kawakami, and M. Hashida (2007). Small interfering RNA delivery to the liver by intravenous administration of galactosylated cationic liposomes in mice, *Biomaterials*. **28**: pp. 1434–1442.

129. Schwarz, D.S., H. Ding, L. Kennington, J.T. Moore, J. Schelter, J. Burchard, P.S. Linsley, N. Aronin, Z. Xu, and P.D. Zamore (2006). Designing siRNA that distinguish between genes that differ by a single nucleotide, *PLoS Genet.* **2**: pp. e140.

130. Schwarz, D.S., G. Hutvagner, T. Du, Z. Xu, N. Aronin, and P.D. Zamore (2003). Asymmetry in the assembly of the RNAi enzyme complex, *Cell*. **115**: pp. 199–208.

131. Shin, J., P. Shum, and D.H. Thompson (2003). Acid-triggered release via dePEGylation of DOPE liposomes containing acid-labile vinyl ether PEG-lipids, *J Control Release* **91**: pp. 187–200.

132. Sioud, M. (2005). Induction of inflammatory cytokines and interferon responses by double-stranded and single-stranded siRNAs is sequence-dependent and requires endosomal localization, *J Mol Biol.* **348**: pp. 1079–1090.

133. Sledz, C.A., M. Holko, M.J. de Veer, R.H. Silverman, and B.R. Williams (2003). Activation of the interferon system by short-interfering RNAs, *Nat Cell Biol.* **5**: pp. 834–839.

134. Sonawane, N.D., F.C. Szoka, Jr., and A.S. Verkman (2003). Chloride accumulation and swelling in endosomes enhances DNA transfer by polyamine-DNA polyplexes, *J. Biol. Chem.* **278**: pp. 44826–44831.

135. Song, E., S.K. Lee, D.M. Dykxhoorn, C. Novina, D. Zhang, K. Crawford, J. Cerny, P.A. Sharp, J. Lieberman, N. Manjunath, and P. Shankar (2003). Sustained small interfering RNA-mediated human immunodeficiency

virus type 1 inhibition in primary macrophages, *J Virol.* **77**: pp. 7174–7181.

136. Song, E., S.K. Lee, J. Wang, N. Ince, N. Ouyang, J. Min, J. Chen, P. Shankar, and J. Lieberman (2003). RNA interference targeting Fas protects mice from fulminant hepatitis, *Nat Med.* **9**: pp. 347–351.

137. Song, E., P. Zhu, S.K. Lee, D. Chowdhury, S. Kussman, D.M. Dykxhoorn, Y. Feng, D. Palliser, D.B. Weiner, P. Shankar, W.A. Marasco, and J. Lieberman (2005). Antibody mediated *in vivo* delivery of small interfering RNAs via cell-surface receptors, *Nat Biotechnol.* **23**: pp. 709–717.

138. Soutschek, J., A. Akinc, B. Bramlage, K. Charisse, R. Constien, M. Donoghue, S. Elbashir, A. Geick, P. Hadwiger, J. Harborth, M. John, V. Kesavan, G. Lavine, R.K. Pandey, T. Racie, K.G. Rajeev, I. Rohl, I. Toudjarska, G. Wang, S. Wuschko, D. Bumcrot, V. Koteliansky, S. Limmer, M. Manoharan, and H.P. Vornlocher (2004). Therapeutic silencing of an endogenous gene by systemic administration of modified siRNAs, *Nature.* **432**: pp. 173–178.

139. Subramanya, S., S.S. Kim, S. Abraham, J. Yao, M. Kumar, P. Kumar, V. Haridas, S.K. Lee, L.D. Shultz, D. Greiner, M. N, and P. Shankar (2010). Targeted delivery of small interfering RNA to human dendritic cells to suppress dengue virus infection and associated proinflammatory cytokine production, *J Virol.* **84**: pp. 2490–2501.

140. Takanashi, M., K. Oikawa, K. Sudo, M. Tanaka, K. Fujita, A. Ishikawa, S. Nakae, R.L. Kaspar, M. Matsuzaki, M. Kudo, and M. Kuroda (2009). Therapeutic silencing of an endogenous gene by siRNA cream in an arthritis model mouse, *Gene Ther.* **16**: pp. 982–989.

141. Tiemann, K., and J.J. Rossi (2009). RNAi-based therapeutics — current status, challenges and prospects, *EMBO Mol Med.* **1**: pp. 142–151.

142. Tuschl, T., P.D. Zamore, R. Lehmann, D.P. Bartel, and P.A. Sharp (1999). Targeted mRNA degradation by double-stranded RNA *in vitro*, *Genes Dev.* **13**: pp. 3191–3197.

143. Umbach, J.L., and B.R. Cullen (2009). The role of RNAi and microRNAs in animal virus replication and antiviral immunity, *Genes Dev.* **23**: pp. 1151–1164.

144. Urban-Klein, B., S. Werth, S. Abuharbeid, F. Czubayko, and A. Aigner (2005). RNAi-mediated gene-targeting through systemic application of polyethylenimine (PEI)-complexed siRNA *in vivo*, *Gene Ther.* **12**: pp. 461–466.

145. Vaishnaw, A.K., J. Gollob, C. Gamba-Vitalo, R. Hutabarat, D. Sah, R. Meyers, T. de Fougerolles, and J. Maraganore (2010) A status report on RNAi therapeutics, *Silence.* **1**: pp. 14.

146. van Rooij, E., L.B. Sutherland, N. Liu, A.H. Williams, J. McAnally, R.D. Gerard, J.A. Richardson, and E.N. Olson (2006). A signature pattern of stress-responsive microRNAs that can evoke cardiac hypertrophy and heart failure, *Proc Natl Acad Sci USA*. **103**: pp. 18255–18260.

147. van Rooij, E., Sutherland, L.B., Thatcher, J.E., DiMaio, J.M., Naseem, R.H., Marshall, W.S., Hill, J.A., Olson, E.N. (2008). Dysregulation of microRNAs after myocardial infarction reveals a role of miR-29 in cardiac fibrosis, *Proc Natl Acad Sci USA*. **105**: pp. 13027–13032.

148. Volkov, A.A., N.S. Kruglova, M.I. Meschaninova, A.G. Venyaminova, M.A. Zenkova, V.V. Vlassov, and E.L. Chernolovskaya (2009). Selective protection of nuclease-sensitive sites in siRNA prolongs silencing effect, *Oligonucleotides*. **19**: pp. 191–202.

149. von Mehren, M., G.P. Adams, and L.M. Weiner (2003). Monoclonal antibody therapy for cancer, *Annu Rev Med*. **54**: pp. 343–369.

150. Wang, X.-L., T. Nguyen, D. Gillespie, R. Jensen, and Z.-R. Lu (2008). A multifunctional and reversibly polymerizable carrier for efficient siRNA delivery, *Biomaterials* **29**: pp. 15–22.

151. Wang, X.-L., R. Xu, and Z.-R. Lu (2009). A peptide-targeted delivery system with pH-sensitive amphiphilic cell membrane disruption for efficient receptor-mediated siRNA delivery, *J Control Release* **134**: pp. 207–213.

152. Wang, X.-L., R. Xu, X. Wu, D. Gillespie, R. Jensen, and Z.-R. Lu (2009). Targeted Systemic Delivery of a Therapeutic siRNA with a multifunctional carrier controls tumor proliferation in mice, *Mol Pharm*. **6**: pp. 738–746.

153. Watts, J.K., G.F. Deleavey, and M.J. Damha (2008). Chemically modified siRNA: tools and applications, *Drug Discov Today*. **13**: pp. 842–855.

154. Weiner, L.M., and G.P. Adams (2000). New approaches to antibody therapy, *Oncogene*. **19**: pp. 6144–6151.

155. Wu, S.Y., and N.A. McMillan (2009). Lipidic Systems for *in vivo* siRNA Delivery, *AAPS J*.

156. Wu, Y., F. Navarro, A. Lal, E. Basar, R.K. Pandey, M. Manoharan, Y. Feng, S.J. Lee, J. Lieberman, and D. Palliser (2009). Durable protection from herpes simplex virus-2 transmission following intravaginal application of siRNAs targeting both a viral and host gene, *Cell Host Microbe*. **5**: pp. 84–94.

157. Yagi, N., I. Manabe, T. Tottori, A. Ishihara, F. Ogata, J.H. Kim, S. Nishimura, K. Fujiu, Y. Oishi, K. Itaka, Y. Kato, M. Yamauchi, and R. Nagai (2009). A nanoparticle system specifically designed to deliver short interfering RNA inhibits tumor growth *in vivo*, *Cancer Res*. **69**: pp. 6531–6538.

158. Yeom, K.H., Y. Lee, J. Han, M.R. Suh, and V.N. Kim (2006). Characterization of DGCR8/Pasha, the essential cofactor for Drosha in primary miRNA processing, *Nucleic Acids Res.* **34**: pp. 4622–4629.

159. Yi, R., B.P. Doehle, Y. Qin, I.G. Macara, and B.R. Cullen (2005). Overexpression of exportin 5 enhances RNA interference mediated by short hairpin RNAs and microRNAs, *RNA.* **11**: pp. 220–226.

160. Zabner, J., A.J. Fasbender, T. Moninger, K.A. Poellinger, and M.J. Welsh (1995). Cellular and molecular barriers to gene transfer by a cationic lipid, *J. Biol. Chem.* **270**: pp. 18997–19007.

161. Zamore, P.D., T. Tuschl, P.A. Sharp, and D.P. Bartel (2000). RNAi: double-stranded RNA directs the ATP-dependent cleavage of mRNA at 21 to 23 nucleotide intervals, *Cell.* **101**: pp. 25–33.

162. Zender, L., and S. Kubicka (2007). Suppression of apoptosis in the liver by systemic and local delivery of small-interfering RNAs, *Methods Mol Biol.* **361**: pp. 217–226.

163. Zhang, X., P. Shan, D. Jiang, P.W. Noble, N.G. Abraham, A. Kappas, and P.J. Lee (2004). Small interfering RNA targeting heme oxygenase-1 enhances ischemia-reperfusion-induced lung apoptosis, *J Biol Chem.* **279**: pp. 10677–10684.

164. Zheng, X., C. Vladau, X. Zhang, M. Suzuki, T.E. Ichim, Z.X. Zhang, M. Li, E. Carrier, B. Garcia, A.M. Jevnikar, and W.P. Min (2009). A novel *in vivo* siRNA delivery system specifically targeting dendritic cells and silencing CD40 genes for immunomodulation, *Blood.* **113**: pp. 2646–2654.

165. Zhou, J., H. Li, S. Li, J. Zaia, and J.J. Rossi (2008). Novel dual inhibitory function aptamer-siRNA delivery system for HIV-1 therapy, *Mol Ther.* **16**: pp. 1481–1489.

166. Zhou, J., P. Swiderski, H. Li, J. Zhang, C.P. Neff, R. Akkina, and J.J. Rossi (2009). Selection, characterization and application of new RNA HIV gp 120 aptamers for facile delivery of Dicer substrate siRNAs into HIV infected cells, *Nucleic Acids Res.* **37**: pp. 3094–3109.

Chapter 7

Novel RNA Interference (RNAi)-Based Nanomedicines for Treating Viral Infections

Nyree Maes,* Skye Zeller,* and Priti Kumar
Department of Internal Medicine, Section for Infectious Diseases, Yale University School of Medicine, New Haven, Connecticut 06520, USA
priti.kumar@yale.edu

The technology of RNA interference (RNAi) allows for the destruction of any RNA in a highly specific manner. This unique feature has enabled scientists to exploit the RNAi machinery for potential therapeutic application in a variety of human diseases. Research aimed at harnessing the endogenous RNAi machinery to treat viral infections has particularly been an area of intense investigation as vaccines and antiviral drugs are lacking for the most pathogenic viruses. A greater understanding of and recent advances in RNAi design and delivery have enabled the faster movement of these therapies from the bench to the bedside. In this chapter, we focus on the use of RNAi as an anti-viral therapeutic modality with special emphasis laid on studies pertaining to preclinical and clinical testing.

* These authors contributed equally to the writing of this chapter.

Handbook of Harnessing Biomaterials in Nanomedicine: Preparation, Toxicity, and Applications
Edited by Dan Peer

ISBN 978-981-4316-46-0 (Hardback), 978-981-4364-27-0 (eBook)
www.panstanford.com

7.1 Introduction

In the 1960s, thanks to the great strides afforded by antibiotics and vaccines, a general opinion that infectious diseases were a problem of the past was beginning to emerge. In fact, then US Surgeon General William H. Stewart has been widely cited as saying that it was "time to close the book on infectious diseases." While it is refuted that Stewart truly made such statements, the irrefutable fact is that the war against infectious diseases is far from over; infectious agents remain unconquered and are now the world's biggest killer of children and young adults. They account for more than 13 million deaths a year — one in two deaths in developing countries [123]. It is estimated that over the next hour alone, 1,500 people will die from an infectious disease—over half of them children under the age of five. For 40 years now, we have been reminded time and time again of the devastation that can be caused by classical re-emerging as well as newly emerging pathogenic viruses. The most well-known examples of this are the ongoing threat of influenza pandemics (estimated death rates of 250,000–500,000/year) [121], the emergence of human immunodeficiency virus (HIV) (a consistent annual death rate of 2 million), and the alarming epidemic caused by the newly emergent severe acute respiratory syndrome (SARS) virus (774 deaths in the 2003 Epidemic) [120]. A plethora of agents of natural, chemical and biological origins have been investigated for their potential to combat these and other viral threats. One method that has been relatively recently added to the arsenal against viral infections is based on the natural biological phenomenon of RNA interference (RNAi).

As recently as 12 years ago, the paramount study of Andrew Fire and Craig Mello [38] described for the first time, the mechanism of RNAi. Using *C. elegans* as a model organism, this study identified the biological mechanism where endogenous small double stranded RNAs (dsRNA) mediated inhibition of gene expression by binding larger messenger RNAs (mRNAs) at homologous sequences and triggering their degradation. A few years later, exogenously added short interfering RNAs (siRNAs) were experimentally shown to trigger the same RNAi machinery in mammalian cells [16, 34]. After extensive research we now know that longer (≥ 70 nucleotides) dsRNAs are cleaved by the enzyme Dicer into the smaller ~19–21 nt-long siRNAs. The resulting siRNA is subsequently loaded onto a RNA-induced silencing complex (RISC), where one strand of the siRNA (called guide or antisense strand) guides the complex to an mRNA with a homologous sequence, resulting in the cleavage of the mRNA by a nuclease Argonaute 2 (AGO2) that is part of the RISC complex (Figure 7.1) (reviewed in [88]). Collectively these studies, along with many others that followed, have unraveled the promise of RNAi as a therapeutic to treat practically any human disease, including those caused by viral infections, through the use of siRNAs designed to shut off expression of only the disease-causing mRNA.

Numerous *in vitro* studies have demonstrated the applicability of RNAi to suppress virtually every class of virus, whether double-stranded, single-positive, or negative-strand RNA or DNA genome (Figure 7.1). The transcribed mRNAs of DNA viruses (such as hepatitis B virus (HBV) and human papilloma virus (HPV)), the uncoated viral genomic RNA of both negative-sense RNA viruses (such as Influenza) and positive-sense RNA viruses (such as hepatitis C (HCV)) as well as processed mRNAs are cytoplasmically located and vulnerable to RNAi-mediated cleavage. Although retroviruses also have positive-sense RNA genomes, they have a unique lifecycle that includes an integration step, and have been discussed separately in this chapter. RNAi targeting of retroviruses can be achieved at two different stages of the viral lifecycle-upon viral uncoating when the linear viral genomic RNA is exposed and following transcription of the integrated proviral DNA when the viral mRNA is again released into the cytoplasm.

RNAi-targeting of these diverse virus species can be accomplished through classical RNAi mechanisms using short hairpin RNAs (shRNAs), long hairpin RNAs (lhRNAs), or siRNAs, all of them leading to RISC-mediated cleavage. Additionally, while not thought of as classical RNAi mediators, antisense oligonucleotides (ASOs) and phosphorodiamidate morpholino oligomers (PMOs) are two additional small RNA molecules that lead to inhibition by RNase H-mediated cleavage and translational inhibition, respectively (see Figure 7.1). All of these inhibitory RNAs can be delivered via several different methods. siRNAs can be delivered in the naked form to some cell types under specialized conditions but mostly require complexation with nanocarriers such as liposomes or nanoparticles (Figure 7.2). shRNAs and lhRNA can be delivered through non-viral plasmid expression vectors encased in nanocarriers or through viral vectors (i.e., adenovirus and lentivirus). Although viral vectors are not classified as "nanomaterials," pioneering work on RNAi-therapeutics utilizes viral vectors and therefore they will also be included in this chapter.

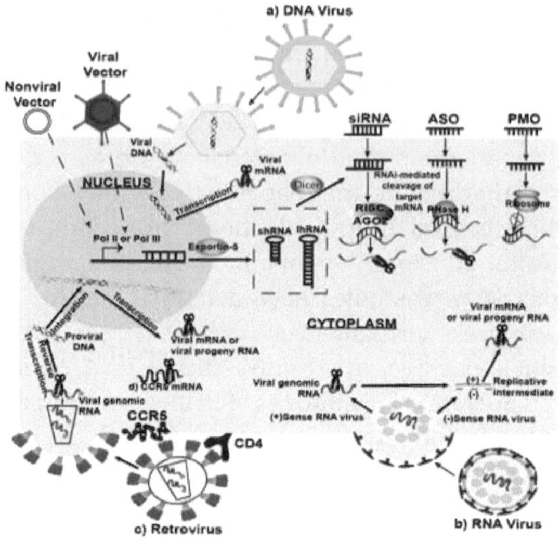

Figure 7.1 The mediators of antiviral RNA interference (RNAi). Mediators of viral suppression can be delivered in multiple formats. Short and long hairpin RNAs (shRNA or lhRNA) can be expressed from viral or non-viral vectors transcribed in the nucleus and are exported into the cytoplasm by association with Exportin-5. The hairpin sequences are processed by Dicer, to yield short interfering RNA (siRNAs). siRNAs can also be delivered directly into the cytoplasm using nanocarriers. The guide strand of the siRNA gets loaded onto the RNA-induce Silencing Complex (RISC); guiding RISC to the target RNA, resulting in cleavage of the target by argonaute (AGO2). Antisense oligonucleotides (ASOs) bind to the target RNA with a complementary sequence and induce RNase H-mediated cleavage. Phosphorodiamidate morpholino oligomers (PMOs) do not mediate cleavage of target RNAs, they bind near the start codon and inhibit translation by blocking ribosome binding.

Virus replication can be inhibited by targeting viral or cellular genes involved in the viral lifecycle at various stages. (**a**) DNA viruses are susceptible to degradation by RNAi machinery when their mRNA exits the nucleus and enters the cytoplasm. (**b**) The (+) sense RNA genome is also the mRNA; therefore upon uncoating it is susceptible to the effects of RNAi. (-) sense RNA viruses must undergo RNA-dependent transcription to generate mRNA, leaving both the negative genomic RNA and the newly generated mRNA vulnerable to RNAi. (**c**) The genomic RNA of Retroviruses is targetable upon uncoating in the cytoplasm. RNA that escapes degradation is reverse transcribed into proviral DNA which enters the nucleus for integration and transcription. The viral mRNA that is released into the cytoplasm can once again be degraded by RNAi mechanisms. (**d**) Host factors essential for the viral life cycle but not essential for the host can also be RNAi targets (i.e., CCR5 coreceptor).

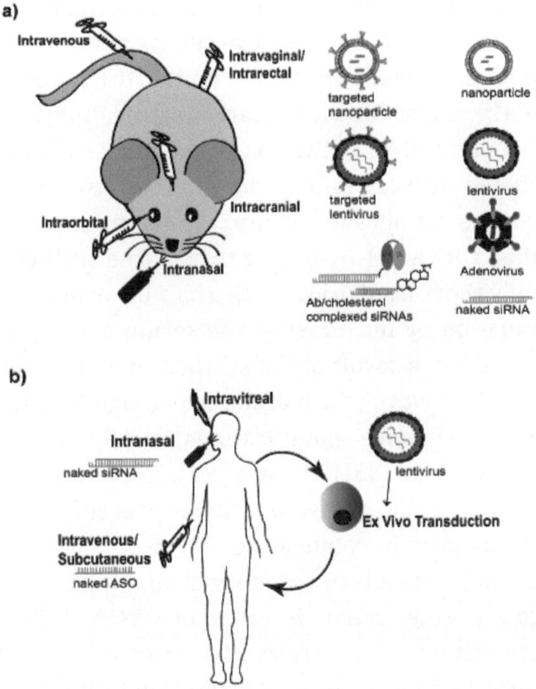

Figure 7.2 Delivery of RNA-inhibition (RNAi)-mediators *in vivo*. (a) RNAi-mediators can be delivered for topical applications (i) into the pulmonary tissue using intranasal aerosols; (ii) intratracheally using a catheter through an incision made near the throat; (iii) intracranially into the ventricular or hippocampal areas using stereotactic techniques ; (iv) intravaginally or intrarectally using blunt rubber tipped needles or; (v) intravitreally in the eye. Systemic delivery is achieved using non-invasive carriers through intraperitoneal and intravenous injections or physical methods like hydrodynamic injections. In the case of systemic routes, delivery has been achieved both non-specifically and through targeting ligands that provide targeting to specific cell types. Long-term effects are achieved using integrating viral vectors or plasmid vectors with a selection marker and short-term effects are achieved with non-integrating viral vectors, plasmid-expression vectors and siRNAs (in the naked form for topical application or carrier-complexed for systemic delivery). (b) RNAi mediators have been administered intravenously (e.g., SPC3549 in treatment of HCV), intranasally (e.g., ALN-RSV0 for treatment of RSV), and intravitreally (e.g., PF-04523655 for the treatment of macular degeneration) to assess efficacy in human subjects in clinical trials. Gene therapeutic methods have also included the *ex vivo* transduction of cells like human stem cells and T cells with lentiviral vectors expressing shRNA followed by transplantation of autologous donors.

Despite the promise of RNAi in *in vitro* studies, for RNAi-based therapies to become viable in a clinical setting many hurdles need to be overcome. These include but are not limited to (i) short *in vivo* half-life of siRNA; (ii) toxicity due to off-targeting resulting in silencing of unintended genes and/or activation of the innate immune system; and (iii) targeted delivery to only the desired tissue/cell types and across the plasma membrane and into the cytoplasm.

Unmodified siRNAs, also referred to as naked siRNAs, are known to be extremely short-lived *in vivo* with a half-life of minutes [28, 106] due to degradation by nucleases in the serum and rapid clearance via kidney filtration, a result of the siRNA's small molecular weight (~7 kilodaltons). However, the half-life can be significantly increased by incorporating chemical modifications and by encapsulation in carriers (Reviewed in [33]) (Figure 7.2). Chemical modifications at the 2′-position of the ribose backbone prevent degradation by RNases [21]. Chemically conjugating siRNAs to cholesterol allows for efficient uptake in cells in the absence of a transfection reagent and significantly slows renal clearance of siRNAs [106]. Similarly, encapsulation within nanocarriers also improves siRNA stability, slows clearance, and improves biodistribution [40].

Off-target effects can never be completely avoided as a stretch of just seven nucleotides is sufficient to achieve translational inhibition; as is seen with targets of microRNAs. A careful design of inhibitory RNAs to minimize unintended sequence matches is very important. Additionally, off-targeting caused by incorporation of the passenger strand, instead of the antisense strand of the siRNA into RISC can be avoided by designing the siRNA ends to thermodynamically favor RISC uptake of the active antisense strand. It has been experimentally shown that certain nucleotide motifs are more likely to induce the innate immune system [62]. Therefore, avoiding these motifs when designing siRNAs can significantly reduce the likelihood of toxicity due to activation of the innate immune response.

Controlled biodistribution is key to increasing efficacy by concentrating RNAi mediators at the site of action and also reducing toxicity of RNAi mediators in unintended cell types. Once the inhibitory RNAs have been administered it is imperative that they encounter the intended tissues/cells. Administering the inhibitory RNAs directly to the intended tissue is sometimes plausible as with intranasal (i.n.) and intraocular inoculations. Further, the impenetrance of several cell types to naked siRNA and impracticality of physical methods like electroporation and hydrodynamic injections for clinical application makes it essential to find a means to target delivery upon systemic administration of inhibitory RNAs. A few approaches have been achieved *in vivo* by encasing siRNAs within lipids that enable delivery to the liver [92] or conjugation to molecules like tetramers, peptides or antibodies that recognize surface receptors on target cells [70, 72, 135]. This also enables uptake of the siRNAs not capable of passive diffusion into cells.

Designing RNAi-therapeutics to treat viral infections faces additional and unique challenges. The high sequence specificity of siRNAs allows mutating viruses to escape under siRNA pressure. Escape can occur by changing just one nucleotide within the target sequence [12]. Further, numerous viruses have evolved efficient suppressors of RNAi that could compromise antiviral RNAi strategies [8, 80]. Targeting an early stage in the viral life cycle before a suppressor accumulates, or directly targeting the suppressor mRNA, may be necessary to circumvent these mechanisms of viral resistance. The use of inhibitory RNAs that target multiple highly conserved regions of the viral RNA where mutations would be associated with a loss in viral fitness or host factors that are immutable and do not cause adverse effects upon being depleted (i.e., the HIV coreceptor CCR5) may prevent escape mutants.

Since RNAi was first described we have been witness to identification of potent problems associated with RNAi therapeutics and several innovations for overcoming them to enable the potential translation of RNAi into a viable clinical therapeutic modality. The first siRNA-based antiviral to successfully enter phase I clinical trials in 2007 used siRNAs to target Respiratory syncytial virus (RSV) infection [29]. Since then several other RNAi-based drugs are being tested in clinical trials, with many more in the pipeline. In this chapter, we lay a special emphasis on the numerous RNAi-based approaches that have shown promise as antivirals in preclinical animal models and clinical trials (summarized in Table 7.1).

Table 7.1 Antiviral RNAi-based therapeutics

Virus	Drug Name	RNAi Type	Delivery Method	Stage	Reference
HBV	N/A	shRNA	Hydrodynamic Tail vein	Murine Model	[86]
	N/A	shRNA	Adeno-associated virus	Murine Model	[45]
	N/A	siRNA	SNALPs	Murine Model	[91, 92]
	N/A	siRNA	Apo A-I cationic nanoparticle	Murine Model	[65]
	N/A	siRNA	Single-chain antibody	Murine Model	[116]
HPV	N/A	shRNA	*Ex vivo* lentiviral transduction	Murine Model	[47]
	N/A	siRNA	Intratumoral	Murine Model	[126]
HSV-2	N/A	siRNA	Intravaginal microbiocide	Murine Model	[98]
	N/A	siRNA	Cholesterol	Murine Model	[124]
WNV	N/A	siRNA	Hydrodynamic tail vein	Murine Model	[5]
JEV/ WNV	N/A	shRNA	Lentivirus pseudotyped with RVG (i.c.)	Murine Model	[71]
	N/A	siRNA	i.c.	Murine Model	[71]
	N/A	siRNA	i.v. complexed to RVG	Murine Model	[72]
YFV	N/A	shRNA	i.c.	Murine Model	[97]
HCV	ISIS 14803	ASO	i.v	Phase II discontinued	[87]
	Miravirsen	ASO	s.c.	Phase II ongoing	[22]
	N/A	siRNA	Cationic liposome	Marmoset GBV-B Model	[129]

Virus	Drug Name	RNAi Type	Delivery Method	Stage	Reference
SARS	N/A	siRNA	Intratracheal/Intranasal	Rhesus Macaque	[77]
HIV	VRX496	asRNA	*Ex vivo* lentiviral transduction	Phase II ongoing	[76]
	rHIV7-shI-TAR-CCR5RZ	shRNA	*Ex vivo* lentiviral transduction	Phase I completed	[31]
HIV	N/A	shRNA	*Ex vivo* lentiviral transduction	Rhesus Macaque	[2]
	CCR5-ZZ-SIN	shRNA	targeted lentiviral transduction	Hu-PBL mouse model	[4]
	scFVCD7-9R	siRNA	i.v.	Hu-PBL, Hu-HSC mouse models	[70]
	N/A	siRNA	i.v. targeted nanoliposomes	BLT humanized mouse	[66]
	N/A	siRNA	i.v. aptamer targeted	RAG-hu	[134]
RSV	ALN-RSV01	siRNA	i.n.	Phase II completed	[30]
	N/A	siRNA	i.n.	Murine model	[11, 130]
EBOV	N/A	PMO	i.p.	Murine, guinea pig, non-human primate models	[42, 115]
	N/A	siRNA	SNALPs	Non-human primate models	[43]
Influenza	N/A	ODN	i.v. liposome	Murine model	[55, 90]
	N/A	siRNA	i.v.	Murine Model	[41, 110, 125, 132]
	N/A	siRNA	i.n.	Chickens	[125]

7.2 DNA Viruses

7.2.1 Hepatitis B Virus (HBV)

HBV, a member of the *Hepadnavirus* family, comprises a partially double-stranded relaxed circular DNA genome. HBV poses a threat to public health worldwide, with an estimated 350 million people being chronically infected with the virus and an estimated 600,000–1,200,000 HBV-related deaths per year [74]. Chronic infection with HBV can lead to significant health problems including cirrhosis of the liver and hepatocellular carcinoma. Although a very effective HBV vaccine exists, therapeutics for individuals infected with HBV are lacking [74]. Currently, chronic HBV infections are treated with interferon-α, often in combination with nucleoside or nucleotide analogues. However, the low overall efficacy, poor compliance and toxicity of these drug regimens [94] have spurred an interest in potential RNAi therapies for chronic HBV infection despite the lack of relevant and reliable small animal models for HBV [105].

One of earliest *in vivo* studies by McAffrey and coworkers [86] tested a panel of seven different U6 promoter driven anti-HBV shRNAs targeting sequences conserved across HBV genotypes for blocking HBV replication from a plasmid expressing the HBV genome. Hydrodynamic transfection of mice via tail vein injections with both the shRNA and HBV expression plasmids resulted in a reduction of serum HBV surface antigen (HBsAg) and liver-associated HBV core antigen (HBcAg). The negative strand of the HBV genome consists of four partially overlapping open-reading frames (ORFs) that encode the viral transcripts [104]. The most effective shRNA mapped to a sequence in the overlapping reading frames enabling the simultaneous targeting of 3 of the 4 viral RNA transcripts [86]. Another study treated mice with hepatocytes transgenic for HBV with hepatotropic recombinant adenoviruses expressing anti-HBV shRNAs targeting the same sequence in the overlapping ORFs. This also led to reduced serum HBsAg and liver HBcAg levels throughout a 26-day period of experimentation [112].

Numerous studies have since demonstrated shRNA-mediated repression of HBV replication in murine models [18, 20, 32, 44, 45, 100–102, 105]. However, the results of one particular *in vivo* study raised concern over the use of shRNAs in human therapy.

Treatment of mice with an adeno-associated viral vector expressing shRNA resulted in fatality by oversaturation of the host's RNAi machinery [45]. Exportin-5, the enzyme responsible for mediating the export of both pre-miRNAs and shRNAs out of the nucleus [128], was determined to be the limiting factor. After this report, several strategies of shRNA expression were developed to address this concern. Use of a tissue-specific vector expressing shRNA from the liver-derived polymerase (Pol) II promoter reduced shRNA levels and restricted shRNA expression and thereby toxic effects, if any, to liver hepatocytes. Remarkably, Pol II expression of shRNA persisted for more than 1 year after injection without any evidence of liver damage [44]. More recently, a tRNA Pol III promoter was used to express shRNAs as pre-miRs. When generated this way the shRNAs get processed by alternative mechanisms that do not require the conventional microprocessor complex and hence do not disrupt the endogenous miRNA pathway. Thus, anti-HBV shRNA expressed from a $tRNA^{Lys3}$ promoter effectively inhibited HBV *in vivo* with minimal toxicity [32]. Additionally, reducing the dosage by using Pol II promoters instead of a U6 promoter for expression as well as shortening the length of the expressed shRNA to a maximum of 19 nucleotides significantly reduces toxicity [45].

A gene therapeutic approach that provides stable shRNA expression is considered as the ideal option for treating a chronic infection such as HBV. However, synthetic siRNAs modified to incorporate 2-fluoro, 2-*O*-methyl, and 2-deoxysugars, phosphorothioate linkages, and terminus capping chemistries displayed extended serum stability of up to 3 days, abrogated immunostimulation through innate immune recognition pathways and were at least 1.5 $\log_{10}$ times more effective than unmodified siRNAs in reducing HBsAg and HBcAg in a HBV vector-based murine model [91, 92]. This approach minimizes the risk of oversaturating the exportin-dependent processing pathway. However, the requirement of three daily doses of 30 mg/kg for several days makes it prohibitively expensive for HBV therapy. Subsequently the same group of investigators developed a novel lipid bilayer containing a mixture of cationic and fusogenic lipids coated with diffusible polyethylene glycol. These 120 nanometer wide biopolymers labeled SNALPs, for Stable-Nucleic-Acid-Lipid-Particles, shielded siRNAs from serum nucleases and allowed cellular endosomal uptake and subsequent cytoplasmic release of siRNAs [91, 92]. Using the SNALP approach, the dosing regimen was reduced 10 fold to 3 mg/kg three times daily and a single weekly injection was sufficient to maintain greater than 10-fold inhibition of HBV antigen production up to 6 weeks.

Complexing siRNAs to the liver-specific protein apolipoprotein A-I (apo A-I) is yet another method that has been utilized to target delivery of anti-HBV siRNAs to the liver. Apo A-I was formulated onto nanoparticles carrying siRNAs, which were then administered i.v. to mice expressing replicating HBV in the liver [65]. *In vivo* experiments with luciferase reporter siRNAs demonstrated that siRNAs delivered by apo A-I nanoparticles are effectively and specifically delivered to the liver. Moreover, delivery of anti-HBV siRNAs with these nanoparticles significantly reduced HBsAg for up to 8 days post-treatment.

Another method for targeting delivery that is gaining in popularity is the use of cell type-specific antibodies. A slight modification of this method has been used to deliver siRNAs specifically to HBV infected hepatocytes. Rather than delivering siRNAs to hepatocytes in general, one group has used a humanized anti-HBV single-chain antibody to deliver siRNAs specifically to HBsAg-positive cells *in vivo* [116]. siRNA delivered with this method were efficiently delivered to HBs-Ag-positive cells and inhibited HBV gene expression in HBV transgenic mice. All of the aforementioned studies suggest that siRNAs are a feasible antiviral therapy for the treatment of HBV and that several methods can be utilized to target delivery of these siRNAs, therefore increasing potency while reducing toxicity.

7.2.2 Human Papillomavirus (HPV)

HPV is one of the most prevalent sexually transmitted diseases in the world [14]. HPV causes cervical cancer; the second leading cause of cancer related deaths in women [122]. A HPV vaccine for immunization of women between 9 and 26 years of age exists; however, there are currently no effective therapies for individuals already infected with HPV and a small fraction of those patients will develop cancer in a decade or two. More than 200 genotypes of HPV exist, but HPV-16 and HPV-18 alone account for approximately 70% of cervical cancers worldwide [122]. HPV is a member of the family *Papovaviridae*, a group of double-stranded circular DNA viruses. The DNA genome of HPV encodes 6 early genes (E1, E2, E4, E5, E6 and E7) and two late genes (L1 and L2) [14]. The oncogenic properties of

E6 and E7 proteins make the corresponding RNA transcripts targets for anti-HPV RNAi therapies. siRNAs targeting the E6 protein of HPV-16 are capable of inhibiting expression of both E6 and E7, as both mRNAs are bicistronically transcribed. HeLa cervical cancer cells transduced with a lentiviral vector-expressing shRNAs targeting the HPV-18 E6 RNA produced significantly smaller tumors in $Rag^{-/-}$ mice. Tumor repression was dosage dependent with high doses of shRNA-expressing vector completely abrogating tumor development [47]. Moreover, systemically delivered lentivirus-shRNA could inhibit the growth of established tumors in a murine lung metastasis model. In an interesting variation to RNAi-based tumor therapy, the RNAi mechanism was used to induce anti-tumor immune responses to HPV proteins. Translation of incomplete protein products from anti-E6 shRNA-cleaved mRNA resulted in increased presentation of the target protein and the generation of immune response that protected mice from a subsequent challenge with tumor cells [46]. More recently, anti-E6/E7 siRNAs designed using the current algorithms for optimal siRNAs were very effective in controlling tumor growth in a therapeutic *in vivo* experimental setup in NOD/SCID mice. siHa HPV16+ cervical cancer cell-derived tumors could be regressed as late as 6 weeks after tumor establishment by daily intratumoral injections of anti-E6/E7 siRNA for a total of 30 days [126]. All these promising data suggest that RNAi therapy may speed up the reduction in rates of HPV incidence and cervical cancer when used in parallel with HPV vaccines.

7.2.3 Herpes Simplex Virus 2 (HSV-2)

HSV-2 is a sexually transmitted viral infection, which often produces painful sores, usually in the genital area. It has been estimated that 536 million people are infected with HSV-2 globally [82]. Suppressive antiviral drugs like valacyclovir effectively minimize symptoms and reduce the risk of viral transmission during a symptomatic outbreak. However, the mostly asymptomatic nature of HSV-2 infections is a huge cause for concern as HSV-2 is also an important cofactor for transmission of the HIV. People infected with HSV-2 are twice as likely to become infected with HIV and four times as likely to transmit HIV to others [19]. A topical microbicide with the ability to protect against HSV-2 at the site of infection is expected to contribute significantly to controlling HSV-2 and HIV transmission.

HSV-2, a member of the *Herpesviridae* family of viruses is a double-stranded DNA virus with a complex genome that encodes more than 80 proteins. In a study conducted to evaluate the use of siRNAs as topical vaginal microbiocides, the HSV-2 genes UL27 (the HSV-2 envelope glycoprotein), and UL29 (the gene encoding ICP8, a DNA binding protein) were targeted [98]. Mice treated intravaginally with the two siRNAs complexed with a transfection lipid prior to lethal challenge with HSV-2 exhibited increased survival rates (60% and 75% with the anti-UL27 and –UL29 siRNAs, respectively, compared with a 25% survival in control groups) and decreased viral shedding. When siRNAs were administered 3 and 6 hours after lethal challenge with HSV-2, only a combination of both UL27 and UL29 siRNAs resulted in protection. This study highlighted that siRNA can be effectively taken up at mucosal surfaces; however, the lipid vehicle used to deliver the siRNA unfortunately also helped transmit the virus nucleic acid.

A subsequent study by the same group investigated the effects of treating mice with cholesterol-conjugated siRNAs that enable direct entry across the cell membrane [124]. A solution made of siRNAs targeting UL29 and the host gene nectin-1 (the HSV-2 cellular receptor) led to rapid but short-lived viral suppression while targeting UL27, and a delayed but long-lasting suppression for up to a week when the host molecule was targeted. This study demonstrated the benefits of using fast-acting-but-short-lived RNAi with the slower-acting-but-long-lived RNAi and underscored the feasibility of treating HSV-2, and possibly other sexually transmitted diseases, by topical application of cholesterol-conjugated siRNAs.

7.3 Positive-Strand RNA Viruses

7.3.1 Flaviviruses

The genus *Flavivirus* comprises approximately 70 species of small, enveloped viruses with ~ 11 kilobase long positive-sense genomic RNA [49] encoding a single ORF of three structural and seven nonstructural (NS) proteins [81] bounded by a 5′ and 3′ untranslated region (UTR). At least 38 flaviviruses (55% of all flaviviruses) are medically important causing severe human disease with different clinical manifestations [52]. The extraordinary ability of flaviviruses to utilize new vectors for transmission and spread to new geographic regions highlights the need for a safe and efficient antiviral therapy for these emergent and recurrent infectious agents [84]. Flaviviruses, like other positive-sense RNA viruses, use their RNA genomes for both replication and translation in the host cell cytoplasm, making them an attractive target for the cytoplasmically located host RNAi machinery.

7.3.1.1 Encephalitic flaviviruses: Japanese encephalitis virus (JEV) and West Nile virus (WNV)

Japanese encephalitis virus (JEV), a mosquito-borne flavivirus, is the major cause of pediatric encephalitis in Asia resulting in up to 50,000 cases reported annually [118]. West Nile virus (WNV) another closely related mosquito-borne encephalitic flavivirus was endemic in Africa, Asia and Europe before 1999 [48]. In 1999 after the first incidence in New York, USA, the virus quickly spread becoming endemic to all the 50 states within 4 years causing thousands of human infections and hundreds of deaths each year [48]. Two prophylactic JEV vaccines are available for human use; however, no antiviral therapies exist for any flavivirus.

The major hurdle for harnessing the therapeutic efficacy of RNAi for flaviviral encephalitis is the presence of a blood brain barrier (BBB) that restricts siRNA delivery into the brain tissue. The very first *in vivo* demonstration of the feasibility of RNAi therapy for encephalitic flaviviruses tested the effects of two different siRNAs targeting the WNV envelope gene in the murine model of WNV infection [5]. Only one of the siRNAs reduced the viral load and afforded partial protection when administered in the naked form by hydrodynamic tail vein injection 24h before lethal challenge with an intraperitoneal (i.p.) inoculum of WNV. The poor *in vivo* efficacy was perhaps due to the inefficient delivery of siRNA to brain tissue.

In 2006, a study by Kumar and coworkers [71] examined the protective effects of RNAi therapies using intracranial (i.c.) injections for the delivery of si/shRNA targeting sequences in the envelope gene of JEV and WNV. Using a lentiviral vector pseudotyped with the rabies virus glycoprotein (RVG) for improved neuronal spread, they achieved complete protection of mice against challenge with both WNV and JEV using shRNAs targeting the corresponding envelope gene sequences. Excellent protection was also observed upon i.c. injection of synthetic siRNA complexed to lipid delivery reagents. The study tested two cationic lipids i-Fect and JetSI/DOPE that varied in their capacity to complex siRNAs. The ability of JetSI/DOPE to package a higher dosage of siRNA improved survival statistics with 60% of the mice treated as late as 18 hrs post challenge recovering from encephalitis. The study demonstrated that short-lived synthetic siRNAs were sufficient to protect against acute neuronal infections like flaviviral encephalitis by persisting for extended periods of time in non-dividing cells like neurons. Perhaps the most notable feature of the study was the ability of a synthetic siRNA designed against the conserved fusion-loop region of the flaviviral envelope to provide cross-protection against both JEV and WNV. 100% of the mice were protected when treated with lipid-siRNA complexes before viral challenge while 80% of mice having an established infection with WNV or JEV were protected. These results emphasized the power of RNAi therapeutics as broad-spectrum antivirals against related viruses with practically indistinguishable clinical manifestations.

Furthering their studies, the same group developed a novel method for the transvascular delivery of siRNAs into the brain tissue across the BBB [72]. A chimeric peptide consisting of a 32 amino acid sequence derived from the RVG for binding of the α7 subunit of the nicotinic actylcholine receptor expressed on neuronal cells and a positively charged D-arginine nonamer for siRNA binding was used as the siRNA nanocarrier. This peptide electrostatically complexed siRNA at a 10:1 M ratio to form particles ~110 nm in diameter and delivered the payload specifically into mouse brain tissue *in vivo* after simple intravenous (i.v.) injection. Treatment with complexes containing siRNA targeting the flaviviral envelope gene protected 80% of mice from a lethal challenge with JEV, without activating an innate interferon response. Taken together, the results from these studies suggested that siRNA-nanocarriers are a viable therapy for treating acute flaviviral encephalitis.

7.3.1.2 Hemorrhagic flaviviruses: Yellow fever virus (YFV) and dengue virus (DENV)

YFV, also a mosquito-borne flavivirus causes severe hepatitis and hemorrhagic fever. Despite the existence of an effective vaccine for more than 70 years now, YFV still results in nearly 200,000 human infections per year, mostly in Africa and South America due to incomplete vaccination of endemic inhabitants [7]. The closely related DENV is a group of four antigenically distinct serotypes (DENV1-4) that cause dengue fever (DF), and in more severe cases dengue hemorrhagic fever (DHF) and dengue shock syndrome (DSS). Annually, DENV infects an estimated 100 million people [49] with 500,000 of these cases resulting in DHF/DSS and 25,000 deaths per year [84]. The high amount of morbidity and mortality associated with this virus makes DENV the most epidemiologically significant arthropod-borne virus [57]. As with most flaviviruses, no vaccines or therapies exist for DENV infections. Small animal models that manifest clinical signs consistent with viscerotropism, acute hepatitis, and hemorrhagic fever upon infection with these viruses have been lacking, limiting evaluation of antiviral RNAi strategies to cell lines and mosquito vectors.

Using an intracerebral acute challenge murine model for YFV, the ability of shRNAs targeting highly conserved sites in the YFV genome to protect from lethal challenge was investigated [97]. I.c. injection with a plasmid expressing the anti-NS1 shRNA but not anti-envelope shRNA provided a small, but significant amount of protection from lethal challenge. The study suggested that RNAi may be a feasible YFV therapy but would likely depend on the sequences targeted.

An adeno-associated virus carrying an siRNA targeting the 3′UTR of DENV resulted in a dose-dependent inhibition of DENV in human dendritic cells (DCs), the primary cell target of the virus [49]. In an effort to target these cells *in vivo*, a DC3 peptide previously identified to bind DCs was modified to incorporate the 9R carrier (as described above in [72]).Treatment with this DC3-9dR nanocarrier complexed to siRNA targeting the DENV envelope gene inhibited DENV replication in both DCs and macrophages [108]. The cytokine TNF-α is believed to be the mediator of plasma leakage seen in DHF/DSS patients [103]. A siRNA targeting TNF-α used in conjunction with the DC3-9R nanocarrier significantly reduced DENV-induced TNF-α expression in DCs *in vitro* and poly-IC-induced TNF-α expression *in vivo*. DENV infected DCs that were simultaneously treated with DENV and TNF-α siRNAs showed decreased TNF-α expression and decreased viral loads. Taken together these results suggest an RNAi-therapy targeting both the virus and a host gene could be developed to control the immunopathology associated with DENV infection.

7.3.3 Hepatitis C Virus (HCV)

HCV is a member of the genus hepacivirus in the family *Flaviviridae* and causes serious liver diseases such as cirrhosis and hepatocellular carcinoma in chronically infected individuals. The World Health Organization (WHO) estimates that 3% of the world's population is infected with HVC, with 170 million being chronically infected [119]. The current treatments for HCV with pegylated IFN-α in combination with ribavirin is only effective in about 50% of the treated individuals and is associated with serious side effects [37, 94]. Therefore, RNAi therapy is being actively investigated as a plausible treatment method for chronic HCV.

The positive-sense RNA genome of HCV is very similar to that of other flaviviruses, but the 5'UTR contains an internal ribosomal entry site (IRES), which controls translation of the genome [75]. The high conservation of the IRES makes it a good target for antisense RNA-based therapies. For instance, i.v. administration of an antisense oligonucleotide (ASO) ISIS 14803 targeting the IRES of the HCV genome completed phase I clinical trials [87] although the phase II trial was discontinued due to unsatisfactory results [50]. Along the same lines, Santaris Pharma is testing an ASO (SPC3649) targeting the cellular microRNA-122 (miR-122) as this miRNA is required for efficient HCV replication [61]. In a recent publication, systemic i.v. administration of SPC3649 at 5mg/kg in chimpanzees chronically infected with HCV resulted in a significant decrease in serum HCV RNA beginning 3 weeks after start of treatment and lasting several weeks after cessation of treatment without inducing mutations in the HCV RNA [73]. This ASO, which has been renamed Miravirsen, completed a phase I clinical trial in September of 2010 [25] and moved on to a phase II clinical trial where it is being administered subcutaneously to chronic HCV patients [22].

Testing of RNAi-based antivirals to HCV has been slowed by the absence of tractable small animal models. One study that came closest to investigating RNAi control of viral hepatitis *in vivo* used non-human primates infected with the closely related GB virus (GBV)-B as a surrogate model for hepatitis C [129]. The significant similarity between HCV and the flavivirus-like virus GBV-B at the genomic and biochemical levels and the fact that intrahepatic inoculation of new world monkeys like tamarins and marmosets with GBV-B RNA establishes persistent infection with chronic hepatic inflammation, both of which are key features of hepatitis C infection, has led to the proposal of the GBV-B/monkey system as a good surrogate model for hepatitis C [85]. Administration into marmosets of cationic liposome-encapsulated siRNA targeting the

5′UTR of GBV-B repressed GBV-B replication in a dose-dependent manner. However, since elevated levels of serum IFNs were observed upon siRNA treatment, the study concluded that the observed antiviral effect was attributable to both RNAi as well as activation of innate immune responses. Nevertheless, the promising results with siRNAs, shRNAs and lhRNAs targeting structural (i.e., core and envelope) and nonstructural proteins, the HCV IRES and CD81, the human receptor for HCV in cell culture assays (reviewed in [56, 64]) indicate that RNAi based approaches is a feasible therapy for HCV infection.

7.3.4 SARS Coronavirus (SARS-CoV)

The SARS epidemic, which started in November 2002 in the People's Republic of China spread to 29 countries, resulted in more than 8,000 cases and 744 reported deaths within a year [114]. By July 2003, a novel coronavirus, SARS-CoV was identified as the etiological agent of SARS [69]. SARS-CoV, like other coronaviruses, has a large positive-sense RNA genome encoding 14 ORFs, including 2 overlapping reading frames ORF 1a and 1b, which account for more than two-thirds of the genome [131]. While vaccine and therapeutic drug development have been an area of ongoing research since the outbreak, neither are currently approved for use [107]. This has highlighted the need for novel treatments like RNAi-based ones.

Two siRNAs targeting the mRNA encoding the spike protein and non-structural protein 12 were identified in a screen for potent conserved RNAi targets conducted in SARS-CoV-infected Rhesus monkey kidney (FRhK-4) cells [131]. These were further validated for the prophylactic and therapeutic treatment of SARS infection in a Rhesus macaque model [77]. Reporter gene assays in mice demonstrated that both siRNAs, administered intratracheally in D5W (5% dextrose/water solution) were effectively delivered to the lungs and were able to effectively reduce luciferase expression from reporters bearing the target sequences. Furthermore, SARS-CoV infected macaques treated intranasally (i.n.) with the two siRNAs individually or in combination showed significantly lower body temperatures when treated prior to or after being infected, although siRNA dosages varied from 30 to 120 mg over a 120h treatment time. The best prognosis was seen in macaques on a prophylactic regimen with the smallest dose of 30mg siRNA. The treatment provided relief from SARS-CoV infection–induced fever, diminished SARS-CoV viral levels, and reduced antiviral IgG titers and acute diffuse alveoli damage; all without siRNA-mediated toxicity or inflammation even at the highest doses of siRNA.

More recently, an *in vitro* study examining the interaction between SARS-CoV and its cellular receptor angiotensin-converting enzyme 2 (ACE2) discovered that interaction between the viral spike protein and ACE2 triggers activation of TNF-α-converting enzyme (TACE) [51]. Knockdown of both ACE2 and TACE by siRNAs inhibited SARS-CoV infection, suggesting that these two cellular proteins may also be vital targets for SARS-CoV treatment. Cumulatively, the studies discussed above reveal the functional ability of siRNAs to inhibit both SARS-CoV replication and infection by targeting viral and/or host RNA, supporting the notion that RNAi can be harnessed to provide a novel antiviral against SARS.

7.4 Retroviruses

7.4.1 Human Immunodeficiency Virus (HIV)

HIV, the retrovirus that causes AIDS, has infected over 34 million people worldwide. The HIV genome is a diploid positive sense RNA genome encoding 9 ORFs that give rise to 15 viral proteins. The ends of the genome have repeats called long terminal repeats (LTRs) that act as the promoter driving HIV gene expression and contain sites for integration into the host genome. Gene expression is biphasic, the early and late, the late genes requiring the presence of a rev protein expressed during the early phase. Highly active antiretroviral therapy (HAART) that involves treatment with over 25 antiretroviral drugs given in combinations of 3 has been very effective at suppressing HIV levels and extending the average life span of the infected by at least 10 years. However, the prohibitive costs, non-compliance and development of viral resistance hinder long-term treatment regimens. RNAi has been seriously considered supportive therapy for the clinical management of HIV-AIDS. Historically, HIV was the first virus against which the inhibitory effects of RNAi were demonstrated in tissue culture [95]. The successful repression of viral replication using combinations of siRNAs targeting multiple conserved sequences in the viral genome or host factors have spurred the evaluation of a number of RNAi-based drugs in *in vivo* preclinical animal models and in clinical trials.

The first clinical trial for gene therapy against HIV used a conditionally-replicating lentiviral vector expressing a LTR-driven long antisense RNA (asRNA), VRX494. This asRNA targeted a large sequence in the envelope gene and showed great promise in cell culture experiments. Mutant viruses generated contained large deletions in the envelope that resulted in a significant loss of fitness [60, 83]. A phase I nonrandomized clinical trial initiated in 2003 recruited five subjects with chronic drug resistant HIV who were transfused with ~10 billion VRX496 transduced autologous CD4+ T cells [76]. Despite low levels of long-term engraftment, three subjects showed strong decline in viral titers (0.75 log to 1.7 logs), four had elevated $CD4^+$ T cell counts at 1 year following engraftment and three had elevated IFN-γ responses and increases in general immune function up to 2 years following treatment. The major safety concerns that were quelled by this study included integration site preferences (integration was random), emergence of replication-competent lentivirus (none was detected at any time point), and vector mobilization into non-target tissues (mobilization was transient and did not appear after day 60). Further clinical trials have been initiated including two phase II trials evaluating multiple doses or a higher single dose and one phase I/II trial, which will stop HAART on patients following infusion of VRX496 treated cells [113].

Unlike asRNAs, the short length and high sequence specificity of siRNAs necessitates targeting multiple highly conserved sequences for suppressing viral escape under siRNA pressure. A recent clinical study utilized a lentiviral vector, rHIV7-shI-TAR-CCR5RZ, encoding a CCR5 targeting ribozyme (R5RZ), a TAR decoy, and shRNA targeting a *tat/rev* exon (shI), [6, 15, 31, 78, 79, 89]. The triple combination vector efficiently transduced human $CD34^+$ hematopoetic stem cells (HSC) and did not affect their ability to differentiate into fully functional immune cells upon engraftment of SCID-hu mice [3]. Transgenic thymoctes isolated from these mice and challenged with $HIV_{NL4\text{-}3}$ showed >1 log reduction in viral loads. This triple combination vector has since been evaluated in a clinical phase I trial [31]. Four patients with AIDS-related lymphoma and on HAART therapy were treated with a single allograft of 7.3×10^5 to 1.6×10^6 autologous $CD34^+$ cells transduced with the triple combination lentiviral vector. At 18 months, all patients remained in remission from lymphoma and had gene marking frequencies between 0.2 and 0.32% of peripheral blood mononuclear cells (PBMCs). Vector expressed RNAs were detectable up to 24 months following infusion and marking was seen in T cells, monocytes, B cells, and Lin^- subsets indicating that HSC were truly transduced. A second pilot study is now recruiting patients who have failed anti-retroviral therapy for infusion of autologous T-cells transduced with the same vector in multiple doses [24].

The natural resistance of CCR5Δ32 homozygous individuals to HIV [27, 58] has made CCR5 a promising target for both small molecule inhibitors, such as the FDA-approved maraviroc, and RNAi based interventions. Clinical proof-of-principle was provided by transplantation of stem cells from a CCR5Δ32 homozygous donor into a HIV^+ leukemic patient [59]. Following transplant, HIV levels have remained undetectable even after discontinuing HAART. As only ~1% of Caucasians are homozygous for the CCR5Δ32 mutation and there is currently no infrastructure to track these individuals, RNAi targeting CCR5 is being explored as an alternative to homozygous donor stem cell transplantation. In a preclinical experiment with non-human primates Rhesus macaque $CD34^+$ HSC transduced *ex vivo* with a lentiviral vector encoding a H1 driven shRNA targeting the macaque CCR5 was stably maintained for up to 14 months after transplantation into autologous recipients with no toxicity [2]. Surface levels of CCR5 decreased 3–10-fold and CCR5 mRNA levels decreased 5–10-fold. Lymphocytes isolated from these animals demonstrated a higher resistance to *in vitro* challenge with SIV_{mac239}.

Viral vectors capable of specifically transducing only the desired cell type after systemic administration have also been investigated to alleviate the high costs and sophisticated manipulations associated with *ex vivo* transduction protocols. Lentiviral vectors expressing shRNA targeting CCR5 were pseudotyped with a Sindbis virus envelope that expresses the Fc binding domain (ZZ) of *S. aureus* protein A [4]. Conjugation of this ZZ-SIN vector to a α-CCR5 monoclonal antibody enabled targeting of CCR5-expressing $CD3^+$ T cells and $CD14^+$ macrophages but not $CD19^+$ B cells upon i.v. administration into NOD-SCID-IL2rγ mice reconstituted with human PBMC.

Synthetic siRNAs allow for varying siRNA sequences to keep pace with the mutating virus if the need arises during the course of treatment unlike lentivirally delivered shRNA. However, the greatest impediment to the use of siRNA for HIV therapy is the intransigence of immune cells, particularly primary T cells to siRNA uptake. Using a single-chain antibody to the human T cell-specific surface molecule CD7 coupled to the siRNA carrier oligo-9-D-arginine (scFVCD7-9R), Kumar and coworkers showed that systemic T cell specific siRNA delivery for the treatment of HIV is a feasible strategy [70]. Binding of the scFv to CD7 induced internalization enabling cytoplasmic delivery of the siRNAs. Weekly treatment with scFVCD7-9R complexed to a combination of siRNAs targeting the viral genes *vif* and *tat* and/or CCR5 enabled control of HIV infection in two different humanized mouse models — NOD-SCID-IL2rγ mice reconstituted with human PBMC or HSC. The treatment was also able to suppress endogenous virus in mice reconstituted with PBMC from a HIV-positive donor. Significantly this approach enabled siRNA delivery into naïve and resting T cells, important reservoirs for latent HIV that develop in NOD-SCID-IL2rγ mice reconstituted with human HSC, and resulted in reduced viral loads and maintenance of normal CD4 T cell numbers with no toxicity or disruption of endogenous RNAi pathway.

One drawback of using scFvCD7 was the inability to target other cells infectable with HIV such as macrophages and dendritic cells. Recently, this group tested a new strategy where neutral lipid based siRNA carriers were surface modified to include an antibody directed against LFA-1, an integrin present on all leukocytes [66]. These nanoliposomes allowed the delivery of a siRNA payload 3 logs greater than the arginine carrier. i.v. treatment of humanized mice with 50 μg encapsulated siRNA targeting CCR5 three times during viral challenge enabled control of viral replication for nearly 2 months and did not require the weekly treatment regimen used in the previous study.

An alternate approach targeted HIV infected cells using RNA aptamers against HIV gp120 that get internalized after binding their target. The gp-120 aptamer was either (i) covalently linked to siRNAs that target the HIV-1 *tat/rev* common exon, or (ii) non-covalently linked to siRNAs via complementary GC-rich sticky bridge sequences attached to the 3′ end of the aptamer and to one of the two siRNA strands, which allowed Watson–Crick base pairing [135]. While the first method allowed delivery of a single siRNA the second facilitated the effective interchange of different siRNAs with a single aptamer. Hence this approach was tested with a combination of siRNAs targeting the *tat/rev* common exon and the HIV host dependency factors CD4 and transportin 3. Further, because both the aptamer and the siRNA can inhibit HIV-1 replication by respectively blocking the gp120-CD4 receptor interaction and silencing target gene expression, this novel anti-gp120 aptamer-siRNA chimera possessed a dual inhibitory function. i.v. injection of these chimeras in the 4th week of infection into humanized mice dramatically decreased viral loads to undetectable levels within a week after administration and completely prevented T-cell depletion (unpublished observations) [134].

Taken together, these studies show that gene therapy using RNAi is a feasible approach to control HIV infection.

7.5 Negative-Sense RNA Viruses

7.5.1 Respiratory Syncytial Virus

Globally, RSV is the leading cause of acute lower respiratory infections with an estimated 33.5 million new episodes and 199,000 deaths in children under five in 2005 [93]. Currently there are only two FDA-approved drugs for the treatment of RSV, a monoclonal antibody Palivizumab for use in high-risk infants and Ribavirin for severe infections though not recommended by the American Academy of Pediatrics due to the limited evidence of benefit, high cost, and potential toxic effects [35]. RSV is a member of the *Paramyxoviridae* family with a negative sense single stranded RNA genome encoding 10 viral proteins. Of these, the G glycoprotein distinguishes the two antigenic subgroups, RSV-A and RSV-B, within the RSV serotype. The virus replicates in the outermost layer of the respiratory epithelium that lines the human respiratory tract that is easily accessible to nasally applied naked siRNA [10]. RNAi is therefore an option for RSV treatment.

ALN-RSV01 is a siRNA directed against a highly conserved sequence in the nucleocapsid (N) protein gene sequence [1]. In a murine prophylaxis model, a 100 μg dose of ALN-RSV01 given i.n. 4 hours prior to infection with RSV A2 highly reduced titers in the lung. ALN-RSV01 also proved efficacious when administered in 40 μg doses on days 1, 2, and 3 post-infection (p.i.). ALN-RSV01 became the first siRNA-based antiviral to be tested in two human clinical trials in 2007 [29]. In both trials no serious adverse events were reported with single doses up to 150 mg or daily doses up to 150 mg daily for 5 days. This provided the foundation for a phase II trial whose promising results were recently reported [30]. Eighty five healthy males ages 18–45 were dosed i.n. two days before and three days after challenge with ~4.7 log PFU RSV A (Memphis 37). The dosages were 75 mg and 150 mg of ALN-RSV01 for the pre- and post infection studies. When compared with placebo-treated group, the ASN-RSV01 treated groups had a statistically lower proportion of subjects infected (44% vs. 71%) and a lower acquisition of infection over time. While not powered to show significance, the ALN-RSV01-treated groups trended toward lower viral loads when compared with placebo. Based on results from this trial, volunteers are now being recruited for a Phase IIb trial to assess efficacy of ALN-RSV01 in lung transplant patients infected with RSV [23].

RSV NS1 is thought to antagonize the host cell IFN response through an unknown mechanism and deletion of NS1 or NS2 attenuates RSV infection both *in vivo* and *in vitro* rendering NS1 a potential therapeutic target for siRNA mediated knockdown [109, 117]. Nanoparticles consisting of siRNA directed against NS1 complexed to a nanochitosan polymer effectively knocked down NS1 expression in mice treated i.n. [130]. This corresponded to significant decreases in viral titer, and a significant increase in IFN-β production for up to 4 days when treated prior to infection and up to 2 days p.i. The RSV phosphoprotein (P) complexes with the large protein (L) to form the viral RNA-dependent RNA polymerase. P protein is an essential transcription factor of L and inhibition of P has been shown to decrease viral transcription and replication [9]. Naked or TransitIT-TKO complexed siRNA against a P gene sequence was administered i.n. to mice prior to infection [11]. The complexed siRNA reduced pulmonary titers of RSV by 99.98% while naked siRNA was ~80% as effective. The advantage of siRNA therapy for lung infections is the reduced side effects in non-targeted tissues as siRNA and the transfection reagents congregate solely in the lung following i.n. administration.

7.5.2 Ebola (EBOV)

EBOV is a filovirus that causes severe hemorrhagic fever in humans and non-human primates. Although outbreaks in human populations are rare, they remain a major public health concern as potential agents of bioterrorism. There are currently no therapies for the treatment of EBOV and fatality rates range from 42–90% [54]. Reducing the rate of replication early in infection is expected to aid a successful immune response against EBOV. Transcription and replication of the filovirus genome relies on viral proteins VP35, VP30, the nucleoprotein (NP), and the viral polymerase (L). In addition to its role in transcription and replication, VP35 is also thought to repress host cell type I interferon responses.

PMOs against VP35 have been developed to suppress EBOV infection. Intracellular delivery of the PMOs was achieved by conjugation to a cell-penetrating arginine rich peptide (P-PMO) [36]. i.p. treatment of mice with 500 μg of P-PMO or unconjugated PMO against VP35 prior to infection with a lethal dose of EBOV ensured high survival rates of 100% and 85%, respectively. A single dose of 500 μg of VP35-specific P-PMO administered 24 hours after infection with a lethal dose of EBOV also resulted in survival rate of 100% [42]. A pool of four siRNAs against the L gene encapsulated in SNALPs and administered to guinea pigs at 1mg/kg i.p. daily for the first 6 days p.i. maintained plasma EBOV levels below the range of detection from day 12 through day 30. Combinatorial targeting with PMOs against VP35, L, and VP24, a membrane associated protein postulated to have interferon suppressing effects, were tested in multiple animal models including murine, guinea pig and non-human primates [115]. In all three models, the results were very promising conferring 75–100% protection against lethal challenge with EBOV and also enabling immune T cell responses in the mouse model that helped counter a repeat challenge with EBOV. Recently, siRNA targeting these same genes were also tested in a non-human primate model [43]. The siRNAs were modified with 2′-*O*-methyl guanosine or uridines to reduce stimulation of IFN and encapsulated in SNALPS. When treated daily with 2mg/kg EBOV SNALPs, rhesus macaques had a 100% survival rate and undetectable viral loads by day 14. The availability of data from large animal studies indicates RNAi could be a plausible treatment for EBOV.

7.5.3 Influenza

Influenza viruses are of the family *Orthomixoviridae* that have a negative sense segmented RNA genome. Influenza A and B contain eight gene segments that are enclosed in an envelope composed of hemagglutanin (HA) neuraminidase (NA) and matrix 2 (M2) proteins. In addition, the genome encodes three components of the viral RNA-dependent RNA polymerase (RdRp): polymerase acidic protein (PA), polymerase basic protein 1 (PB1) and PB2, nucleoprotein (NP), and two non-structural proteins: NS1A and NS2. While Influenza B and C have a limited host tropism, Influenza A can infect a variety of mammals and is thus a major public health concern. Categorization of Influenza A is determined by the antigenic HA and NA subtypes that drift in prevalence from year to year escaping existing immune defenses and limiting the effectiveness of prophylactic vaccines. Approaches targeting conserved regions of Influenza A genes, such as those afforded by RNAi, could provide broad protection from potentially pandemic strains.

The first *in vivo* studies evaluated antisense phosphorothioate oligonucleotides (s-ODN) targeting PB-2 and PA against the H1N1 A/PR/8/34 strain. i.v. administration of ODNs encapsulated in the cationic liposome Tfx [55, 90] prior to infection reduced target mRNA levels and viral titers in mouse lungs resulting in reduced neutrophil infiltration and fewer bronchiolar and alveolar edemas thus significantly increasing the time of survival. Interestingly, i.n. or i.p. administration of liposomally encapsulated s-ODNs failed to promote uptake into lung tissues.

In 2004, two groups reported the results of *in vivo* administration of siRNAs that targeted NP and components of the RdRp. siRNAs directed against NP and/or PA were complexed with either PEI [41] or lipofectamine [110] and delivered to mice i.v. prior to infection. In both studies large reductions in viral titers up to 100-fold were observed against several strains of influenza including H1N1, H5N1, H7N7 and H9N2 and survival rates of mice were significantly increased. Treatment with a combination of these siRNAs was more potently inhibitory. Combinations of PEI complexed siRNAs targeting NP and M2 [132] or 2′*O*-methyl modified siRNAs complexed to lipofectamine targeting NP and NS1 [125] have also been explored *in vivo* with similar results. Treatment prior to infection increased survival of mice (i.v. treatment) or chickens (i.n. treatment) following challenge with lethal dose of H5N1 with significant reductions in viral titers.

7.6 Conclusions

The studies discussed above have definitely cleared apprehensions about engineering RNAi for the *in vivo* control of viral infections. As these technologies continue to advance, the main focus no longer remains proof-of-principle experimentation in animal models, but making it a feasible and cost-effective treatment option for clinical application.

The ease and speed of synthesis of siRNAs confers upon them a higher ground in comparison with the conventional protein, peptide and antibody therapies. Even with chemical drugs, the complexity involved in developing a new one for a particular malady is dissuasive when considering the ease and speed of siRNA design although the associated costs could be higher with the RNAi therapeutics. RNAi therapeutics appear to be perfectly suited for controlling fast and acute viral infections making it a particularly smart choice for combating epidemics and pandemics like the 2009 H1N1 outbreak or as a weapon against a bioterror attack. Another niche for these drugs would be in topical applications like microbicide formulations for the prevention of sexually transmitted infections where rapid kinetics of drug action is warranted.

While the use of RNAi for treating chronic ailments is debatable in the face of viral ability to mutate under shRNA pressure, aiming at the immutable host factors that viruses rely on seem to be a good strategy. While the search is on for expandable host targets, the enormous data gleaned from high-throughput screening for human factors promoting viral infections like HIV, [13, 67, 127, 133], Influenza [53, 63], HCV [99] and WNV [68], have revealed a plethora of targets for investigation.

Finally, another approach to combating viral infections that is being actively pursued is to attack non-human viral reservoirs using antiviral RNAi in an effort to prevent transmission to the human hosts. This approach has been explored in the mosquito vector to limit replication of flaviviruses [17, 39, 111] and has proven efficacious in laboratory-controlled studies. More recently, this approach is being examined in the poultry reservoir of influenza by testing siRNAs in drinking water or in aerosol sprays and also developing chickens transgenic for antiviral shRNAs [26, 96]. While these alternate avenues are being explored for RNAi implementation, it appears inevitable that a RNAi-based drug will hit the market not too far in the future.

References

1. Alvarez, R., Elbashir, S., Borland, T., Toudjarska, I., Hadwiger, P., John, M., Roehl, I., Morskaya, S. S., Martinello, R., Kahn, J., Van Ranst, M., Tripp, R. A., DeVincenzo, J. P., Pandey, R., Maier, M., Nechev, L., Manoharan, M., Kotelianski, V. and Meyers, R. (2009). RNA interference-mediated silencing of the respiratory syncytial virus nucleocapsid defines a potent antiviral strategy. *Antimicrob Agents Chemother,* **53,** pp. 3952–3962.

2. An, D. S., Donahue, R. E., Kamata, M., Poon, B., Metzger, M., Mao, S. H., Bonifacino, A., Krouse, A. E., Darlix, J. L., Baltimore, D., Qin, F. X. and Chen, I. S. (2007). Stable reduction of CCR5 by RNAi through hematopoietic stem cell transplant in non-human primates. *Proc Natl Acad Sci U S A,* **104,** pp. 13110–13115.

3. Anderson, J., Li, M. J., Palmer, B., Remling, L., Li, S., Yam, P., Yee, J. K., Rossi, J., Zaia, J. and Akkina, R. (2007). Safety and efficacy of a lentiviral vector containing three anti-HIV genes — CCR5 ribozyme, tat-rev siRNA, and TAR decoy — in SCID-hu mouse-derived T cells. *Mol Ther,* **15,** pp. 1182–1188.

4. Anderson, J. S., Walker, J., Nolta, J. A. and Bauer, G. (2009). Specific transduction of HIV-susceptible cells for CCR5 knockdown and resistance to HIV infection: a novel method for targeted gene therapy and intracellular immunization. *J Acquir Immune Defic Syndr,* **52,** pp. 152–161.

5. Bai, F., Wang, T., Pal, U., Bao, F., Gould, L. H. and Fikrig, E. (2005). Use of RNA interference to prevent lethal murine West Nile virus infection. *J Infect Dis,* **191,** pp. 1148–1154.

6. Banerjea, A., Li, M. J., Bauer, G., Remling, L., Lee, N. S., Rossi, J. and Akkina, R. (2003). Inhibition of HIV-1 by lentiviral vector-transduced siRNAs in T lymphocytes differentiated in SCID-hu mice and CD34+ progenitor cell-derived macrophages. *Mol Ther,* **8,** pp. 62–71.

7. Barnett, E. D. (2007). Yellow Fever: Epidemiology and Prevention. *Clin Infect Dis,* **44,** pp. 850–856.

8. Bennasser, Y., Le, S. Y., Benkirane, M. and Jeang, K. T. (2005). Evidence that HIV-1 encodes an siRNA and a suppressor of RNA silencing. *Immunity,* **22,** pp. 607–619.

9. Bitko, V. and Barik, S. (2001). Phenotypic silencing of cytoplasmic genes using sequence-specific double-stranded short interfering RNA and its application in the reverse genetics of wild type negative-strand RNA viruses. *BMC Microbiol,* **1,** p. 34.

10. Bitko, V. and Barik, S. (2008). Nasal delivery of siRNA. *Methods Mol Biol,* **442,** pp. 75–82.

11. Bitko, V., Musiyenko, A., Shulyayeva, O. and Barik, S. (2005). Inhibition of respiratory viruses by nasally administered siRNA. *Nat Med,* **11,** pp. 50–55.

12. Boden, D., Pusch, O., Lee, F., Tucker, L. and Ramratnam, B. (2003). Human immunodeficiency virus type 1 escape from RNA interference. *J Virol,* **77,** pp. 11531–11535.

13. Brass, A. L., Dykxhoorn, D. M., Benita, Y., Yan, N., Engelman, A., Xavier, R. J., Lieberman, J. and Elledge, S. J. (2008). Identification of host proteins required for HIV infection through a functional genomic screen. *Science,* **319,** pp. 921–926.

14. Burd, E. M. (2003). Human papillomavirus and cervical cancer. *Clin Microbiol Rev,* **16,** pp. 1–17.

15. Cagnon, L. and Rossi, J. J. (2000). Downregulation of the CCR5 beta-chemokine receptor and inhibition of HIV-1 infection by stable VA1-ribozyme chimeric transcripts. *Antisense Nucleic Acid Drug Dev,* **10,** pp. 251–261.

16. Caplen, N. J., Parrish, S., Imani, F., Fire, A. and Morgan, R. A. (2001). Specific inhibition of gene expression by small double-stranded RNAs in invertebrate and vertebrate systems. *Proc Natl Acad Sci U S A,* **98,** pp. 9742–9747.

17. Caplen, N. J., Zheng, Z., Falgout, B. and Morgan, R. A. (2002). Inhibition of viral gene expression and replication in mosquito cells by dsRNA-triggered RNA interference. *Mol Ther,* **6,** pp. 243–251.

18. Carmona, S., Ely, A., Crowther, C., Moolla, N., Salazar, F. H., Marion, P. L., Ferry, N., Weinberg, M. S. and Arbuthnot, P. (2006). Effective inhibition of HBV replication *in vivo* by anti-HBx short hairpin RNAs. *Mol Ther,* **13,** pp. 411–421.

19. Celum, C., Levine, R., Weaver, M. and Wald, A. (2004). Genital herpes and human immunodeficiency virus: double trouble. *Bull World Health Organ,* **82,** pp. 447–453.

20. Chen, Y., Du, D., Wu, J., Chan, C. P., Tan, Y., Kung, H. F. and He, M. L. (2003). Inhibition of hepatitis B virus replication by stably expressed shRNA. *Biochem Biophys Res Commun,* **311,** pp. 398–404.

21. Chiu, Y. L. and Rana, T. M. (2003). siRNA function in RNAi: a chemical modification analysis. *RNA,* **9,** pp. 1034–1048.

22. ClinicalTrials.gov (2010). Multiple Ascending Dose Study of Miravirsen in Treatment-Naive Chronic Hepatitis C Subjects. Available from: http://clinicaltrials.gov/ct2/show?term=SPC3649&rank=3.

23. ClinicalTrials.gov (2010). Phase 2b Study of ALN-RSV01 in Lung Transplant Patients Infected With Respiratory Syncytial Virus (RSV).

24. ClinicalTrials.gov (2010). Gene Transfers for HIV Using Autologous T cells. Available from: http://clinicaltrials.gov/ct2/show/NCT01153646.

25. ClinicalTrials.gov (2010). SPC3649 Multiple Dose Study in Healthy Volunteers. Available from: http://clinicaltrials.gov/ct2/show/NCT00979927?term=SPC3649&rank=1.

26. CSIRO (2008). Avian influenza activities at CSIRO's Australian Animal Health Laboratory. Available from: http://www.csiro.au/science/Avian-Influenza-At-AAHL.html#5.

27. Dean, M., Carrington, M., Winkler, C., Huttley, G. A., Smith, M. W., Allikmets, R., Goedert, J. J., Buchbinder, S. P., Vittinghoff, E., Gomperts, E., Donfield, S., Vlahov, D., Kaslow, R., Saah, A., Rinaldo, C., Detels, R. and O'Brien, S. J. (1996). Genetic restriction of HIV-1 infection and progression to AIDS by a deletion allele of the CKR5 structural gene. Hemophilia Growth and Development Study, Multicenter AIDS Cohort Study, Multicenter Hemophilia Cohort Study, San Francisco City Cohort, ALIVE Study. *Science,* **273,** pp. 1856–1862.

28. Deng, L., Li, G., Xi, L., Yin, A., Gao, Y., You, W., Wang, X. and Sun, B. (2009). Hepatitis B virus inhibition in mice by lentiviral vector mediated short hairpin RNA. *BMC Gastroenterol,* **9,** p. 73.

29. DeVincenzo, J., Cehelsky, J. E., Alvarez, R., Elbashir, S., Harborth, J., Toudjarska, I., Nechev, L., Murugaiah, V., Van Vliet, A., Vaishnaw, A. K. and Meyers, R. (2008). Evaluation of the safety, tolerability and pharmacokinetics of ALN-RSV01, a novel RNAi antiviral therapeutic directed against respiratory syncytial virus (RSV). *Antiviral Res,* **77,** pp. 225–231.

30. DeVincenzo, J., Lambkin-Williams, R., Wilkinson, T., Cehelsky, J., Nochur, S., Walsh, E., Meyers, R., Gollob, J. and Vaishnaw, A. (2010). A randomized, double-blind, placebo-controlled study of an RNAi-based therapy directed against respiratory syncytial virus. *Proc Natl Acad Sci U S A,* **107,** pp. 8800–8805.

31. DiGiusto, D. L., Krishnan, A., Li, L., Li, H., Li, S., Rao, A., Mi, S., Yam, P., Stinson, S., Kalos, M., Alvarnas, J., Lacey, S. F., Yee, J. K., Li, M., Couture, L., Hsu, D., Forman, S. J., Rossi, J. J. and Zaia, J. A. (2010). RNA-based gene therapy for HIV with lentiviral vector-modified CD34(+) cells in patients undergoing transplantation for AIDS-related lymphoma. *Sci Transl Med,* **2,** p. 36ra43.

32. Dyer, V., Ely, A., Bloom, K., Weinberg, M. and Arbuthnot, P. (2010). tRNA(Lys3) promoter cassettes that efficiently express RNAi-activating antihepatitis B virus short hairpin RNAs. *Biochem Biophys Res Commun,* **398**(4), pp. 640–646.

33. Dykxhoorn, D. M., Palliser, D. and Lieberman, J. (2006). The silent treatment: siRNAs as small molecule drugs. *Gene Ther,* **13,** pp. 541–552.

34. Elbashir, S. M., Harborth, J., Lendeckel, W., Yalcin, A., Weber, K. and Tuschl, T. (2001). Duplexes of 21-nucleotide RNAs mediate RNA interference in cultured mammalian cells. *Nature,* **411,** pp. 494–498.

35. Empey, K. M., Peebles, R. S., Jr. and Kolls, J. K. (2010). Pharmacologic advances in the treatment and prevention of respiratory syncytial virus. *Clin Infect Dis,* **50,** pp. 1258–1267.

36. Enterlein, S., Warfield, K. L., Swenson, D. L., Stein, D. A., Smith, J. L., Gamble, C. S., Kroeker, A. D., Iversen, P. L., Bavari, S. and Mühlberger, E. (2006). VP35 knockdown inhibits Ebola virus amplification and protects against lethal infection in mice. *Antimicrob Agents Chemother,* **50,** pp. 984–993.

37. Feld, J. J. and Hoofnagle, J. H. (2005). Mechanism of action of interferon and ribavirin in treatment of hepatitis C. *Nature,* **436,** pp. 967–972.

38. Fire, A., Xu, S., Montgomery, M. K., Kostas, S. A., Driver, S. E. and Mello, C. C. (1998). Potent and specific genetic interference by double-stranded RNA in Caenorhabditis elegans. *Nature,* **391,** pp. 806–811.

39. Franz, A. W., Sanchez-Vargas, I., Adelman, Z. N., Blair, C. D., Beaty, B. J., James, A. A. and Olson, K. E. (2006). Engineering RNA interference-based resistance to dengue virus type 2 in genetically modified Aedes aegypti. *Proc Natl Acad Sci U S A,* **103,** pp. 4198–4203.

40. Gao, S., Dagnaes-Hansen, F., Nielsen, E. J., Wengel, J., Besenbacher, F., Howard, K. A. and Kjems, J. (2009). The effect of chemical modification and nanoparticle formulation on stability and biodistribution of siRNA in mice. *Mol Ther,* **17,** pp. 1225–1233.

41. Ge, Q., Filip, L., Bai, A., Nguyen, T., Eisen, H. N. and Chen, J. (2004). Inhibition of influenza virus production in virus-infected mice by RNA interference. *Proc Natl Acad Sci U S A,* **101,** pp. 8676–8681.

42. Geisbert, T. W., Hensley, L. E., Kagan, E., Yu, E. Z., Geisbert, J. B., Daddario-DiCaprio, K., Fritz, E. A., Jahrling, P. B., McClintock, K., Phelps, J. R., Lee, A. C., Judge, A., Jeffs, L. B. and MacLachlan, I. (2006). Postexposure protection of guinea pigs against a lethal ebola virus challenge is conferred by RNA interference. *J Infect Dis,* **193,** pp. 1650–1657.

43. Geisbert, T. W., Lee, A. C., Robbins, M., Geisbert, J. B., Honko, A. N., Sood, V., Johnson, J. C., de Jong, S., Tavakoli, I., Judge, A., Hensley, L. E. and Maclachlan, I. (2010). Postexposure protection of non-human primates against a lethal Ebola virus challenge with RNA interference: a proof-of-concept study. *Lancet,* **375,** pp. 1896–1905.

44. Giering, J. C., Grimm, D., Storm, T. A. and Kay, M. A. (2008). Expression of shRNA from a tissue-specific pol II promoter is an effective and safe RNAi therapeutic. *Mol Ther,* **16,** pp. 1630–1636.

45. Grimm, D., Streetz, K. L., Jopling, C. L., Storm, T. A., Pandey, K., Davis, C. R., Marion, P., Salazar, F. and Kay, M. A. (2006). Fatality in mice due to oversaturation of cellular microRNA/short hairpin RNA pathways. *Nature,* **441,** pp. 537–541.

46. Gu, W., Cochrane, M., Leggatt, G. R., Payne, E., Choyce, A., Zhou, F., Tindle, R. and McMillan, N. A. J. (2009). Both treated and untreated tumors are eliminated by short hairpin RNA-based induction of target-specific immune responses. *Proc Natl Acad Sci U S A,* **106,** pp. 8314–8319.

47. Gu, W., Putral, L., Hengst, K., Minto, K., Saunders, N. A., Leggatt, G. and McMillan, N. A. (2006). Inhibition of cervical cancer cell growth *in vitro* and *in vivo* with lentiviral-vector delivered short hairpin RNA targeting human papillomavirus E6 and E7 oncogenes. *Cancer Gene Ther,* **13,** pp. 1023–1032.

48. Gubler, D. J. (2007). The Continuing Spread of West Nile virus in the Western Hemisphere. *Clin Infect Dis,* **45,** pp. 1039–1046.

49. Gubler, D. J., Kuno, G. and Markoff, L. (2007) *Fields Virology* **1,** eds. Knipe, D. M. and Howley, P. M., Chapter 34 "Flaviviruses" (Lippincott Williams & Wilkins, Philadelphia) pp. 1154–1252.

50. Haasnoot, J., Westerhout, E. M. and Berkhout, B. (2007). RNA interference against viruses: strike and counterstrike. *Nat Biotechnol,* **25,** pp. 1435–1443.

51. Haga, S., Yamamoto, N., Nakai-Murakami, C., Osawa, Y., Tokunaga, K., Sata, T., Yamamoto, N., Sasazuki, T. and Ishizaka, Y. (2008). Modulation of TNF-alpa converting enzyme by the spike protein of SARS-CoV and ACE2 induces TNF-alpa production and facilitates viral entry. *Proc Natl Acad Sci U S A,* **105,** pp. 7809–7814.

52. Hanley, K. A. and Weaver, S. C. (2008) *Origin and Evolution of Viruses,* eds. Domingo, E., Webster, R. G. J. and Holland, J. F., Chapter "Arbovirus Evolution," (Elsevier Inc., St. Louis) pp. 351–392.

53. Hao, L., Sakurai, A., Watanabe, T., Sorensen, E., Nidom, C. A., Newton, M. A., Ahlquist, P. and Kawaoka, Y. (2008). Drosophila RNAi screen identifies host genes important for influenza virus replication. *Nature,* **454,** pp. 890–893.

54. Hartman, A. L., Towner, J. S. and Nichol, S. T. (2010). Ebola and marburg hemorrhagic fever. *Clin Lab Med,* **30,** pp. 161–177.

55. Hatta, T., Ishikawa, M., Takai, K., Nakada, S., Yokota, T., Hata, T., Miura, K. and Takaku, H. (1998). Inhibition of influenza virus RNA polymerase by 5′-capped short RNA fragments. *Biochem Biophys Res Commun,* **249,** pp. 103–106.

56. Henry, S. D., van der Wegen, P., Metselaar, H. J., Tilanus, H. W., Scholte, B. J. and van der Laan, L. J. (2006). Simultaneous targeting of HCV replication and viral binding with a single lentiviral vector containing multiple RNA interference expression cassettes. *Mol Ther,* **14,** pp. 485–493.

57. Hotez, P. J., Remme, J. H. F., Buss, P., Alleyne, G., Morel, C. and Breman, J. G. (2004). Combating Tropical Infectious Diseases: Report of the Disease Control Priorities in Developing Countries Project. *Clin Infect Dis,* **38,** pp. 871–878.

58. Huang, Y., Paxton, W. A., Wolinsky, S. M., Neumann, A. U., Zhang, L., He, T., Kang, S., Ceradini, D., Jin, Z., Yazdanbakhsh, K., Kunstman, K., Erickson, D., Dragon, E., Landau, N. R., Phair, J., Ho, D. D. and Koup, R. A. (1996). The role of a mutant CCR5 allele in HIV-1 transmission and disease progression. *Nat Med,* **2,** pp. 1240–1243.

59. Hütter, G., Nowak, D., Mossner, M., Ganepola, S., Müssig, A., Allers, K., Schneider, T., Hofmann, J., Kücherer, C., Blau, O., Blau, I. W., Hofmann, W. K. and Thiel, E. (2009). Long-term control of HIV by CCR5 Delta32/Delta32 stem-cell transplantation. *N Engl J Med,* **360,** pp. 692–698.

60. Humeau, L. M., Binder, G. K., Lu, X., Slepushkin, V., Merling, R., Echeagaray, P., Pereira, M., Slepushkina, T., Barnett, S., Dropulic, L. K., Carroll, R., Levine, B. L., June, C. H. and Dropulic, B. (2004). Efficient lentiviral vector-mediated control of HIV-1 replication in CD4 lymphocytes from diverse HIV+ infected patients grouped according to CD4 count and viral load. *Mol Ther,* **9,** pp. 902–913.

61. Jopling, C. L., Yi, M., Lancaster, A. M., Lemon, S. M. and Sarnow, P. (2005). Modulation of hepatitis C virus RNA abundance by a liver-specific MicroRNA. *Science,* **309,** pp. 1577–1581.

62. Judge, A. D., Sood, V., Shaw, J. R., Fang, D., McClintock, K. and MacLachlan, I. (2005). Sequence-dependent stimulation of the mammalian innate immune response by synthetic siRNA. *Nat Biotechnol,* **23,** pp. 457–462.

63. Karlas, A., Machuy, N., Shin, Y., Pleissner, K. P., Artarini, A., Heuer, D., Becker, D., Khalil, H., Ogilvie, L. A., Hess, S., Mäurer, A. P., Müller, E., Wolff, T., Rudel, T. and Meyer, T. F. (2010). Genome-wide RNAi screen identifies human host factors crucial for influenza virus replication. *Nature,* **463,** pp. 818–822.

64. Khaliq, S., Khaliq, S. A., Zahur, M., Ijaz, B., Jahan, S., Ansar, M., Riazuddin, S. and Hassan, S. (2010). RNAi as a new therapeutic strategy against HCV. *Biotechnol Adv,* **28,** pp. 27–34.

65. Kim, S. I., Shin, D., Choi, T. H., Lee, J. C., Cheon, G. J., Kim, K. Y., Park, M. and Kim, M. (2007). Systemic and specific delivery of small interfering

RNAs to the liver mediated by apolipoprotein A-I. *Mol Ther,* **15,** pp. 1145–1152.

66. Kim, S. S., Peer, D., Kumar, P., Subramanya, S., Wu, H., Asthana, D., Habiro, K., Yang, Y. G., Manjunath, N., Shimaoka, M. and Shankar, P. (2010). RNAi-mediated CCR5 silencing by LFA-1-targeted nanoparticles prevents HIV infection in BLT mice. *Mol Ther,* **18,** pp. 370–376.
67. König, R., Zhou, Y., Elleder, D., Diamond, T. L., Bonamy, G. M., Irelan, J. T., Chiang, C. Y., Tu, B. P., De Jesus, P. D., Lilley, C. E., Seidel, S., Opaluch, A. M., Caldwell, J. S., Weitzman, M. D., Kuhen, K. L., Bandyopadhyay, S., Ideker, T., Orth, A. P., Miraglia, L. J., Bushman, F. D., Young, J. A. and Chanda, S. K. (2008). Global analysis of host-pathogen interactions that regulate early-stage HIV-1 replication. *Cell,* **135,** pp. 49–60.
68. Krishnan, M. N., Ng, A., Sukumaran, B., Gilfoy, F. D., Uchil, P. D., Sultana, H., Brass, A. L., Adametz, R., Tsui, M., Qian, F., Montgomery, R. R., Lev, S., Mason, P. W., Koski, R. A., Elledge, S. J., Xavier, R. J., Agaisse, H. and Fikrig, E. (2008). RNA interference screen for human genes associated with West Nile virus infection. *Nature,* **455,** pp. 242–245.
69. Kuiken, T., Fouchier, R. A., Schutten, M., Rimmelzwaan, G. F., van Amerongen, G., van Riel, D., Laman, J. D., de Jong, T., van Doornum, G., Lim, W., Ling, A. E., Chan, P. K., Tam, J. S., Zambon, M. C., Gopal, R., Drosten, C., van der Werf, S., Escriou, N., Manuguerra, J. C., Stöhr, K., Peiris, J. S. and Osterhaus, A. D. (2003). Newly discovered coronavirus as the primary cause of severe acute respiratory syndrome. *Lancet,* **362,** pp. 263–270.
70. Kumar, P., Ban, H. S., Kim, S. S., Wu, H., Pearson, T., Greiner, D. L., Laouar, A., Yao, J., Haridas, V., Habiro, K., Yang, Y. G., Jeong, J. H., Lee, K. Y., Kim, Y. H., Kim, S. W., Peipp, M., Fey, G. H., Manjunath, N., Shultz, L. D., Lee, S. K. and Shankar, P. (2008). T cell-specific siRNA delivery suppresses HIV-1 infection in humanized mice. *Cell,* **134,** pp. 577–586.
71. Kumar, P., Lee, S. K., Shankar, P. and Manjunath, N. (2006). A Single siRNA Suppresses Fatal Encephalitis Induced by Two Different Flaviviruses. *PLoS Med,* **3,** p. e96.
72. Kumar, P., Wu, H., McBride, J. L., Jung, K.-E., Hee Kim, M., Davidson, B. L., Kyung Lee, S., Shankar, P. and Manjunath, N. (2007). Transvascular delivery of small interfering RNA to the central nervous system. *Nature,* **448,** pp. 39–43.
73. Lanford, R. E., Hildebrandt-Eriksen, E. S., Petri, A., Persson, R., Lindow, M., Munk, M. E., Kauppinen, S. and Ørum, H. (2010). Therapeutic silencing of microRNA-122 in primates with chronic hepatitis C virus infection. *Science,* **327,** pp. 198–201.
74. Lavanchy, D. (2008). Chronic viral hepatitis as a public health issue in the world. *Best Pract Res Clin Gastroenterol,* **22,** pp. 991–1008.

75. Lemon, S. M., Walker, C., Alter, M. J. and Yi, M. (2007) *Fields Virology* **1,** eds. Knipe, D. M. and Howley, P. M., Chapter 35 "Hepatitis C Virus" (Lippincott Williams & Wilkins, Philadelphia) pp. 1253–1304.

76. Levine, B. L., Humeau, L. M., Boyer, J., MacGregor, R. R., Rebello, T., Lu, X., Binder, G. K., Slepushkin, V., Lemiale, F., Mascola, J. R., Bushman, F. D., Dropulic, B. and June, C. H. (2006). Gene transfer in humans using a conditionally replicating lentiviral vector. *Proc Natl Acad Sci U S A,* **103,** pp. 17372–17377.

77. Li, B. J., Tang, Q., Cheng, D., Qin, C., Xie, F. Y., Wei, Q., Xu, J., Liu, Y., Zheng, B. J., Woodle, M. C., Zhong, N. and Lu, P. Y. (2005). Using siRNA in prophylactic and therapeutic regimens against SARS coronavirus in Rhesus macaque. *Nat Med,* **11,** pp. 944–951.

78. Li, M. J., Bauer, G., Michienzi, A., Yee, J. K., Lee, N. S., Kim, J., Li, S., Castanotto, D., Zaia, J. and Rossi, J. J. (2003). Inhibition of HIV-1 infection by lentiviral vectors expressing Pol III-promoted anti-HIV RNAs. *Mol Ther,* **8,** pp. 196–206.

79. Li, M. J., Kim, J., Li, S., Zaia, J., Yee, J. K., Anderson, J., Akkina, R. and Rossi, J. J. (2005). Long-term inhibition of HIV-1 infection in primary hematopoietic cells by lentiviral vector delivery of a triple combination of anti-HIV shRNA, anti-CCR5 ribozyme, and a nucleolar-localizing TAR decoy. *Mol Ther,* **12,** pp. 900–909.

80. Li, W.-X., Li, H., Lu, R., Li, F., Dus, M., Atkinson, P., Brydon, E. W. A., Johnson, K. L., Garcia-Sastre, A., Ball, L. A., Palese, P. and Ding, S.-W. (2004). Interferon antagonist proteins of influenza and vaccinia viruses are suppressors of RNA silencing. *Proc Natl Acad Sci U S A,* **101,** pp. 1350–1355.

81. Lindenbach, B. D., Thiel, H.-J. R. and Rice, C. M. (2007) *Fields Virology* **1,** eds. Knipe, D. M. and Howley, P. M., Chapter 33 "Flaviviridae: The Viruses and Their Replication" (Lippincott Williams & Wilkins Philadelphia) pp. 1101–1152.

82. Looker, K. J., Garnett, G. P. and Schmid, G. P. (2008). An estimate of the global prevalence and incidence of herpes simplex virus type 2 infection. *Bull World Health Organ,* **86,** pp. 805–812.

83. Lu, X., Humeau, L., Slepushkin, V., Binder, G., Yu, Q., Slepushkina, T., Chen, Z., Merling, R., Davis, B., Chang, Y. N. and Dropulic, B. (2004). Safe two-plasmid production for the first clinical lentivirus vector that achieves >99% transduction in primary cells using a one-step protocol. *J Gene Med,* **6,** pp. 963–973.

84. Mackenzie, J. S., Gubler, D. J. and Petersen, L. R. (2004). Emerging flaviviruses: the spread and resurgence of Japanese encephalitis, West Nile and dengue viruses. *Nature Medicine,* **10,** pp. S90–109.

85. Martin, A., Bodola, F., Sangar, D. V., Goettge, K., Popov, V., Rijnbrand, R., Lanford, R. E. and Lemon, S. M. (2003). Chronic hepatitis associated with GB virus B persistence in a tamarin after intrahepatic inoculation of synthetic viral RNA. *Proc Natl Acad Sci U S A,* **100,** pp. 9962–9967.

86. McCaffrey, A. P., Nakai, H., Pandey, K., Huang, Z., Salazar, F. H., Xu, H., Wieland, S. F., Marion, P. L. and Kay, M. A. (2003). Inhibition of hepatitis B virus in mice by RNA interference. *Nat Biotechnol,* **21,** pp. 639–644.

87. McHutchison, J. G., Patel, K., Pockros, P., Nyberg, L., Pianko, S., Yu, R. Z., Dorr, F. A. and Kwoh, T. J. (2006). A phase I trial of an antisense inhibitor of hepatitis C virus (ISIS 14803), administered to chronic hepatitis C patients. *J Hepatol,* **44,** pp. 88–96.

88. Meister, G. and Tuschl, T. (2004). Mechanisms of gene silencing by double-stranded RNA. *Nature,* **431,** pp. 343–349.

89. Michienzi, A., Li, S., Zaia, J. A. and Rossi, J. J. (2002). A nucleolar TAR decoy inhibitor of HIV-1 replication. *Proc Natl Acad Sci U S A,* **99,** pp. 14047–14052.

90. Mizuta, T., Fujiwara, M., Hatta, T., Abe, T., Miyano-Kurosaki, N., Shigeta, S., Yokota, T. and Takaku, H. (1999). Antisense oligonucleotides directed against the viral RNA polymerase gene enhance survival of mice infected with influenza A. *Nat Biotechnol,* **17,** pp. 583–587.

91. Morrissey, D. V., Blanchard, K., Shaw, L., Jensen, K., Lockridge, J. A., Dickinson, B., McSwiggen, J. A., Vargeese, C., Bowman, K., Shaffer, C. S., Polisky, B. A. and Zinnen, S. (2005). Activity of stabilized short interfering RNA in a mouse model of hepatitis B virus replication. *Hepatology,* **41,** pp. 1349–1356.

92. Morrissey, D. V., Lockridge, J. A., Shaw, L., Blanchard, K., Jensen, K., Breen, W., Hartsough, K., Machemer, L., Radka, S., Jadhav, V., Vaish, N., Zinnen, S., Vargeese, C., Bowman, K., Shaffer, C. S., Jeffs, L. B., Judge, A., MacLachlan, I. and Polisky, B. (2005). Potent and persistent *in vivo* anti-HBV activity of chemically modified siRNAs. *Nat Biotechnol,* **23,** pp. 1002–1007.

93. Nair, H., Nokes, D. J., Gessner, B. D., Dherani, M., Madhi, S. A., Singleton, R. J., O'Brien, K. L., Roca, A., Wright, P. F., Bruce, N., Chandran, A., Theodoratou, E., Sutanto, A., Sedyaningsih, E. R., Ngama, M., Munywoki, P. K., Kartasasmita, C., Simões, E. A., Rudan, I., Weber, M. W. and Campbell, H. (2010). Global burden of acute lower respiratory infections due to respiratory syncytial virus in young children: a systematic review and meta-analysis. *Lancet,* **375,** pp. 1545–1555.

94. Negro, F. (2010). Adverse effects of drugs in the treatment of viral hepatitis. *Best Pract Res Clin Gastroenterol,* **24,** pp. 183–192.

95. Novina, C. D., Murray, M. F., Dykxhoorn, D. M., Beresford, P. J., Riess, J., Lee, S. K., Collman, R. G., Lieberman, J., Shankar, P. and Sharp, P. A. (2002). siRNA-directed inhibition of HIV-1 infection. *Nat Med,* **8,** pp. 681–686.

96. O'Neill, G. (2007). Australia tackles bird flu using RNAi. *Nat Biotechnol,* **25,** pp. 605–606.

97. Pacca, C. C., Severino, A. A., Mondini, A., Rahal, P., D'Avila, S. G., Cordeiro, J. A., Nogueira, M. C., Bronzoni, R. V. and Nogueira, M. L. (2009). RNA interference inhibits yellow fever virus replication *in vitro* and *in vivo.* *Virus Genes,* **38,** pp. 224–231.

98. Palliser, D., Chowdhury, D., Wang, Q. Y., Lee, S. J., Bronson, R. T., Knipe, D. M. and Lieberman, J. (2006). An siRNA-based microbicide protects mice from lethal herpes simplex virus 2 infection. *Nature,* **439,** pp. 89–94.

99. Randall, G., Panis, M., Cooper, J. D., Tellinghuisen, T. L., Sukhodolets, K. E., Pfeffer, S., Landthaler, M., Landgraf, P., Kan, S., Lindenbach, B. D., Chien, M., Weir, D. B., Russo, J. J., Ju, J., Brownstein, M. J., Sheridan, R., Sander, C., Zavolan, M., Tuschl, T. and Rice, C. M. (2007). Cellular cofactors affecting hepatitis C virus infection and replication. *Proc Natl Acad Sci U S A,* **104,** pp. 12884–12889.

100. Ren, G. L., Fang, Y., Ma, H. H., Lei, Y. F., Wang, D., Xu, M. C., Wang, P. Z., Huang, C. X., Nie, O. H., Sun, Y. T. and Bai, X. F. (2007). The short hairpin RNA driven by polymerase II suppresses both wild-type and lamivudine-resistant hepatitis B virus strains. *Antivir Ther,* **12,** pp. 865–876.

101. Ren, X., Luo, G., Xie, Z., Zhou, L., Kong, X. and Xu, A. (2006). Inhibition of multiple gene expression and virus replication of HBV by stable RNA interference in 2.2.15 cells. *J Hepatol,* **44,** pp. 663–670.

102. Ren, X. R., Zhou, L. J., Luo, G. B., Lin, B. and Xu, A. (2005). Inhibition of hepatitis B virus replication in 2.2.15 cells by expressed shRNA. *J Viral Hepat,* **12,** pp. 236–242.

103. Restrepo, B. N., Isaza, D. M., Salazar, C. L., Ramírez, R., Ospina, M. and Alvarez, L. G. (2008). Serum levels of interleukin-6, tumor necrosis factor-alpha and interferon-gamma in infants with and without dengue. *Rev Soc Bras Med Trop,* **41,** pp. 6–10.

104. Seeger, C., Zoulim, F. and Mason, W. S. (2007) *Fields Virology* **1,** eds. Knipe, D. M. and Howley, P. M., Chapter 76 "Hepadnaviruses" (Lippincott Williams & Wilkins, Philadelphia) pp. 2977–3029.

105. Shlomai, A. and Shaul, Y. (2003). Inhibition of hepatitis B virus expression and replication by RNA interference. *Hepatology,* **37,** pp. 764–770.

106. Soutschek, J., Akinc, A., Bramlage, B., Charisse, K., Constien, R., Donoghue, M., Elbashir, S., Geick, A., Hadwiger, P., Harborth, J., John, M., Kesavan, V., Lavine, G., Pandey, R. K., Racie, T., Rajeev, K. G., Röhl, I., Toudjarska, I., Wang, G., Wuschko, S., Bumcrot, D., Koteliansky, V., Limmer, S., Manoharan, M. and Vornlocher, H. P. (2004). Therapeutic silencing of an endogenous gene by systemic administration of modified siRNAs. *Nature,* **432,** pp. 173–178.

107. Stockman, L. J., Bellamy, R. and Garner, P. (2006). SARS: systematic review of treatment effects. *PLoS Med,* **3,** p. e343.

108. Subramanya, S., Kim, S. S., Abraham, S., Yao, J., Kumar, M., Kumar, P., Haridas, V., Lee, S. K., Shultz, L. D., Greiner, D., N, M. and Shankar, P. (2010). Targeted delivery of small interfering RNA to human dendritic cells to suppress dengue virus infection and associated proinflammatory cytokine production. *J Virol,* **84,** pp. 2490–2501.

109. Teng, M. N., Whitehead, S. S., Bermingham, A., St Claire, M., Elkins, W. R., Murphy, B. R. and Collins, P. L. (2000). Recombinant respiratory syncytial virus that does not express the NS1 or M2-2 protein is highly attenuated and immunogenic in chimpanzees. *J Virol,* **74,** pp. 9317–9321.

110. Tompkins, S. M., Lo, C. Y., Tumpey, T. M. and Epstein, S. L. (2004). Protection against lethal influenza virus challenge by RNA interference *in vivo. Proc Natl Acad Sci U S A,* **101,** pp. 8682–8686.

111. Travanty, E. A., Adelman, Z. N., Franz, A. W., Keene, K. M., Beaty, B. J., Blair, C. D., James, A. A. and Olson, K. E. (2004). Using RNA interference to develop dengue virus resistance in genetically modified Aedes aegypti. *Insect Biochem Mol Biol,* **34,** pp. 607–613.

112. Uprichard, S. L., Boyd, B., Althage, A. and Chisari, F. V. (2005). Clearance of hepatitis B virus from the liver of transgenic mice by short hairpin RNAs. *Proc Natl Acad Sci U S A,* **102,** pp. 773–778.

113. Virxsys Corporation (2009). HIV RNA Therapy. Available from: http://www.virxsys.com/pages/human-therapies/hiv-rna-therapy.php.

114. Wang, M. D. and Jolly, A. M. (2004). Changing virulence of the SARS virus: the epidemiological evidence. *Bull World Health Organ,* **82,** pp. 547–548.

115. Warfield, K. L., Swenson, D. L., Olinger, G. G., Nichols, D. K., Pratt, W. D., Blouch, R., Stein, D. A., Aman, M. J., Iversen, P. L. and Bavari, S. (2006). Gene-specific countermeasures against Ebola virus based on antisense phosphorodiamidate morpholino oligomers. *PLoS Pathog,* **2,** p. e1.

116. Wen, W. H., Liu, J. Y., Qin, W. J., Zhao, J., Wang, T., Jia, L. T., Meng, Y. L., Gao, H., Xue, C. F., Jin, B. Q., Yao, L. B., Chen, S. Y. and Yang, A. G. (2007). Targeted inhibition of HBV gene expression by single-chain antibody mediated small interfering RNA delivery. *Hepatology,* **46,** pp. 84–94.

117. Whitehead, S. S., Bukreyev, A., Teng, M. N., Firestone, C. Y., St Claire, M., Elkins, W. R., Collins, P. L. and Murphy, B. R. (1999). Recombinant respiratory syncytial virus bearing a deletion of either the NS2 or SH gene is attenuated in chimpanzees. *J Virol,* **73,** pp. 3438–3442.

118. Wong, S. C., Ooi, M. H., Abdullah, A. R., Wong, S. Y., Krishnan, S., Tio, P. H., Pek, P. C., Lai, B. F., Mohan, A., Muhi, J., Kiyu, A., Arif, M. T. and Cardosa, M. J. (2008). A decade of Japanese encephalitis surveillance in Sarawak, Malaysia: 1997–2006. *Trop Med Int Health,* **13,** pp. 52–55.

119. World Health, O. (2002). WHO|Hepatitis C. Available from: http://www.who.int/csr/disease/hepatitis/whocdscsrlyo2003/en/index.html .

120. World Health Organization (2003). WHO|Summary of probable SARS cases with onset of ilness from 1 November 2002 to 31 July 2003. Available from: http://www.who.int/csr/sars/country/table2004_04_21/en/index.html.

121. World Health Organization (2009). WHO|Influenza (Seasonal) Fact Sheet. Available from: http://www.who.int/mediacentre/factsheets/fs211/en/index.html .

122. World Health Organization (2010). WHO|Viral Cancers. Available from: http://www.who.int/vaccine_research/diseases/viral_cancers/en/print.html.

123. World Health Organization (2008). Hepatitis B Fact Sheet. Available from: http://www.who.int/mediacentre/factsheets/fs204/en/.

124. Wu, Y., Navarro, F., Lal, A., Basar, E., Pandey, R. K., Manoharan, M., Feng, Y., Lee, S. J., Lieberman, J. and Palliser, D. (2009). Durable protection from Herpes Simplex Virus-2 transmission following intravaginal application of siRNAs targeting both a viral and host gene. *Cell Host Microbe,* **5,** pp. 84–94.

125. Wu, Y., Zhang, G., Li, Y., Jin, Y., Dale, R., Sun, L. Q. and Wang, M. (2008). Inhibition of highly pathogenic avian H5N1 influenza virus replication by RNA oligonucleotides targeting NS1 gene. *Biochem Biophys Res Commun,* **365,** pp. 369–374.

126. Yamato, K., Yamada, T., Kizaki, M., Ui-Tei, K., Natori, Y., Fujino, M., Nishihara, T., Ikeda, Y., Nasu, Y., Saigo, K. and Yoshinouchi, M. (2008). New highly potent and specific E6 and E7 siRNAs for treatment of HPV16 positive cervical cancer. *Cancer Gene Ther,* **15,** pp. 140–153.

127. Yeung, M. L., Houzet, L., Yedavalli, V. S. and Jeang, K. T. (2009). A genome-wide short hairpin RNA screening of jurkat T-cells for human proteins contributing to productive HIV-1 replication. *J Biol Chem,* **284,** pp. 19463–19473.

128. Yi, R., Qin, Y., Macara, I. G. and Cullen, B. R. (2003). Exportin-5 mediates the nuclear export of pre-microRNAs and short hairpin RNAs. *Genes Dev,* **17,** pp. 3011–3016.

129. Yokota, T., Iijima, S., Kubodera, T., Ishii, K., Katakai, Y., Ageyama, N., Chen, Y., Lee, Y. J., Unno, T., Nishina, K., Iwasaki, Y., Maki, N., Mizusawa, H. and Akari, H. (2007). Efficient regulation of viral replication by siRNA in a non-human primate surrogate model for hepatitis C. *Biochem Biophys Res Commun,* **361,** pp. 294–300.

130. Zhang, W., Yang, H., Kong, X., Mohapatra, S., San Juan-Vergara, H., Hellermann, G., Behera, S., Singam, R., Lockey, R. F. and Mohapatra, S. S. (2005). Inhibition of respiratory syncytial virus infection with intranasal siRNA nanoparticles targeting the viral NS1 gene. *Nat Med,* **11,** pp. 56–62.

131. Zheng, B. J., Guan, Y., Tang, Q., Du, C., Xie, F. Y., He, M. L., Chan, K. W., Wong, K. L., Lader, E., Woodle, M. C., Lu, P. Y., Li, B. and Zhong, N. (2004). Prophylactic and therapeutic effects of small interfering RNA targeting SARS-coronavirus. *Antivir Ther,* **9,** pp. 365–374.

132. Zhou, H., Jin, M., Yu, Z., Xu, X., Peng, Y., Wu, H., Liu, J., Liu, H., Cao, S. and Chen, H. (2007). Effective small interfering RNAs targeting matrix and nucleocapsid protein gene inhibit influenza A virus replication in cells and mice. *Antiviral Res,* **76,** pp. 186–193.

133. Zhou, H., Xu, M., Huang, Q., Gates, A. T., Zhang, X. D., Castle, J. C., Stec, E., Ferrer, M., Strulovici, B., Hazuda, D. J. and Espeseth, A. S. (2008). Genome-scale RNAi screen for host factors required for HIV replication. *Cell Host Microbe,* **4,** pp. 495–504.

134. Zhou, J. and Rossi, J. J. (2010). Aptamer-targeted cell-specific RNA interference. *Silence,* **1,** p. 4.

135. Zhou, J., Swiderski, P., Li, H., Zhang, J., Neff, C. P., Akkina, R. and Rossi, J. J. (2009). Selection, characterization and application of new RNA HIV gp 120 aptamers for facile delivery of Dicer substrate siRNAs into HIV infected cells. *Nucleic Acids Res,* **37,** pp. 3094–3109.

Chapter 8

Detection and Description of Tissue Disease: Advances in the Use of Nanomedicine for Medical Imaging

Jason L.J. Dearling and Alan B. Packard
Division of Nuclear Medicine and Molecular Imaging, Department of Radiology, Children's Hospital, Boston and Harvard Medical School, Boston, Massachusetts, USA
jason.dearling@childrens.harvard.edu

Medical imaging offers a powerful tool for the detection and characterization of disease. In order to take full advantage of the possibilities offered, imaging agents with specific uptake in the target tissue are required. The development of these agents presents several challenges, as the agents must have sufficient absolute uptake at the target site to be detectable, must clear from other tissues to achieve contrast, and should be non-toxic and non-immunogenic.

In this chapter, we discuss how the use of biomaterials has advanced the development of novel nanoparticles as contrast agents for computed tomography (CT) and ultrasound (US).

8.1 Introduction

An essential role of medical imaging is the ability to discriminate between normal and diseased tissue. This discrimination can be

Handbook of Harnessing Biomaterials in Nanomedicine: Preparation, Toxicity, and Applications
Edited by Dan Peer

ISBN 978-981-4316-46-0 (Hardback), 978-981-4364-27-0 (eBook)
www.panstanford.com

achieved by using contrast agents that selectively accumulate in the diseased tissue, increasing the signal from that tissue, thus distinguishing it from adjacent, normal, tissue. The increasing ability of therapies to address specific subtypes of disease as well as the associated increases in the cost of these therapies demands a corresponding improvement in the ability to define disease, preferably non-invasively, and to assess response to therapy in near real time. Medical imaging has the ability to answer these demands through increasingly specific contrast agents.

In the spectrum of available molecular imaging technologies, nuclear medicine, using either single-photon or positron-emitting tracers, provides the greatest sensitivity, with the ability to detect targets that are present at the nanomolar level. The trade-off for this high sensitivity is relatively lower resolution (5–10 mm) than is available with magnetic resonance imaging (MRI), computed tomography (CT), or ultrasound (US), all of which can achieve anatomic resolution of 1 mm or less. However, MRI, CT, and US require a much greater mass of contrast agent at the imaging site to provide adequate differentiation between normal and diseased tissue. An obvious way to provide this increase in mass is through the use of targeted nanoparticles, which by their very nature deliver a large mass of material to the target, assuming that the technical challenges associated with delivering such a massive particle to an *in vivo* target can be overcome. These challenges include evading the body's defenses against particulate contaminants (including the reticuloendothelial system), developing a particle that is small enough not to be trapped in the capillary bed while still large enough to provide an adequate signal once it reaches the target, and overcoming the toxicological challenge inherent in administering a significant mass of material intravenously. The development of novel biomaterials offers a great opportunity to overcome these challenges. The aim of this review is to discuss the role of biomaterials in development of contrast agents in two fields, CT and US, their similarities and differences, and how the novel properties of nanoparticles have facilitated this development.

Owing to the breadth of this subject and space limitations, this review is not intended to be comprehensive, but rather to provide an introduction to the requirements of the field, as well as an overview of how advances in nanotechnology have exploited the unique properties of biomaterials to address the challenges outlined above.

8.2 Contrast Media for Computed Tomography

Computed tomography (CT) is an imaging modality in which x-rays are projected through the subject at different angles and the resulting data are then reconstructed into three-dimensional images. X-rays are able to pass through the different types of tissue to varying degrees, with bone being relatively radiodense, air being essentially radiotransparent, and water lying between these two extremes. The attenuation of the x-rays is measured in Hounsfield Units (HU), with air and water arbitrarily set to 0 and 1000, respectively. As soft tissues tend to have very similar radiodensities, CT imaging can be significantly improved by injecting radiopaque compounds intravenously, improving the definition of vascular structures and providing some degree of soft tissue targeting and differentiation.

There is both a need and an opportunity for new CT contrast agents that target specific tissues or provide prolonged imaging times. Magnetic resonance imaging (MRI) can also provide high-resolution anatomic images as well as quantitative information on blood flow, but CT offers both technical and pragmatic advantages compared with MRI: There is a direct proportionality between x-ray absorption and contrast agent concentration, simplifying quantitative studies, and CT is less expensive and more widely available than MRI. The primary disadvantage of CT compared with MRI is that CT scans involve exposure to ionizing radiation, but the radiation dose can be minimized by only imaging the region of interest and by careful selection of imaging parameters (i.e., power (kvp) and x-ray current (mA)).

CT contrast media must be very water soluble because of the large quantities that are injected. The solubility requirement results in rapid clearance from the blood, which in turn limits the available imaging time. Prolonging the clearance time, by means such as increasing the molecular weight of the agent, has, therefore, been an important research focus. A second research focus is the development of CT contrast agents that target specific tissues. This objective has proved difficult to achieve because a significant mass of the contrast agent must accumulate in the target tissue before the tissue density increases enough to improve the contrast of the image. This requirement, in turn, increases the risk of toxicity. While iodine is the primary element used in CT contrast agents, primarily because of its low cost and minimal toxicity, a third research focus is the evaluation of radiodense elements other than iodine (e.g., barium).

8.2.1 Macromolecular Contrast Agents

To address the problem of increasing the time available for imaging, the most straightforward approach is to increase the size of the contrast agent to the nanoparticle range (typically 1–100 nM), which slows its clearance from the blood (for more detailed discussion, see Hallouard *et al.* [1]). If one adopts this approach, the choices that must be made are: (1) What type of nanoparticle to use and how this choice affects the particle's *in vivo* behavior, (2) What radiopaque element will be used and how will it be attached to the nanoparticle, and (3) What other steps are required for *in vivo* use? In terms of which nanoparticle is optimal, there has been a progression in the field from use of the relatively simple micelles, to more complex but also more efficacious liposomes, to dendrimers, and finally to the use of microcrystalline or particulate forms of radiopaque elements. We will consider each of these in turn.

8.2.1.1 Micelles

Micelles are single-layer vesicles that form spontaneously in surfactant solutions when the surfactant concentration exceeds the critical micelle concentration (CMC). The CMC varies with the surfactant, so the materials used in the manufacture of intravenously administered micellar drugs must be chosen so that the CMC is low enough that the micelle does not collapse when the drug is diluted upon injection, achieving the desired goal of remaining intact in the circulatory system for a prolonged period of time.

Micelles can be used as contrast agents in two ways: The micelle can be used as a carrier, with the radiopaque element transported in the hydrophobic core of the micelle, or the radiopaque element can be covalently attached to the polymer constituents of the micelle, to either the hydrophilic outer "head" or the hydrophobic inner "tail." Covalent attachment of the radiopaque element to the constituents of the micelle is ideal as it improves retention of the element by the micelle, increasing specificity, and also reducing toxicity.

For a micellar CT contrast agent to be effective, it must deliver sufficient mass of the radiopaque element to the tissue of interest to allow increase the tissue density versus that of adjacent tissue. Improved carrying capacity can be achieved through using larger hydrophobic molecules, but with the downside that this increases the CMC, which in turn means that a higher micelle concentration is required to achieve adequate *in vivo* stability. Therefore, the use of micelles in CT imaging is inherently limited.

In early studies of the use of micelles as CT contrast agents, micelles were used as carriers for iodinated molecules. However, a significant weakness of this approach was the loss of the iodinated molecules from the core of the micelle. In a more recent study of micelles as CT contrast agents, Torchilin *et al.* [2] used amphipathic block-polymers containing iodine. These compounds form micelles with an average diameter of 80 nm and an iodine content of 33.8%. Detectable organ opacification was observed from 5 min to 3 h post-injection in rats; attenuation increased from 85 HU to 253 HU in the aorta and from 92 HU to 156 HU in the liver post-micelle injection over this 3 h window. The authors note that while this was a significant achievement in the use of micelles as CT contrast agents, much more work must be carried out before these materials are ready for clinical use. For recent reviews, see Ref. [3].

8.2.1.2 Liposomes

As candidate nanoparticles, liposomes have several advantages over micelles: Their manufacture is more controllable, they are mechanically stronger, they are less susceptible to collapse on dilution, they can be used as carriers for hydrophilic and hydrophobic molecules, and they can be derivatized with targeting moieties more easily.

Liposomes, first described by Bangham in 1964 [4], consist of amphipathic phospholipids that form bilayered vesicles in aqueous solutions. In contrast to micelles, the core of liposomes is hydrophilic. They can, therefore, act as vehicles for either hydrophilic compounds (in the core) or hydrophobic compounds, for example iodinated polymers, in the lipid bilayer. Early liposomes comprised phosphatidyl choline (PC) from egg and cholesterol. These "conventional," or "C," liposomes have been superseded by sterically stabilized, or "S," liposomes (see Ref. [5] for further discussion). Improvements have also been made in the combinations of fatty acids and lipids used in the manufacture of liposomes and in surface modification of the particles so as to evade *in vivo* clearance mechanisms, thereby extending the circulation time and improving uptake at the site of interest.

The materials used in the preparation of liposomes must provide structural strength and stability while at the same time reducing interactions with proteins in order to extend the circulation time. The stability and mechanical strength of liposomes is based on a rigid bilayer that requires lipids with a high phase-transition temperature. The bilayer is typically comprised of a common lipid such as phosphatidyl choline and a mixture of the fatty acids stearate and oleate. Addition of a small amount of cholesterol increases the fluidity of the bilayer by modifying its crystalline nature. Keeping the formulation simple is also beneficial, as mixtures of lipids with different phase transition temperatures can lead to instability *in vivo*.

The rapid loss of liposomes from the blood in early studies was attributed to both their size and interaction with clearing mechanisms. Since larger liposomes (> 100 nm) are cleared more quickly than smaller ones, maintaining diameters below this threshold during the manufacturing process is critical. On the other hand, larger liposomes can carry more payload, increasing their potential efficacy as contrast agents. Reducing their interaction with clearing mechanisms has required several iterations. The primary clearance mechanism is the mononuclear phagocyte system (MPS), also known as the reticuloendothelial system (RES). One early attempt to evade this system was to replicate the outer coatings of red blood cells by incorporating molecules such as the monosialoganglioside GM1 into the liposome [6]. GM1 carries a negative charge, and it was found that inclusion of other negatively charged molecules, such as phosphatidylserine (PS) or phosphatidyl glycerol (PG), on the outer shell of the liposome also reduced RES clearance, though at high levels this advantage was offset by increased liver uptake, possibly through interaction with Kupffer cells [7]. An additional consideration is that directly accessible negative charges, such as those provided by PS and PG, can increase interaction with proteins whereas shielded negative charges, such as those on GM1, increase the zeta potential of the nanoparticle but are not accessible to direct interaction with proteins [8]. This proves to be a double advantage as increasing the zeta potential also reduces aggregation, improving the stability of the liposomes during manufacture, storage, and after injection. More recently, GM1 has been replaced by polyethylene glycol (PEG), which also reduces interactions with the RES and is chemically well defined, as well as being much less expensive than GM1. While PEG does reduce opsonization, there is evidence that PEG-coated liposomes still induce a complement-based immune response [9].

A range of sizes of PEG has been evaluated. With higher MW PEGs (e.g., 5 kDa) there is steric hindrance of the ability of ligands attached to the liposome to bind to their targets [10], while for lower MW PEGs (e.g., 750 Da) the circulation time is shorter [11], leading to use of PEGs in 2 kDa range. Alternatively, the targeting ligand, which could be an antibody, peptide, or other targeting molecule, can be attached to the PEG so that it is held outside the PEG coating, reducing steric hindrance while simultaneously increasing circulation time [12].

Current methods of encapsulating small-molecule, water-soluble, iodinated compounds in the liposome core still leave a significant amount of contrast agent in the bulk formulation medium resulting in uptake of the non-encapsulated material in the kidney shortly after injection. This can confound quantitative studies as it suggests a triphasic clearance of the nanoparticle or a faster initial clearance phase than is actually the case. However, the presence of this excess material in the bulk formulation solution has the advantage of reducing the rate of loss of the contrast agent from the core of the nanoparticle *in vitro*, which results in a longer shelf life and more consistent imaging results [13]. This problem arises because the rate of loss of the iodinated contrast agent from the liposome core is related to the concentration difference across the lipid bilayer and also to the osmotic pressure difference. This can be avoided by using the iodinated-polymer method where the iodine is covalently bound to the lipid itself, effectively precluding loss of the iodine from the liposome. Another approach to avoiding this problem was discussed by Wei *et al* [14] who developed a multilamellar (rather than unilamellar) liposomal construct. This had the advantage of entrapping high concentrations of iodohexol (50 mg/ml) within the liposomal core while reducing the loss of the iodine by diffusion through the bilayer. A further development of this approach was reported by Kweon *et al.* [15], who used a mixture of water-soluble and oil-based iodinated compounds. The water-soluble material is trapped in the hydrophilic core while the oil-based material is trapped in the hydrophobic bilayer, resulting in a significant increase in radioopacity in the target organ. Encapsulating iopamidol, a water-soluble iodine contrast agent, in liposomes (giving an iodine concentration of 13.8 mg/ml in the formulation) resulted in a relatively small improvement in contrast. However, loading the liposomes with both iopamidol and lipiodol, an iodinated oil, resulted in iodine concentrations as high as 49.2 mg/ml in the combined formulation, and the lipiodol did not disrupt the liposomal structure. A limitation of this approach is that increasing the amount of lipiodol in the liposome resulted in a mixture that was too viscous to produce a liposomal dispersion. This formulation included cholesterol in addition to 1,2-dimyristoyl-sn-glycero-3-phosphocholine (DMPC), which increased the rigidity of the liposomal structure, reducing leakage of entrapped iopamidol and increasing its concentration within the liposomes by 1.6-fold. The *in vivo* performance of these liposomes was encouraging, with an increase of 30 HU, and the material also showed delayed clearance from the circulation. For comparison, iopamidol, which is commonly used as a contrast agent by itself, produces an increase of <7 HU when used at the same iodine concentration.

8.2.1.3 Dendrimers

Dendrimers are large, synthetic, branched molecules made from repeats of chemical units built around an inner core. The attraction of these materials as imaging agents is that the structure is highly defined and the size can be precisely controlled by controlling the number of repeats (generations). The outer face of these molecules can be chemically modified, so they can be targeted relatively simply. One of the drawbacks of the dendrimers is the synthesis, which can require up to several days depending on the formulation.

Fu *et al.* [16] reported the synthesis, characterization, and initial imaging studies with a dendrimer-based CT contrast agent. This compound was composed of a PEG core derivatized at each end with polylysine dendrimers. Different lengths of PEG and numbers of generations of polylysine were used to construct molecules of differing sizes with a large number of sites available for iodination. The resulting compounds had molecular weights ranging from 21.7 kDa to 66.4 kDa (compared with 0.82 kDa for iodohexol). An initial imaging study with PEG12000-carbamate-Gen4-IOB showed good contrast in the liver of a rat, including the visualization of the blood vessels. The 35 min blood half-life of this compound meant that contrast was still evident 30+ min after intravenous injection, much longer than is seen with conventional tracers which have blood half-lives of <5 min. This agent was used to measure the plasma volume and endothelial permeability of subcutaneous xenograft breast cancer xenograft tumors [17].

8.2.2 Other Radioopaque Elements

In addition to iodine, a number of other elements have desirable characteristics for CT contrast agents and are being developed for use. For example, in work by Rabin *et al.* [18], nanocrystals of Bi_2S_3 were coated with the polymer polyvinylpyrrolidone (PVP). (The uncoated crystals could not be used as imaging agents because of aggregation and rapid clearance.) When these nanoparticles were tested *in vivo*, sufficient increases in contrast were achieved for clear imaging of vascular structures. The blood half-life was 140 ± 15 min, which is significantly longer than that of commercial iodinated agents (typically <10 min). At later time points, the enhancement of tissues involved in the RES was observed, leading to the suggestion that the agent could be used to image the liver and detect tumor metastases in that organ. The toxicity of these nanoparticles was tested *in vivo* and found to be much lower than the free bismuth ions (LD_{50}'s of 8 mM and 100 mM for bismuth ions and Bi_2S_3 nanoparticles, respectively).

Gold nanoparticles (AuNPs) also have potential application in this field, with gold's higher atomic number (79) than iodine (53) resulting in greater attenuation of x-rays. As with bismuth particles, AuNPs have to be coated, for example with gum Arabic, to reduce their hematological and renal toxicity [19]. They have been shown to be stable *in vivo* and to produce good contrast in CT applications [19, 20]. Another advantage of AuNPs is that they have a large surface-area-to-volume ratio, providing more opportunity for surface modification. For example, Aydogan *et al.* reported the modification of AuNPs with a structural analogue of glucose, 2-deoxy-D-glucose (2DG) [21]. This modification increased their uptake by tumor cells *in vitro* by a factor of 4 compared with unmodified AuNPs, although the exact mechanism of uptake has yet to be fully defined. In another example, targeting was achieved by entrapping AuNPs in dendrimers, then targeting the combined nanoparticle using folate attached to the outside of the dendrimer, resulting in improved binding to KB cells (human epithelial carcinoma cells) *in vitro* [22].

8.2.3 Targeting

These last examples introduce the topic of targeting contrast nanoparticles to tissues or diseases of interest. Some degree of tumor targeting by nanoparticles is achieved passively because of differences in tumor blood vessel structure compared with that of normal tissues, through what is known as the enhanced permeability and retention (EPR) effect [23]. More specific targeting can be achieved either by designing the materials so that they are sensitive to differences in environmental conditions, such as pH, or by attaching targeting molecules such as peptides or antibodies to the exterior of the macromolecule.

Optimal targets for nanoparticle targeting are on the luminal side of blood vessels, as extravasation of macromolecules can be slow. One case where this would be of great value is the detection and description of atherosclerosis. The two following examples demonstrate different methods of identifying atherosclerotic plaques with potential to rupture. Currently, atherosclerotic plaques can be imaged using intravascular ultrasound (IV-US) or by MRI. However, both of these methods have drawbacks, including the invasive nature of IV-US and the long time required for MRI, because tissue movement reduces the image quality. CT is faster and less expensive than both of these techniques and the resolution is high enough to detect the biological features of atherosclerosis. Danila *et al.* [24] encapsulated iohexol in liposomes and then attached anti-ICAM-1 antibodies to the liposomes to target them to inflamed vasculature. This resulted in immunoliposomes that bind specifically to activated human coronary artery endothelial cells *in vitro*. In another example, Wyss *et al.* [25] coated liposomes with a peptide that binds E-selectin with high affinity and measured their *in vitro* and *in vivo* selectivity. In an ischemia-reperfusion injury model, increased uptake by activated endothelial cells was observed compared with controls. In a tumor imaging study, targeting the liposomes did not affect their blood half-lives, but it did extend tumor residence of the particles.

8.2.4 CT Contrast Agent Summary

In this section, we considered the properties required of CT contrast agents and how appropriate biomaterials are being selected. A primary requirement for the development of targeted CT contrast agents is that sufficient mass of radiodense material must accumulate at the site of interest to cause a corresponding change in the attenuation of the incident x-ray beam. Sufficient mass is also necessary for ultrasound contrast agents, except that they must also possess echogenicity for detection, placing a further developmental constraint on these nanoparticles. It is also necessary that there be a change in the attenuation of the incident x-ray beam or that sufficient radiodense material accumulate at the site of interest. Neither (x-rays or radiodensity) is applicable to US. We will now consider how these imaging probes are being developed.

8.3 Ultrasound

Medical ultrasonography uses reflected sound waves with frequencies above 20 MHz to construct images. This technology has been used for several decades to visualize a range of anatomic features in the human body. Ultrasound can be used to evaluate cardiac abnormalities, such as blood vessel wall inflammation, as an early indicator of heart disease. It can also be used to detect blood clots, such as deep-vein thromboses. More intense US beams can also be used therapeutically. Thus, one of the more interesting features of ultrasound is that, in some cases, it can be used both to detect and to treat disease.

Ultrasound has a number of advantages over other imaging modalities: It is relatively inexpensive and portable and has a low risk profile, with no exposure to ionizing radiation and no inherent toxicity associated with the potential contrast agents (i.e., no iodine or gadolinium is required). The primary disadvantage is that imaging is confined to a relatively small area of interest. Advantages over MRI include high resolution (of the order of 10's of microns, enabling imaging of small blood vessels) and that repeat scans can be made immediately, which is difficult with MRI if repeated administration of contrast agents is required.

Until relatively recently, all US was carried out without the use of contrast agents. The past 10 years, however, have witnessed the introduction of the first US contrast agents. The agents enhance the US image by creating differences in the sound reflection, or echogenicity, between different anatomic compartments. For example, intravenous administration of encapsulated air bubbles ("microbubbles") results in an increased difference in echogenicity between the lumen of the vessel and its surroundings. Ultrasound contrast agents (UCAs) have a number of desirable characteristics that they share with CT contrast agents, such as low toxicity and ease of formulation and administration. Additionally, as with CT contrast agents, the mass of imaging agent concentrating at the site of disease is important in achieving a good signal-to-noise ratio. However, the nature of the imaging modality adds additional constraints above those required for CT contrast agents. For example, large bubbles are required for good echogenicity, but if they are too large, they become trapped in microvasculature, especially in the lung. Initially, the microbubbles that were used were of the order of 100 μm, while the current microbubbles are <5 μm in diameter. The microbubbles must flex to produce signal, but at the same time, they must be strong enough to withstand the pressures in the left side of the heart without rupturing if they are to have a long circulation time, a requirement for optimal concentration at the site of interest. As with all contrast agents, the optimal UCA will depend on the purpose of the imaging study. It must have adequate echogenicity to produce a high-contrast image and also strong enough to withstand the US beam used for detection, but if it is designed to be susceptible to rupture by more intense US radiation, then local signal can be artificially reduced to enable repeated studies. Another way in which the ability of microbubbles to be "fractured on demand" can be exploited is as targeted drug delivery vehicles. A drug can be encapsulated in the microbubbles, the bubbles are then administered intravenously, and an US beam can be used to fracture the bubbles at the target site, delivering the drug specifically to that site.

In the development of UCAs, three components must be optimized: the shell, the core, and the targeting moiety. We will discuss each of these in turn.

8.3.1 Shell

The composition of the UCA's shell determines its physical properties, most important, its mechanical elasticity. If it is too brittle, then it will fracture too easily, but if it is too elastic, then it will not produce an adequate signal (see McCulloch *et al.* [26]). The optimal UCA for each purpose varies — for example, a more brittle shell might be used as a drug delivery vehicle so that it can be ruptured more easily at the target site.

The shell can be made of protein, galactose, lipid, or polymers (see Ref. [27]). Following early studies with a range of water-based solutions, encouraging results were obtained with microbubbles consisting of air trapped in a denatured albumin shell made by sonication of an albumin solution. This was an important development because it provided the first useful US contrast agent, but the method of manufacture produced a wide range of particle sizes. This is a significant issue in UCA development because different sized bubbles have different echogenicities. Also, as noted previously, larger bubbles are trapped in small blood vessels, especially in the lungs, hindering transition from the venous injection to arterial distribution, and reducing the circulation time of a significant fraction of the particles. On the other hand, smaller microbubbles also have poor persistence, because they can be damaged by ultrasound radiation.

Lipid-based shells have a number of desirable properties. They are smaller (<5 μm), it is easier to control their size, they are mechanically much more robust than microbubbles, and the composition of the shell can be altered to optimize their properties. Alkan-Onyuksel and colleagues [28] systematically investigated the echogenicity of liposomes produced from combinations of phosphatidylcholine (PC), phosphatidylglycerol (PG), phosphatidylethanolamine (PE) and cholesterol, selected because they are the main constituent of cell membranes (PC), confer a negative charge (PG), provide options for conjugation (PE), and increase rigidity (cholesterol). They found that high concentrations of PE (e.g., 4%), low concentrations of PG (1%), and constant cholesterol (30%) gave highest echogenicity. These findings were confirmed by *in vitro* and *in vivo* studies. It was also found that echogenicity was related to the structure of the liposomes. More echogenic liposomes tended to have multilamellar structures, while the less echogenic liposomes had thick, unseparated, unilamellar structures. It was suggested that the formulation of the liposomes caused these differences, with, for example, the negative charge of PG preventing aggregation and the small head of PE affecting the formation of the multiwalled structures. In later work by the same group [29], it was found that entrapment of air in the liposomes during the lyophilization step in their manufacture was a requirement for their echogenicity. The inclusion of mannitol in the formulation as a cryoprotectant resulted in the exposure of hydrophobic regions to air during lyophilization and then its subsequent retention in the rehydrated form.

8.3.2 Core

In addition to the above-described issues of size, etc., the nature of the fluid entrapped within the microbubble also influences its imaging characteristics. Air is easily incorporated into microbubbles, but is soluble in blood, so it escapes from the bubble and shortens the potential imaging time. The rate of diffusion of air from microbubbles can be reduced by, for example, using biopolymer shells. Heavy gases have lower solubility in blood and so lead to the UCAs having longer persistence. Polyfluorinated carbon gases (PFCs) are also poorly soluble in water and are liquids at room temperature, and their non-toxicity, stability, and low acoustic impedance make them attractive fluids to use as the core of microbubble contrast agents.

Marsh *et al.* [30] systematically investigated the echogenicity of seven PFCs at a range of temperatures between 25°C and 45°C. Their conclusion was that perfluorohexane had the lowest acoustic impedance within this temperature range (the acoustic impedance of distilled water at 37°C is approximately 1.5 g/cm^2-s, while perfluorohexane is approximately 0.8 g/cm^2-s), and therefore would provide a good enhancement agent as it has a very different impedance compared with water, resulting in good contrast. The group then extended this work by investigating the suitability of various fluids as the core of targeted microbubbles *in vitro* [31]. This study investigated the observation that targeting the microbubbles to a surface improved their impedance. The authors suggested that this improvement was due to the development of a reflective interface between the targeted surface and the medium surrounding it.

The introduction of fluids into nanoparticles and then ensuring their entrapment, at least for the duration of scanning, presents a challenge that can be met in various ways. One interesting method of introducing the gas *in vivo* was reported by Kang *et al.* [32], who used polyesters with carbonate side-chains to produce nanoparticles, which, when injected intravenously, produce nanobubbles that coalesce into microbubbles. Water diffuses into the microbubbles and cleaves the carbonate side-chain forming carbon dioxide *in situ*. The viability of this approach was confirmed by ultrasound imaging *in vivo*. Another advantage of this technology is that the nanobubbles are themselves not visible at 100 μm US resolution, but once they arrive at the target tissue and coalesce into microbubbles, the size increases and the bubbles become visible by US.

The transition of UCAs from protein-based microbubbles to optimized liposomal particles containing gases that further enhance the US signal also provides a greatly improved platform for derivatization using specific ligands to facilitate targeting. The two main areas that have been investigated for UCA targeting are inflammation and cancer.

8.3.3 Targeting Inflammation

UCAs can be actively targeted to specific tissues in two ways, by inclusion of a targeting moiety on the one or more of the chemical constituents of the UCA or by chemical attachment of a targeting ligand, such as a peptide or antibody, to one of its constituents. The size and the composition of the shell, especially in the case of protein-based shells, will also affect the distribution *in vivo*, providing additional biological information. This "passive" targeting can provide information on blood flow, the lymphatic system, or the systems that interact with foreign agents in the body, such as phagocytic lymphocytes. It could be argued that microbubbles with a shell consisting of denatured albumin represent both passive and active targeting of inflammation because the microbubble itself provides a marker of increased vascular permeability while the albumin shell interacts with activated endothelial cells. It has also been noted that in some cases albumin-based microbubbles are retained in the myocardium, leading to an enhanced US signal. It was hypothesized that this was due to interaction between the microbubbles and the inflamed endothelial tissue. Villanueva *et al.* [33] tested this hypothesis in an *in vitro* study in which they found that albumin-based microbubbles adhered strongly to the exposed inflamed extracellular matrix of endothelial cells. In related work also targeting inflammation, Unger *et al.* [34] coupled a hexapeptide representing the minimum functional unit from fibrinogen (amino acid sequence KQAGDV) to a lipid, incorporated the functionalized lipid into a PFC-containing liposome, and observed increased binding of this UCA to blood clots *in vitro*. Similarly, Christiansen *et al.* [35] used phosphatidylserine (PS)-containing lipid microbubbles to target leukocytes in order to quantify inflammation from myocardial reperfusion injury. Including PS in the lipid composition increased complement-mediated microbubble attachment to the activated leukocytes involved in inflammation. The authors report both quantitative and qualitative agreement between the localization of microbubbles in infarcted inflamed tissue and reference methods used to detect and quantify inflammation: ^{99m}Tc-RP517 was used to detect neutrophils and TTC staining to describe viable tissue. This method has also been used to detect inflammation in renal ischemia-reperfusion injury [36].

8.3.4 Targeting Cancer

Ellegala *et al.* [37] used the peptide echistatin to target microbubbles to neovasculature expressing the integrin $\alpha_v\beta_3$. The targeted microbubbles were retained preferentially within the microvasculature of intracerebrally implanted U87MG tumors (i.e., orthotopic) as detected by confocal microscopy of fluorescently labeled microbubbles. Ultrasound imaging was carried out 10 min after bolus injection of targeted microbubbles and increased contrast was observed between 14 and 28 days post tumor inoculation. Leong-Poi *et al.* [38] also reported targeting of angiogenesis for ultrasound detection using both echistatin and an anti-α_v integrin antibody to achieve significant increases in US contrast compared with controls. The animal model used by these investigators was based on the injection of the proangiogenic factor FGF into the cremaster muscle to stimulate vessel development. FGF can also be used to stimulate vessel development in infarcted myocardial muscle, presenting the opportunity to monitor the response of injured tissue to this therapeutic agents using ultrasound. In another example, Lui *et al.* [39] demonstrated *in vitro* targeting of polylactic-acid-based UCAs using the anti-HER2 antibody Herceptin as the targeting agent and observed an increase in echogenicity by HER2-antigen-positive cells.

8.4 Summary

The increasing personalization of medicine and its increasing ability to specifically target appropriate medicines to ever-smaller populations of patients demands a corresponding improvement in our ability to more precisely characterize and describe disease. Medical imaging offers the opportunity to detect, describe, and, in some cases, treat disease, as well as the ability to monitor the response of diseased tissue to therapy. Here we have briefly considered some aspects of the development of contrast agents for both computed tomography and ultrasound imaging. Both modalities have advantages as well as limitations, depending on the specific application. Through the appropriate use of biomaterials within the field of nanotechnology, these challenges are gradually being addressed.

References

1. Hallouard, F., et al., Iodinated blood pool contrast media for preclinical X-ray imaging applications — a review. *Biomaterials*, 2010. **31**(24): p. 6249–6268.
2. Torchilin, V.P., M.D. Frank-Kamenetsky, and G.L. Wolf, CT visualization of blood pool in rats by using long-circulating, iodine-containing micelles. *Acad Radiol*, 1999. **6**(1): p. 61–65.
3. Torchilin, V.P., Micellar nanocarriers: pharmaceutical perspectives. *Pharm Res*, 2007. **24**(1): p. 1–16.
4. Bangham, A.D. and R.W. Horne, Negative staining of phospholipids and their structural modification by surface-active agents as observed in the electron microscope. *J Mol Biol*, 1964. **8**: p. 660–668.
5. Allen, T.M., Long-circulating (sterically stabilized) liposomes for targeted drug delivery. *Trends Pharmacol Sci*, 1994. **15**(7): p. 215–220.
6. Gabizon, A. and D. Papahadjopoulos, Liposome formulations with prolonged circulation time in blood and enhanced uptake by tumors. *Proc Natl Acad Sci U S A*, 1988. **85**(18): p. 6949–6953.
7. Dijkstra, J., et al., Interaction of liposomes with Kupffer cells *in vitro*. *Exp Cell Res*, 1984. **150**(1): p. 161–176.
8. Lasic, D.D., et al., Sterically stabilized liposomes: a hypothesis on the molecular origin of the extended circulation times. *Biochim Biophys Acta*, 1991. **1070**(1): p. 187–192.
9. Moghimi, S.M. and J. Szebeni, Stealth liposomes and long circulating nanoparticles: critical issues in pharmacokinetics, opsonization and protein-binding properties. *Prog Lipid Res*, 2003. **42**(6): p. 463–478.
10. Mori, A., et al., Influence of the steric barrier activity of amphipathic poly(ethyleneglycol) and ganglioside GM1 on the circulation time of liposomes and on the target binding of immunoliposomes *in vivo*. *FEBS Lett*, 1991. **284**(2): p. 263–266.
11. Woodle, M.C., et al., Versatility in lipid compositions showing prolonged circulation with sterically stabilized liposomes. *Biochim Biophys Acta*, 1992. **1105**(2): p. 193–200.
12. Koning, G.A., et al., Interaction of differently designed immunoliposomes with colon cancer cells and Kupffer cells. An *in vitro* comparison. *Pharm Res*, 2003. **20**(8): p. 1249–1257.

13. Leander, P., et al., A new liposomal liver-specific contrast agent for CT: first human phase-I clinical trial assessing efficacy and safety. *Eur Radiol*, 2001. **11**(4): p. 698–704.
14. Wei, X., et al., Liposomal contrast agent for CT imaging of the liver. *Conf Proc IEEE Eng Med Biol Soc*, 2005. **6**: p. 5702–5705.
15. Kweon, S., et al., Liposomes coloaded with iopamidol/lipiodol as a RES-targeted contrast agent for computed tomography imaging. *Pharm Res.*, 2010. **27**(7): p. 1408–1415.
16. Fu, Y., et al., Dendritic iodinated contrast agents with PEG-cores for CT imaging: synthesis and preliminary characterization. *Bioconjug Chem*, 2006. **17**(4): p. 1043–1056.
17. Simon, G.H., et al., Initial computed tomography imaging experience using a new macromolecular iodinated contrast medium in experimental breast cancer. *Invest Radiol*, 2005. **40**(9): p. 614–620.
18. Rabin, O., et al., An X-ray computed tomography imaging agent based on long-circulating bismuth sulphide nanoparticles. *Nat Mater*, 2006. **5**(2): p. 118–122.
19. Kattumuri, V., et al., Gum arabic as a phytochemical construct for the stabilization of gold nanoparticles: *in vivo* pharmacokinetics and X-ray-contrast-imaging studies. *Small*, 2007. **3**(2): p. 333–341.
20. Boote, E., et al., Gold nanoparticle contrast in a phantom and juvenile swine: models for molecular imaging of human organs using x-ray computed tomography. *Acad Radiol*, 2011. **17**(4): p. 410–417.
21. Aydogan, B., et al., AuNP-DG: deoxyglucose-labeled gold nanoparticles as X-ray computed tomography contrast agents for cancer imaging. *Mol Imaging Biol*, 2010. **12**(5): p. 463–467.
22. Shi, X., et al., Dendrimer-entrapped gold nanoparticles as a platform for cancer-cell targeting and imaging. *Small*, 2007. **3**(7): p. 1245–1252.
23. Matsumura, Y. and H. Maeda, A new concept for macromolecular therapeutics in cancer chemotherapy: mechanism of tumoritropic accumulation of proteins and the antitumor agent smancs. *Cancer Res*, 1986. **46**(12 Pt 1): p. 6387–6392.
24. Danila, D., et al., Antibody-labeled liposomes for CT imaging of atherosclerotic plaques: *in vitro* investigation of an anti-ICAM antibody-labeled liposome containing iohexol for molecular imaging of atherosclerotic plaques via computed tomography. *Tex Heart Inst J*, 2009. **36**(5): p. 393–403.
25. Wyss, C., et al., Molecular imaging by micro-CT: specific E-selectin imaging. *Eur Radiol*, 2009. **19**(10): p. 2487–2494.
26. McCulloch, M., et al., Ultrasound contrast physics: A series on contrast echocardiography, article 3. *J Am Soc Echocardiogr*, 2000. **13**(10): p. 959–967.

27. Lindner, J.R., Microbubbles in medical imaging: current applications and future directions. *Nat Rev Drug Discov*, 2004. **3**(6): p. 527–532.

28. Alkan-Onyuksel, H., et al., Development of inherently echogenic liposomes as an ultrasonic contrast agent. *J Pharm Sci*, 1996. **85**(5): p. 486–90.

29. Huang, S.L., et al., Physical correlates of the ultrasonic reflectivity of lipid dispersions suitable as diagnostic contrast agents. *Ultrasound Med Biol*, 2002. **28**(3): p. 339–48.

30. Marsh, J.N., et al., Temperature dependence of acoustic impedance for specific fluorocarbon liquids. *J Acoust Soc Am*, 2002. **112**(6): p. 2858–2862.

31. Marsh, J.N., et al., Improvements in the ultrasonic contrast of targeted perfluorocarbon nanoparticles using an acoustic transmission line model. *IEEE Trans Ultrason Ferroelectr Freq Control*, 2002. **49**(1): p. 29–38.

32. Kang, E., et al., Nanobubbles from gas-generating polymeric nanoparticles: ultrasound imaging of living subjects. *Angew Chem Int Ed Engl*, 2010. **49**(3): p. 524–528.

33. Villanueva, F.S., et al., Albumin microbubble adherence to human coronary endothelium: implications for assessment of endothelial function using myocardial contrast echocardiography. *J Am Coll Cardiol*, 1997. **30**(3): p. 689–693.

34. Unger, E.C., et al., *In vitro* studies of a new thrombus-specific ultrasound contrast agent. *Am J Cardiol*, 1998. **81**(12A): p. 58G–61G.

35. Christiansen, J.P., et al., Noninvasive imaging of myocardial reperfusion injury using leukocyte-targeted contrast echocardiography. *Circulation*, 2002. **105**(15): p. 1764–1767.

36. Lindner, J.R., et al., Microbubble persistence in the microcirculation during ischemia/reperfusion and inflammation is caused by integrin- and complement-mediated adherence to activated leukocytes. *Circulation*, 2000. **101**(6): p. 668–675.

37. Ellegala, D.B., et al., Imaging tumor angiogenesis with contrast ultrasound and microbubbles targeted to alpha(v)beta3. *Circulation*, 2003. **108**(3): p. 336–341.

38. Leong-Poi, H., et al., Noninvasive assessment of angiogenesis by ultrasound and microbubbles targeted to alpha(v)-integrins. *Circulation*, 2003. **107**(3): p. 455–460.

39. Liu, J., et al., Biodegradable nanoparticles for targeted ultrasound imaging of breast cancer cells *in vitro*. *Phys Med Biol*, 2007. **52**(16): p. 4739–4747.

Chapter 9

Image-Based High-Content Analysis, Stem Cells and Nanomedicines: A Novel Strategy for Drug Discovery

Leonardo J. Solmesky, Yonatan Adalist, and Miguel Weil
Laboratory for Personalized Medicine and Neurodegenerative Diseases, Department of Cell Research and Immunology, The George S. Wise Faculty of Life Sciences, Tel Aviv University, Ramat Aviv 69978, Israel
miguelw@tauex.tau.ac.il

Image-based high content screening (HCS) is rapidly gaining recognition as the future of drug discovery. The ability to screen vast amounts of possible therapeutic agents in a relatively short time, while obtaining various levels of information about each target cell's biology, has an immense potential. Moreover, since the screening is done using cells, it is possible to look for a broader phenotype than, for example, when focusing on the activity of an isolated enzyme. This allows the search for new drugs for diseases with unknown molecular hallmarks or with multifactorial causes. The recently achieved advances in human stem cell research have opened the way to a new horizon in medical technology. Our ability to manipulate these cells will allow us to change the focus of drug development from generic to personal. Consequently, it will be possible to characterize

Handbook of Harnessing Biomaterials in Nanomedicine: Preparation, Toxicity, and Applications
Edited by Dan Peer

ISBN 978-981-4316-46-0 (Hardback), 978-981-4364-27-0 (eBook)
www.panstanford.com

the effect of a repertoire of available therapies for a certain disease using the cells obtained from a certain individual. This would offer an unparalleled achievement, and its contribution to the success rate of treatments could prove truly astronomical. Similarly to the way high-content screening is revolutionizing the process of drug discovery, the application of these methods using human stem cells together with nanotechnology for improving targeted drug delivery, is expected to produce the next major breakthrough for personalized medicine in the pharmaceutical industry.

9.1 Introduction

Drug discovery and development is an extremely dynamic process and the challenges it involves are constantly changing. As in most commercial industries, there are numerous external aspects that affect the pharmaceutical industry. Thus, the process of constructing a successful research and development strategy that is cost-effective includes components such as focus on diseases with the highest potential return on investment, increased R&D productivity, and the achievement of unquestionable benefit versus risk.

During recent years, the pharmaceutical industry has been struggling with dwindling R&D productivity. A few of the causes of this lower productivity are the prolonged R&D cycles, immensely prolonged approval times, and staggering rates of drug attrition. For example, over 90% of the drugs entered into clinical trials fail to gain FDA approval [1]. Whereas due to the regulatory authorities it would appear difficult to speed up the approval times, the long R&D cycles and high attrition rates are factors that could be addressed by the pharmaceutical companies through using novel or improved technologies for drug discovery. Technological improvements that would allow a more cost-efficient R&D process would also open the way for development of drugs that would treat those diseases that, under the current conditions, may not receive the funding and attention necessary for significant progress to be made. It is quite clear that by improving the screening technologies used in this industry, it will be possible to revolutionize an industry that has been falling short of fulfilling its true potential for quite some time.

9.2 Image-Based High-Content Screening

Image-based HCS is rapidly gaining recognition as the future of drug discovery. The ability to screen vast amounts of possible therapeutic agents in a relatively short time, while obtaining various levels of information about the biology of each cell under the influence of each tested compound, seems to offer immense potential [2].

In addition, the high content of this technology facilitates increased robustness of the employed assays. In screening, the most commonly used parameter for monitoring assay quality is the Z' factor, which is based on one selected readout. However, biological assays are able to monitor multiple readouts when using image-based HCS. It has been suggested that an extension of the Z' factor, which integrates multiple readouts for assay quality assessment, will enable increased robustness of the assay [3].

Furthermore, since the screening is performed with cells rather than using a specific target, such as a protein, it allows the filtering of those compounds that are most likely to pass the pharmacokinetic tests during the process of drug testing (i.e., only compounds that have suitable solubility, permeability and stability for the target cells will be able to produce a hit in the screening). This technology thereby optimizes the process of drug discovery, allowing the discarding of those molecules that, while possibly optimal for effective influence of the protein involved in the disease, would not be suitable for therapy in a cellular context due to pharmacokinetic barriers [4]. Moreover, also due to the screening is employing cells, it is possible to look for a broader phenotype in the process (i.e., rescue from induced apoptosis by a compound) than, for example, when focusing on the activity of an isolated enzyme, thus allowing the process of drug discovery to be applied to diseases with unknown molecular hallmarks or multifactorial causes [5]. Such diseases have until recently been very far from being curable. Now, however, image-based HCS brings hope for a change in this situation.

The introduction of advances in microscopy, like z-autofocus and x and y axes sample positioning has allowed the use of image-based analysis for high-throughput screenings. Until the introduction of such advances, these screenings were generally carried out by end-point reactions, showing only a global outcome from any well (i.e., change in fluorescence intensity). The introduction of these new features has allowed the automation of microscopy and its incorporation into the field of high-throughput screening [6].

In addition, developments in liquid handling automation now enable the preparation of samples in a high-throughput approach, allowing easy screening of collections of thousands of compounds [7]. Furthermore, the software tools for analyzing the output of the screening have been further developed to optimize object segmentation [8] in the images and to allow the extraction of information at all the cellular and intracellular levels [9]. Moreover, many of the applications for biological analysis are even already preset in the software of the HCS systems, in increasingly friendly program interfaces for the operator. Some of these typically used biological software applications are listed in Table 9.1.

Table 9.1 Typical applications for biological analysis using image based HCS technology

Some pre-set biological applications in HCS systems
Cell count
Nuclear size
Cell size
Cell cycle
Cell perimeter
Neurite analysis (number, length, branching)
Protein expression or reporter expression (intensity, localization)
Organelles (number, size, morphology, distance to nuclei, etc.)
Texture

The possibility to obtain an almost unlimited quantity of biological parameters from a large number of cell images taken from multi-well plates poses a challenge for informatics and data management, which needs to be addressed by every HCS core facility. Some of these use their own homemade programs for solving all their customary needs, while others use commercially available software able to deal with the chemistry of the compounds, hit identification, library management, and visualization of the results [10, 11].

Since the field first began to evolve and continues to do so, several companies have inundated the market with instruments suitable for HCS analysis. Table 9.2 lists the most representative instruments currently available for image-based HCS and their type of optics. Their characteristics differ regarding light source, the feasibility of carrying out kinetic assays, autofocus technology, resolution, dynamic range of the camera, and software for analysis, among several other features. Moreover, almost every brand offers its own proprietary algorithms for cell analysis and there are even companies that also offer kits for developing the assays [4].

Table 9.2 Current commercially available instruments for image based HCS and their optics

Company	HCS system	Optics	Website
Amnis	ImageStream	Wide field	www.amnis.com
BD Biosciences	BD Pathway 855	Wide Field/ confocal	www.bdbiosciences.com
BD Biosciences	BD Pathway 435	Wide Field/ confocal	www.bdbiosciences.com
GE Healthcare	IN Cell Analyzer 2000	Wide field	www.biacore.com
Intelligent Imaging Innovations	3i Marianas	Wide field	www.intelligent-imaging.com
Leica Microsystems	TCS SP5	Confocal	www.leica-microsystems.com
Molecular Devices	ImageXpressULTRA	Confocal	www.moleculardevices.com
Molecular Devices	ImageXpressMICRO	Wide field	www.moleculardevices.com
Olympus	Scan^R	Wide field	www.olympus.com
Perkin Elmer	Opera	Confocal	www.perkinelmer.com
Perkin Elmer	Operetta	Wide Field/ confocal	www.perkinelmer.com
Thermo Scientific	Cellomics ArrayScan VTI	Wide field/ confocal	www.cellomics.com

High-throughput screening technologies are widely used in the early stages of drug discovery in order to rapidly evaluate the properties of thousands of compounds. In most cases, pre-existing libraries of compounds are used, although in some cases customized libraries are employed [12]. In addition, before large naive libraries are tested, many companies will use a library that consists of compounds that have already been approved as drugs. If a compound that has already been FDA approved shows potential for a particular target, R&D departments will save enormous amounts of both time and money [13]. Altogether, high-throughput screening technologies are paving the way to the development of novel strategies that will enable the discovery of drugs at affordable commercial risks for as yet incurable and rare diseases.

9.3 Stem Cells Used for Lead Discovery

Unmet medical needs are essentially the stimulus behind the development of new therapies. Drug discovery is driven by the need to add medical value while concomitantly limiting the costs for the pharmaceutical industry. Understanding and treatment of the pathology, rather than symptomatic relief, is the cardinal factor in drug discovery. This approach necessitates model systems that will emulate the pathological conditions as faithfully as possible. An excellent way to achieve this is to rely on human-derived cells rather than animal-derived cell lines that express specific proteins to mimic a human disease or condition. The use of animal-derived cells or tissues to develop selective drugs is problematic, since their success in treatment of animals or animal models does not always translate into efficacy in humans. There are vast differences in the biological background between the animal model and humans. These differences are believed to be major factors in the difficulty of matching treatment success in these models to the actual beneficial use of such drugs for human clinical trials [14]. Another approach taken is to use immortalized or cancerous human cells to obtain unlimited number of cells for drug-testing trials compared with primary cells directly isolated from human tissue. These are in many cases better models than the animal equivalent, but they still do not necessarily provide an accurate indication of the effects of compounds on normal human cells. This is due to the fact that any immortalized or cancerous cell could have vast differences in its gene expression pattern and, in turn, in its biochemistry, when compared with its non-immortalized counterpart. Recent advances in stem cell (SC) technology have the potential to allow production of a virtually limitless supply of normal human cells that can be differentiated into any specific cell type, except those cell types that make up the extra-embryonic tissues such as the placenta [15]. If this potential is realized, we may witness a leap in our ability to screen for new cell type specific drugs.

SC can differentiate into clinically relevant cell types with uniform physiological characteristics that allow improved target validation decisions [16]. Additionally, SC may allow inclusion of previously unavailable cell types to be used to screen the libraries of therapeutic candidates [17].

These reasons make the use of SC for image-based high-content screening a very valuable option for novel drug discovery.

9.3.1 Stem Cells

During the first stages of life for multi-cellular organisms, a fertilized oocyte is the progenitor for an entire organism. This single cell creates all the different tissues and cell types with all their various characteristics and functions needed to perform as a multicellular organism. During embryogenesis, cells both proliferate and differentiate, thus enabling the growth of tissues and organs.

In an adult organism, most tissues and organs maintain a homeostasis wherein cells continually die and are continually replenished. The extent of this ability varies considerably among organisms and among different types of tissues. Some flatworms are capable of regenerating most of their bodies and even use this as a method of reproduction by splitting into two parts, with each half subsequently repairing itself into a whole [18–21]. While mammals in general and humans specifically do have regenerative capabilities, they do not enjoy anything similar to this spectacular level of plasticity. The liver, epidermis, small intestine and hematopoietic system are a few examples of relatively replenishable cells in mammals [22–25]. We owe this fantastic and necessary capability to SC.

SC are capable of undergoing both self-renewal and differentiation into specific specialized cell types. Embryonic stem cells (ESC) are pluripotent; hence, they bear the potential to produce all the cell types of an embryo [26], while the slightly more specialized multipotent cells that reside in the tissues and organs of multi-cellular organisms are much more restricted in their "choice" of cellular fate. Recently, it has been shown that some adult stem cells, under certain culture conditions, are able to differentiate into other cell types unusual to their tissue of origin [27].

9.3.2 Human Embryonic Stem Cells

Exploiting the great potential that lies in human ESC (hESC) would be an immense advantage in our attempt to improve the drug discovery process.

The ESC research started with seminal studies in murine embryos obtained by *in vitro* fertilization in the 1970s and 1980s [26, 28]. This conduced to the current ability to generate and maintain human ESC in culture by the late 1990s [29]. Since hESCs are the progenitors of all the cells in the human body, we can deduce that they have the capability, under the correct conditions, to be "guided" to form the cells needed for any potential drug screening.

This unlimited potential is in fact both a blessing and a curse for our purposes. Clearly it is a blessing in the sense that ESCs can eventually be used to differentiate into virtually any cell type that, in turn, can be employed as a screening tool for almost any disease. As a result of their pluripotency, however, it is also an immensely complex task to direct such cells homogenously to a specific desired fate [30]. Difficult as this may be, in recent years great leaps have, nonetheless, been made in this area and more and more protocols are being developed [31–34]. Other problems that arise when considering wide-scale use of hESCs are the ethical concerns of some financing and federal bodies in funding research using these types of cells [35]. However, the way in which hESC are currently being obtained is slowly producing a gain in the number of supporters, or at least is allowing the possibility to obtain these cells from *in vitro* fertilized embryos with serious genetic diseases, since it is based on the use of embryos discarded following pre-implantation genetic diagnosis (PGD) procedures. In such procedures, the embryos selected for research (at the early blastocyst stage) were found positive for a genetic disorder and would never be implanted into the mother's uterus [36, 37]. These offer good platform tools by which to study basic cellular and molecular mechanisms of inheritable diseases such as Huntington's disease [38],

Fragile x syndrome [39], cystic fibrosis, and numerous other diseases [38, 40]. Obviously, these hESC lines will be of great importance for drug-screening purposes for such incurable diseases.

These difficulties aside, there is a general consensus that given the time and funding to develop the proper protocols, hESCs will constitute the basis for countless innovations on a long list of various medical fields. Drug discovery is one of the top issues on that list.

9.3.3 Adult Mesenchymal Stem Cells

Any adult tissue that harbors regenerative or self-repairing capabilities on some level is highly likely to contain stem cells that, despite their slightly more differentiated state, retain the aptitude to reproduce the variety of cells that form that tissue.

Mesenchymal stem cells (MSCs) are one of the several types of adult stem cells. This specific type of adult stem cell has received great attention due to its potential in regenerative medicine [41].

In the early 1970s, the first adult MSCs were isolated and were shown to retain the capability to create bone and reproduce an hematopoietic microenvironment [42]. These cells have shown the capability to differentiate into osteoblasts, chondrocytes, adipocytes, myoblasts, and other mesenchymal cell types [43–46] and thus are prime candidates as screening tools for a variety of conditions that involve such cell types. A unique advantage of hMSC that makes them highly useful for HCS methodologies resides in the fact that they are able to survive for prolonged periods of time under serum-free culture conditions without altering their stem cell properties described above. Properties like the pattern of surface markers and the ability to differentiate to either osteoblasts or adipocytes are retained under these conditions [47].

The serum-free conditions allow direct identification of the biological effects of compounds on these cells without possible serum interference [48]. This fact will certainly present hMSC from bone marrow as a valuable platform for drug screenings and personalized medicine.

9.3.4 Induced Pluriputent Stem Cells

Another prospect by which to circumvent the problems embodied in the use of hESCs is the use of a new and extremely promising technology that is capable of returning somatic cells to a nearly embryonic state of pluripotency.

Induced pluripotent stem cells (iPSC) are derived from somatic cells and have the ability to differentiate to almost every type of tissue (like ESC) by the co-overexpression of specific transcription factors (Oct3/4, Sox2, Klf4, and c-Myc) using retroviral vectors [49]. Researchers have found that iPSC share similar characteristics to those of ES cells, such as cell morphology, self-renewal, surface marker antigens, pattern of gene expression, telomerase activity, and the epigenetic status of pluripotent cell-specific genes [50].

Clearly, the principal advantage of iPSC is that they can be derived from a patient with a certain disease, constituting a platform from which to produce any required cell type in order to study the etiology of the disease [51]. Most interestingly, this approach can be used as a model of the disease that has the identical genetic traits of the individual that donated the tissue sample. Today iPSC can also be generated from readily available tissues such as blood [52], skin, or even hair [53]. This advantage makes IPSC ideal candidates to produce neurons and glia from living individuals suffering from neurodegenerative diseases, constituting a remarkable platform for translational research and personalized medicine [54].

9.4 Personalized Medicine Platforms

Personalized medicine refers to the tailoring of strategies to detect, treat, and prevent disease based on an individual's molecular characteristics [55].

Over the past century, medical care has been based on epidemiological studies of large cohorts. However, this type of medicine does not consider the genetic variability of individuals within a population. Consequently, failure in the treatment or unwanted side effects may arise in certain individuals. The incorporation of pharmacogenomics into clinical drug development offers the opportunity for pharmaceutical companies to evaluate drugs with a better understanding of the effects that specific genetic variants will have on drug response [56]. The goal of personalized medicine is to provide consideration to such individual differences in order to optimize the treatment.

Traditionally, this approach has been limited to the consideration of a patient's family history, environment, behaviors, and clinical parameters (such as cholesterol levels and blood pressure) for tailoring individual care [57, 58].

Several advances in a number of molecular profiling technologies, such as proteomics, metabolomics, or genomics, now allow the personalization of the treatment of a given individual. In addition, HCS of drugs using the cells derived from an individual as target may allow for a greater degree of personalized medicine than is currently available.

The advances achieved with hMSCs and iPSCs have opened the way to a new horizon in medical technology. These stem cells, and more specifically our ability to manipulate them, will allow us to change the focus of drug development from generic to personal. Thus, it will be possible to characterize the effect of a repertoire of therapies available for a certain disease in the cells obtained from a certain individual. This can be an unparalleled achievement and its contribution to the success rate of treatments may be truly astronomical. For example, effective treatment for cancer is far from a certainty. Large numbers of chemo-therapeutic drugs are available, but many patients are unresponsive to a large portion of the various treatments. If the stem cell technique is used, it may be possible to improve the effectivity of the treatments by individual selection of treatment choices using the autologous stem cell based approach.

9.5 Stem Cells as Tools for Improvement of Safety and Toxicology

While lack of efficacy is the main cause of failure in clinical testing, toxicity accounts for approximately 30% of the attrition rate [59]. Traditional safety studies in animals are resource- and time consuming. As a consequence, in order to predict adverse clinical effects at a lower cost, cell-based assays have been introduced at earlier stages of the drug discovery process [60]. These assays allow monitoring of the known mechanisms of drug toxicity, such as apoptosis, oxidative stress, mitochondrial dysfunction, micronuclei, phospholipidosis [61], and steatosis [62].

Micronuclei are small, stainable bodies outside the nucleus that form when a chromosome or its fragment is not incorporated into one of the daughter nuclei during cell division, constituting a hallmark of genetic toxicity. Therefore, it is widely used as an assay for risk assessment of the cancer-inducing potential of a new drug, which is required by regulatory agencies for drug approval. The image-based high-content analysis of micronuclei has been shown to have good correlation with *in vivo* micronucleus assays [63].

Since hepatotoxicity is one of the major reasons for drug non-approval, the development of an assay predictive of drug-induced liver toxicity has been considered imperative. Individual conventional assays in animals have not been reliable in predicting human hepatotoxicity. However, when cellular assays are used in combination, as it is possible using the HCS approach, the level of hepatotoxicity prediction is improved for these assays (e.g., mitochondrial activity, glutathione and cell proliferation). Furthermore, the predictive value can be dramatically increased in HCS assays that use human hepatocyte cell lines. Thus, the assessment of multiple pre-lethal hepatotoxic effects of a potential drug on individual live cells, including mitochondrial toxicity, oxidative stress, deregulation of calcium homeostasis, phospholipidosis, apoptosis, and antiproliferative effects, can be well predicted [64].

Despite these achievements, considerable challenges remain with regard to the design of the toxicity assays and the cell source used. The low proliferation rate of primary human hepatocytes makes them less suitable for cytotoxic assessment. Furthermore, primary human hepatocytes are phenotypically unstable under current cell culture conditions, and de-differentiate rapidly. Therefore, stem cells could be used for deriving hepatocyte cells in order to provide the cell numbers required for toxicity screenings.

9.6 Advances in Nanomedicine for Drug Discovery Using HCS

Nanotechnologies employ materials that have a functional organization in at least one dimension on the nanometer scale [65]. Many of these engineered polymeric devices are capable of interacting with biological systems on a molecular level [66].

Great potential for their use arises from the fact that nanotechnological applications exhibit bulk macro-scale chemical properties that are unique to the engineered material, while not necessarily possessed by the molecules if not arranged in a specific fashion [67, 68]. By utilizing this trait, it is possible to develop entities capable of multiple specific functions either concomitantly or even in a predefined order [69]. A prevalent example of this lies in the emerging field of drug targeting.

Drug targeting is defined as selective drug delivery to specific physiological sites, organs, tissues, or cells where a drug's pharmacological activities are required. In principle, a drug distributes uniformly throughout the whole body when it is injected into the bloodstream, and when it arrives at sites other than the therapeutic sites, this may cause toxic side effects. By increasing delivery to the targeted therapeutic sites, and reducing delivery to the untargeted sites, an improved therapeutic index can be obtained with enhanced and reduced drug action at the desired and the undesired sites, respectively. The essence of this concept lies in a separation of functions for the selective pharmacological action: The carrier plays a role in delivery to the designated sites; while the drug plays a role in the pharmacological activity [70, 71].

There are multiple carriers used as drug delivery systems (e.g., liposomes, micelles, microspheres, nanoparticles, nanogels, and bionanocapsules) [72–76]. These are generally colloidal molecules that vary in size from 1 to 1000 nm, which are utilized to direct drugs to a specific tissue or organ due to their possessing a molecular structure to which therapeutic drugs can be attached, entrapped or adsorbed [72, 77, 78].

While nanomedicines are rising in popularity all around, the area of neurodegenerative diseases is seizing center stage. This is a result of nanomedicine's ability to improve delivery of drugs to the central nervous system (CNS) [79–81]. One of the main difficulties in administering drugs to the CNS is that of infiltrating the blood–brain barrier (BBB). The BBB is essentially a physical barrier that regulates the passage of substances between the bloodstream and the brain. It does this by inhibiting unsupervised molecule entry to the CNS via both paracellular and via transcellular pathways [82].

The endothelial membrane has a large surface area that creates an effective transcellular passive diffusion pathway for small gaseous molecules and lipid-soluble agents. On the other hand, hydrophilic molecules are generally not let through. Owing to extremely tight junctions between the cells that constitute the endothelium, passive paracellular diffusion of soluble molecules through the BBB is also inhibited. Additionally, there are specific transporters that allow the entry of many nutrients, such as amino acids, nucleosides, and glucose [83–85].

Nano-carriers can facilitate passage beyond the BBB in various ways. Some nanoparticles have a local toxic effect at the brain vasculature, which leads to a partial permeability of the endothelial cells [86]. Some nanoparticles can open the tight junctions between endothelial cells and allow the drug to penetrate either in free form or together with the carrier [87]. There are also nanoparticles that mediate transcytosis through the endothelial cell layer [88].

Not only are there high numbers of possible carriers, but each carrier type can usually be constructed by a variety of molecules as long as these molecules have similar characteristics. For example, a liposome can be constructed from a huge variety of naturally occurring or modified phospholipids, or even a combination of different phospholipids in a single liposome. To add an additional level of complexity, each carrier is capable of transporting a huge variety of therapeutic agents.

Because of the immense combinatory options in this promising field, we suggest a novel approach by which to hasten the much-needed progress in this area. In a similar fashion to how high-throughput and high-content screening have revolutionized the way in which we search for standard drugs, the application of these methods using human stem cells to the developing field of nanomedicines has the potential to lead to the next big breakthrough in the pharmaceutical industry.

9.7 Concluding Remarks

The common denominator in most *in vitro* drug discovery applications is the biological component whose functionalities and responses to a battery of compounds are being assayed. There is a substantial need for physiological cell models and, in particular, for efficacy and safety studies. The properties of stem cells that make them so attractive for use for these studies too lie in their ability to produce a variety of specific cell types that can be used for cell-specific assays.

Concomitantly, the introduction of nanomolecules may conduce to improving therapies by allowing, for example, the delivery of drugs directly to the desired target. The combination of both technologies, image-based HCS and nanomolecules, using stem cells as target for the study, is expected to contribute to improve current therapy efficacies, finding new drugs for currently incurable diseases and also to the designing of personalized medicine platforms.

References

1. Kola I, Landis J. Can the pharmaceutical industry reduce attrition rates? *Nat Rev Drug Discov*. 2004 Aug; 3(8):711–715.
2. Zock J. Applications of high content screening in life science research. *Comb Chem High Throughput Screen*. 2009 Nov; 12(9):870–876.
3. Kümmel A, Gubler H, Gehin P, Beibel M, Gabriel D, Parker C. Integration of multiple readouts into the z' factor for assay quality assessment. *J Biomol Screen*. 2010 Jan; 15(1):95–101.
4. Zanella F, Lorens J, Link W. High content screening: seeing is believing. *Trends Biotechnol*. 2010 May; 28(5):237–245.
5. Tárnok A, Pierzchalski A, Valet G. Potential of a cytomics top-down strategy for drug discovery. *Curr Med Chem*. 2010; 17(16):1719–1729.
6. Conrad C, Gerlich D. Automated microscopy for high-content RNAi screening. *J Cell Biol*. 2010 Feb; 188(4):453–461.
7. Pepperkok R, Ellenberg J. High-throughput fluorescence microscopy for systems biology. Nat Rev Mol Cell Biol. 2006 Sep; 7(9):690–696.
8. Fenistein D, Lenseigne B, Christophe T, Brodin P, Genovesio A. A fast, fully automated cell segmentation algorithm for high-throughput and high-content screening. *Cytometry A*. 2008 Oct; 73(10):958–964.
9. Rabal O, Link W, Serelde B, Bischoff J, Oyarzabal J. An integrated one-step system to extract, analyze and annotate all relevant information from image-based cell screening of chemical libraries. *Mol Biosyst*. 2010 Apr; 6(4):711–720.
10. Jackson D, Lenard M, Zelensky A, Shaikh M, Scharpf J, Shaginaw R, et al. HCS road: an enterprise system for integrated HCS data management and analysis. *J Biomol Screen*. 2010 Aug; 15(7):882–891.
11. Kozak K, Bakos G, Hoff A, Bennett E, Dunican D, Davies A, et al. Workflow-based software environment for large-scale biological experiments. *J Biomol Screen*. 2010 Aug; 15(7):892–899.
12. Korn K, Krausz E. Cell-based high-content screening of small-molecule libraries. *Curr Opin Chem Biol*. 2007 Oct; 11(5):503–510.
13. Ou H, Cunningham L, Francis S, Brandon C, Simon J, Raible D, et al. Identification of FDA-approved drugs and bioactives that protect hair cells in the zebrafish (Danio rerio) lateral line and mouse (Mus musculus) utricle. *J Assoc Res Otolaryngol*. 2009 Jun; 10(2):191–203.

14. Wendler A, Wehling M. The translatability of animal models for clinical development: biomarkers and disease models. *Curr Opin Pharmacol.* 2010 Oct; 10(5):601–606.

15. Li W, Ding S. Small molecules that modulate embryonic stem cell fate and somatic cell reprogramming. *Trends Pharmacol Sci.* 2010 Jan; 31(1):36–45.

16. McNeish J, Roach M, Hambor J, Mather R, Weibley L, Lazzaro J, et al. High-throughput screening in embryonic stem cell-derived neurons identifies potentiators of alpha-amino-3-hydroxyl-5-methyl-4-isoxazolepropionate-type glutamate receptors. *J Biol Chem.* 2010 May; 285(22):17209–17217.

17. Zweigerdt R. Large scale production of stem cells and their derivatives. *Adv Biochem Eng Biotechnol.* 2009; 114:201–235.

18. Saló E, Baguñà J. Regeneration in planarians and other worms: new findings, new tools, and new perspectives. *J Exp Zool.* 2002 May; 292(6):528–539.

19. Reddien P, Sánchez Alvarado A. Fundamentals of planarian regeneration. *Annu Rev Cell Dev Biol.* 2004; 20:725–757.

20. Saló E. The power of regeneration and the stem-cell kingdom: freshwater planarians (Platyhelminthes). *Bioessays.* 2006 May; 28(5):546–559.

21. Sánchez Alvarado A. Planarian regeneration: its end is its beginning. *Cell.* 2006 Jan; 124(2):241–245.

22. Schwartz R, Verfaillie C. Hepatic stem cells. Methods Mol Biol. 2010; 640:167–179.

23. Schreder A, Pierard G, Paquet P, Reginster M, Pierard-Franchimont C, Quatresooz P. Facing towards epidermal stem cells (Review). *Int J Mol Med.* 2010 Aug; 26(2):171–174.

24. Garrison A, Helmrath M, Dekaney C. Intestinal stem cells. *J Pediatr Gastroenterol Nutr.* 2009 Jul; 49(1):2–7.

25. Loutit J. Versatile haemopoietic stem cells. *Br J Haematol.* 1968 Oct; 15(4):333–336.

26. Martin G. Isolation of a pluripotent cell line from early mouse embryos cultured in medium conditioned by teratocarcinoma stem cells. *Proc Natl Acad Sci U S A.* 1981 Dec; 78(12):7634–7638.

27. Wu X, Wang S, Chen B, An X. Muscle-derived stem cells: isolation, characterization, differentiation, and application in cell and gene therapy. *Cell Tissue Res.* 2010 Jun; 340(3):549–567.

28. Evans M, Kaufman M. Establishment in culture of pluripotential cells from mouse embryos. *Nature.* 1981 Jul; 292(5819):154–156.

29. Thomson J, Itskovitz-Eldor J, Shapiro S, Waknitz M, Swiergiel J, Marshall V, et al. Embryonic stem cell lines derived from human blastocysts. *Science.* 1998 Nov; 282(5391):1145–1147.

30. Keller G. *In vitro* differentiation of embryonic stem cells. *Curr Opin Cell Biol.* 1995 Dec; 7(6):862–869.

31. Kleger A, Seufferlein T, Malan D, Tischendorf M, Storch A, Wolheim A, et al. Modulation of calcium-activated potassium channels induces cardiogenesis of pluripotent stem cells and enrichment of pacemaker-like cells. *Circulation.* 2010 Nov; 122(18):1823–1836.

32. Roelandt P, Pauwelyn K, Sancho-Bru P, Subramanian K, Ordovas L, Vanuytsel K, et al. Human embryonic and rat adult stem cells with primitive endoderm-like phenotype can be fated to definitive endoderm, and finally hepatocyte-like cells. *PLoS One.* 2010; 5(8):e12101.

33. Rezania A, Riedel M, Wideman R, Karanu F, Ao Z, Warnock G, et al. Production of Functional Glucagon-Secreting Alpha Cells from Human Embryonic Stem Cells. *Diabetes.* 2011 Jan; 60(1):239–247. Epub 2010 Oct 22.

34. Valensi-Kurtz M, Lefler S, Cohen M, Aharonowiz M, Cohen-Kupiec R, Sheinin A, et al. Enriched population of PNS neurons derived from human embryonic stem cells as a platform for studying peripheral neuropathies. *PLoS One.* 2010; 5(2):e9290.

35. Cash G. Embryonic stem cells: court decision a threat to science itself. *Nature.* 2010 Sep; 467(7313):271.

36. Tuffs A. German MPs are to vote on allowing preimplantation genetic diagnosis. *BMJ.* 2010; 341:c6017.

37. Adiga S, Kalthur G, Kumar P, Girisha K. Preimplantation diagnosis of genetic diseases. *J Postgrad Med.* 2010 Oct–Dec; 56(4):317–320.

38. Ben-Yosef D, Malcov M, Eiges R. PGD-derived human embryonic stem cell lines as a powerful tool for the study of human genetic disorders. *Mol Cell Endocrinol.* 2008 Jan; 282(1–2):153–158.

39. Eiges R, Urbach A, Malcov M, Frumkin T, Schwartz T, Amit A, et al. Developmental study of fragile X syndrome using human embryonic stem cells derived from preimplantation genetically diagnosed embryos. *Cell Stem Cell.* 2007 Nov; 1(5):568–577.

40. Löser P, Schirm J, Guhr A, Wobus A, Kurtz A. Human embryonic stem cell lines and their use in international research. *Stem Cells.* 2010 Feb; 28(2):240–246.

41. Parekkadan B, Milwid J. Mesenchymal stem cells as therapeutics. *Annu Rev Biomed Eng.* 2010 Aug; 12:87–117.

42. Friedenstein A, Chailakhjan R, Lalykina K. The development of fibroblast colonies in monolayer cultures of guinea-pig bone marrow and spleen cells. *Cell Tissue Kinet.* 1970 Oct; 3(4):393–403.
43. Bianco P, Robey P, Simmons P. Mesenchymal stem cells: revisiting history, concepts, and assays. *Cell Stem Cell.* 2008 Apr; 2(4):313–319.
44. Caplan A. Adult mesenchymal stem cells for tissue engineering versus regenerative medicine. *J Cell Physiol.* 2007 Nov; 213(2):341–347.
45. Kolf C, Cho E, Tuan R. Mesenchymal stromal cells. Biology of adult mesenchymal stem cells: regulation of niche, self-renewal and differentiation. *Arthritis Res Ther.* 2007; 9(1):204.
46. Prockop D. Marrow stromal cells as stem cells for nonhematopoietic tissues. *Science.* 1997 Apr; 276(5309):71–74.
47. Solmesky L, Abekasis M, Bulvik S, Weil M. Bone morphogenetic protein signaling is involved in human mesenchymal stem cell survival in serum-free medium. *Stem Cells Dev.* 2009 Nov; 18(9):1283–1292.
48. Solmesky L, Lefler S, Jacob-Hirsch J, Bulvik S, Rechavi G, Weil M. Serum free cultured bone marrow mesenchymal stem cells as a platform to characterize the effects of specific molecules. PLoS One. 2010; 5(9).
49. Takahashi K, Yamanaka S. Induction of pluripotent stem cells from mouse embryonic and adult fibroblast cultures by defined factors. *Cell.* 2006 Aug; 126(4):663–676.
50. Liu S, Fu R, Huang Y, Chen S, Chien Y, Hsu C, et al. Induced pluripotent stem (iPS) cell research overview. *Cell Transplant.* 2011; 20(1):15–19. Epub 2010 Sep 30.
51. Dimos J, Rodolfa K, Niakan K, Weisenthal L, Mitsumoto H, Chung W, et al. Induced pluripotent stem cells generated from patients with ALS can be differentiated into motor neurons. *Science.* 2008 Aug; 321(5893):1218–1221.
52. Ye Z, Cheng L. Potential of human induced pluripotent stem cells derived from blood and other postnatal cell types. *Regen Med.* 2010 Jul; 5(4):521–530.
53. Aasen T, Belmonte J. Isolation and cultivation of human keratinocytes from skin or plucked hair for the generation of induced pluripotent stem cells. *Nat Protoc.* 2010; 5(2):371–382.
54. Chakraborty C, Shah K, Cao W, Hsu C, Wen Z, Lin C. Potentialities of Induced Pluripotent Stem (iPS) Cells for Treatment of Diseases. *Curr Mol Med.* 2010 Nov; 10(8):756–762.
55. Committee on State of the Science of Nuclear Medicine, Council NR. *Advancing Nuclear Medicine Through Innovation.* Washington, DC: National Academy Press; 2007.

56. Murphy M. Current pharmacogenomic approaches to clinical drug development. *Pharmacogenomics.* 2000 May; 1(2):115–123.

57. Foster M, Sharp R, Mulvihill J. Pharmacogenetics, race, and ethnicity: social identities and individualized medical care. *Ther Drug Monit.* 2001 Jun; 23(3):232–238.

58. Kernan W, Launer L, Goldstein L. What is the future of stroke prevention?: Debate: polypill versus personalized risk factor modification. *Stroke.* 2010 Oct; 41(10 Suppl):S35–S38.

59. Whitebread S, Hamon J, Bojanic D, Urban L. Keynote review: *in vitro* safety pharmacology profiling: an essential tool for successful drug development. *Drug Discov Today.* 2005 Nov; 10(21):1421–1433.

60. Schoonen W, Westerink W, Horbach G. High-throughput screening for analysis of *in vitro* toxicity. *EXS.* 2009; 99:401–452.

61. Gum R, Hickman D, Fagerland J, Heindel M, Gagne G, Schmidt J, et al. Analysis of two matrix metalloproteinase inhibitors and their metabolites for induction of phospholipidosis in rat and human hepatocytes(1). *Biochem Pharmacol.* 2001 Dec; 62(12):1661–1673.

62. McMillian M, Grant E, Zhong Z, Parker J, Li L, Zivin R, et al. Nile Red binding to HepG2 cells: an improved assay for *in vitro* studies of hepatosteatosis. *In Vitr Mol Toxicol.* 2001; 14(3):177–190.

63. Fenech M. *In vitro* micronucleus technique to predict chemosensitivity. *Methods Mol Med.* 2005; 111:3–32.

64. Diaz D, Scott A, Carmichael P, Shi W, Costales C. Evaluation of an automated *in vitro* micronucleus assay in CHO-K1 cells. *Mutat Res.* 2007 Jun; 630(1–2):1–13.

65. Kreuter, J. Nanoparticles, J. Swarbrick, J.C. Boylan, Editors, *Encyclopedia of Pharmaceutical Technology,* New York (1994).

66. Singh R, Lillard JJ. Nanoparticle-based targeted drug delivery. *Exp Mol Pathol.* 2009 Jun; 86(3):215–223.

67. Iijima S. Helical microtubules of graphitic carbon. Nature. 1991; 354(6348):56–58.

68. Adler-Abramovich L, Aronov D, Beker P, Yevnin M, Stempler S, Buzhansky L, et al. Self-assembled arrays of peptide nanotubes by vapour deposition. *Nat Nanotechnol.* 2009 Dec; 4(12):849–854.

69. Wagner E. Programmed drug delivery: nanosystems for tumor targeting. *Expert Opin Biol Ther.* 2007 May; 7(5):587–593.

70. Barratt G. Therapeutic applications of colloidal drug carriers. *Pharm Sci Technolo Today.* 2000 May; 3(5):163–171.

71. Gregoriadis G. Targeting of drugs. *Nature.* 1977 Feb; 265(5593): 407–411.

72. Juliano R, McCullough H. Controlled delivery of an antitumor drug: localized action of liposome encapsulated cytosine arabinoside administered via the respiratory system. *J Pharmacol Exp Ther.* 1980 Aug; 214(2):381–387.

73. Takada K, Yoshimura H, Shibata N, Masuda Y, Yoshikawa H, Muranishi S, et al. Effect of administration route on the selective lymphatic delivery of cyclosporin A by lipid-surfactant mixed micelles. *J Pharmacobiodyn.* 1986 Feb; 9(2):156–160.

74. Widder K, Senyel A, Scarpelli G. Magnetic microspheres: a model system of site specific drug delivery *in vivo*. *Proc Soc Exp Biol Med.* 1978 Jun; 158(2):141–146.

75. Vinogradov S, Bronich T, Kabanov A. Nanosized cationic hydrogels for drug delivery: preparation, properties and interactions with cells. *Adv Drug* Deliv Rev. 2002 Jan; 54(1):135–147.

76. Burger K, Staffhorst R, de Vijlder H, Velinova M, Bomans P, Frederik P, et al. Nanocapsules: lipid-coated aggregates of cisplatin with high cytotoxicity. *Nat Med.* 2002 Jan; 8(1):81–84.

77. Weckenmann H, Matzku S, Stricker H. Optimisation of the covalent binding of monoclonal antibodies to liposomes. *Arzneimittelforschung.* 1988 Nov; 38(11):1556–1563.

78. Hagiwara A, Takahashi T. A new drug-delivery-system of anticancer agents: activated carbon particles adsorbing anticancer agents. *In Vivo.* 1987 1987 Jul–Aug; 1(4):241–252.

79. Begley D. Delivery of therapeutic agents to the central nervous system: the problems and the possibilities. *Pharmacol Ther.* 2004 Oct; 104(1):29–45.

80. Pignatello R, Pantò V, Salmaso S, Bersani S, Pistarà V, Kepe V, et al. Flurbiprofen derivatives in Alzheimer's disease: synthesis, pharmacokinetic and biological assessment of lipoamino acid prodrugs. *Bioconjug Chem.* 2008 Jan; 19(1):349–357.

81. Deguchi Y, Hayashi H, Fujii S, Naito T, Yokoyama Y, Yamada S, et al. Improved brain delivery of a nonsteroidal anti-inflammatory drug with a synthetic glyceride ester: a preliminary attempt at a CNS drug delivery system for the therapy of Alzheimer's disease. *J Drug Target.* 2000; 8(6):371–381.

82. Reese T, Karnovsky M. Fine structural localization of a blood–brain barrier to exogenous peroxidase. *J Cell Biol.* 1967 Jul; 34(1):207–217.

83. Ermisch A. Peptide receptors of the blood–brain barrier and substrate transport into the brain. *Prog Brain Res.* 1992; 91:155–161.

84. Chishty M, Begley D, Abbott N, Reichel A. Functional characterisation of nucleoside transport in rat brain endothelial cells. *Neuroreport*. 2003 May; 14(7):1087–1090.

85. Pardridge W. Transport of insulin-related peptides and glucose across the blood–brain barrier. *Ann N Y Acad Sci*. 1993 Aug; 692:126–137.

86. Olivier J, Fenart L, Chauvet R, Pariat C, Cecchelli R, Couet W. Indirect evidence that drug brain targeting using polysorbate 80-coated polybutylcyanoacrylate nanoparticles is related to toxicity. *Pharm Res*. 1999 Dec; 16(12):1836–1842.

87. Gummerloch MKaN, E.A. *Drug Entry into the Brain and Its Pharmacologic Manipulation*. Berlin: Springer; 1992.

88. Wang Y, Lui P, Li J. Receptor-mediated therapeutic transport across the blood-brain barrier. *Immunotherapy*. 2009 Nov; 1(6):983–993.

Chapter 10

Wrong Resemblance? Role of the Immune System in the Biocompatibility of Nanostructured Materials

Thomas Vorup-Jensen
Biophysical Immunology Laboratory, Department of Medical Microbiology and Immunology and The Lundbeck Foundation Nanomedicine Center for Individualized Management of Tissue Damage and Regeneration, Aarhus University, The Bartholin Building (1240), Wilhelm Meyers Allé 4, DK-8000 Aarhus C, Denmark
vorup-jensen@microbiology.au.dk

Considerable evidence points to the immune system as a formidable barrier to the proper function of nanomaterials in the body. Results from both experimental models and clinical applications suggest that one of the major current challenges in nanomedicine is to permit unhindered circulation of vehicles for drug delivery or tissue repair. Biocompatibility of these vehicles has been sought out by using materials with a biological origin that ensure low toxicity and biodegradability. However, as discussed in this chapter, the resemblance between physicochemical properties of such materials and products from microbial organisms prompts a diversified response from the immune system.

Handbook of Harnessing Biomaterials in Nanomedicine: Preparation, Toxicity, and Applications
Edited by Dan Peer

ISBN 978-981-4316-46-0 (Hardback), 978-981-4364-27-0 (eBook)
www.panstanford.com

10.1 Introduction

A critical property of devices applied in the human body is their compatibility with human tissues. Such "biocompatibility" can be achieved in a number of ways that depends on the chemical composition, surface topology, and size. The area of nanomedicine is taking advantage of strategies for controlling these characteristics with the aim of improving the function of medical devices and pharmacological treatments. This has led to the manufacture of a new range of materials that hold promise to solve at least some of the problems associated with introducing foreign substances into the body. This chapter focuses on the aspects of the immune response to materials with structural features on the nanometer scale ("nanomaterials") and with applications in biomedicine. While biocompatibility depends on the regulation of a number of physiologic responses other than those supported by the immune system, it is clear from many studies that the immune system forms a major barrier to the successful application of nanomaterials in the body. Indeed, as discussed in detail below, the choice of materials used for the formation of nanomaterials in combination with the structural properties of these materials may pose a special challenge with regard to avoiding an immune response. When such a response leads to uncontrolled inflammation, serious damage to the body or death may be the outcome. Low-grade inflammation may also constitute a health risk when inflammatory nanomaterials are part of a repeated or frequent exposure. Finally, in cases where the immune response to nanomaterials itself presents no risk to the health of exposed individuals, the immune response may inactivate or clear the nanomaterial from the targeted tissues. This way, the desired effect of the nanomaterial, and hence the medical therapy, may be curtailed or attenuated.

10.2 Basic Functions of the Immune System

It is beyond the scope of the present chapter to give a detailed description of the immune system, in particular as the interested reader easily finds several excellent accounts elsewhere [1, 2]. Below, selected mechanisms are discussed with the intention to support a basic understanding of functions of the immune system relevant in the body's response to nanomaterials.

Although it is important to stress that the immune system comprises a highly integrated set of molecular and cellular mechanisms, in the past couple of decades researchers have found it useful to group these mechanisms into "adaptive" and "innate" immunity, respectively.

Adaptive immunity (often also referred to as acquired immunity) comprises complex cellular mechanisms that permit a highly diversified immune response to microbial or other stimulating challenges and includes a recall response upon repeated exposure. Adaptive immunity has been the focus of intense research, mainly because this part of the immune system in consequence of the recall response can be manipulated by vaccination. Injection of microbial proteins or carbohydrates, in the context of vaccination referred to as the antigen, will stimulate an immune response that may protect vaccinated individuals against future infection with viruses. We now have a detailed picture of the processes delivering this protection, which mainly depend on the formation of so-called antibodies. As discussed below, a similar response may also be encountered following the introduction of nanomaterials in the body.

Innate immunity comprises cellular and molecular mechanisms that act as a first line of defense against infection. Proteins of the innate immune system take a structure that permits efficient binding to potential microbial pathogens. The binding of these molecules to microbial surfaces initiates a number of immunological effector mechanisms involving leukocytes as well as plasma proteins, which leads to the elimination of the microbe. Unlike adaptive immunity, the functional properties of innate immunity are largely unaltered throughout life and comprise no known mechanisms that would permit a recall response. With the similarity between certain microbial molecules and those utilized for the manufacture of nanomaterials, innate immunity plays a major role in the immune response evoked by these materials.

10.2.1 Antigen Recognition by Antibodies

Antibodies belong to immunoglobulin (Ig) superfamily of proteins and are exclusively synthesized by B cells in the lymph nodes or by plasma cells, a more differentiated state of B cells, which is able to produce approximately 3200 secreted Ig molecules per cell per second [3]. The ability of B cells to bind antigens is regulated by the B cell receptor, which is a membrane-bound form of antibody. During the maturation of B cell, the gene encoding the B cell receptor is rearranged and mutated in a random fashion, which leads to expression of a receptor with a unique ligand, i.e., antigen, recognizing potential. It is estimated that the resulting repertoire of unique B cell receptors are in the order of 10^{11}, which is further expanded during B cell division by a high frequency of mutations in the antigen-recognizing part of the receptor [1]. This explains the astonishing ability of the immune system to produce antibodies to nearly any antigen introduced in the body. Before secreted antibody to protein antigens is produced, B cell maturation is required, which involves another subset of human immune cells, the T cells. The T cell is an important, albeit not the only, source of soluble factors ("cytokines") that regulate the function of B cells and other leukocytes.

There are four types of secreted antibodies, namely the IgA, IgG, IgM, and IgE isotypes. All immunoglobulins are built from a common structural unit consisting of two covalently linked heavy chains with three or four constant domains (C_H) and one domain containing the variable antigen recognition site (V_H). The heavy chains are covalently linked with two light chains each with one constant (C_L) and variable domain (V_L). IgG and IgE are monomers of this subunit with three and four C_H domains, respectively. In blood, IgA is monomeric. On mucosal surfaces in gastrointestinal tract, IgA is the dominant immunoglobulin and forms a dimeric complex also containing the J chain, which links IgA molecules, and a proteolytic fragment of the poly Ig receptor designated the secretory component. IgM is the largest molecule among the isotypes with a cross-sectional diameter of approximately 35 nm [4]. Secreted IgM consists of a planar pentamer of the structural unit together with the J chain or as a hexamer of the structural unit without the J chain (Figure. 10.1).

Following the initial recognition of an antigen a B cell produces mainly IgM antibody. Further B cell stimulation in the lymph node may change the isotype of the secreted antibody ("class switching") to either IgA, IgG, or IgE, all with the same antigen specificity as the initially produced IgM. There is conflicting data concerning the role of T cells in this process, probably due to that the cytokines required for class switching may be produced by other cells than T cells [5, 6]. This is important since it implies that class-switching also occurs for antibodies directed to T-cell independent antigens, i.e., antibodies

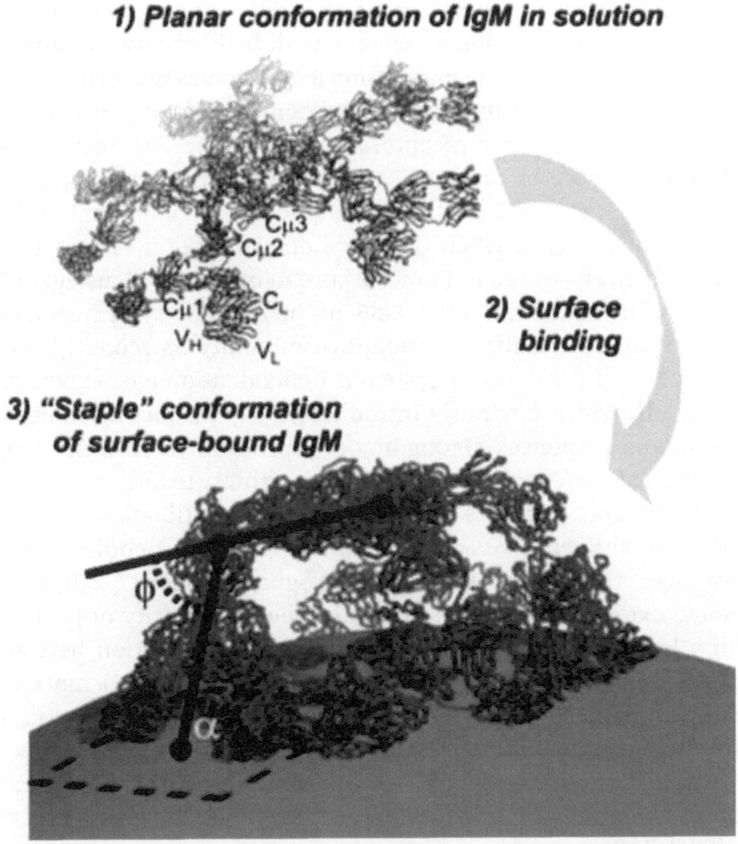

Figure 10.1 Three-step model for the binding of IgM to target surfaces. In solution IgM is a planar structure of five structural units each containing four constant (Cμ1-4) domains and one variable (V_H) domain in the heavy chain and one constant (C_L) and one variable (V_L) domain in the light chain. In 1) the planar structure described by Perkins et al. [4] is shown with indications of the approximate position of some of the structural domains. The dynamics of binding of IgM to target surfaces (2) is not well understood, but suggestions were [71] made that the process brings IgM into the "staple" conformation, which permits binding of the C1 complex and hence initiates complement activation. Perkins et al. suggested that the specific requirement would be that the angle ϕ takes a value of 60°. Pedersen et al. recently suggested that IgM binding to curved surfaces would regulate ϕ according to the curvature by assuming that the contact between epitopes and the variable domains in IgM is geometrically well defined with a characteristic angle α [70]. In (3), IgM is shown drawn to scale and bound to a sphere with a diameter of 66 nm (modified from [70]). The artwork was kindly made by Dr. T. Boesen, Aarhus University. See also Color Insert.

produced without the involvement of T cells. Equally important is that the B cells expressing a receptor with high affinity for antigen are expanded and that the maturation also involves the formation of so-called memory B cells. Thus, the recognition of antigen selects B cell clones that express a receptor appropriate for such recognition and hence is able to produce secreted antibody also recognizing that antigen. Memory B cells enable a quick formation of antibodies to microbial antigens when these are encountered a second time, which effectively serves to limit the spread of an infectious agent in the body. The observation that cells of the immune system support recall response is a hallmark of adaptive immunity. As a consequence, the function of the immune system is dependent on past exposures to antigens, which obviously introduces a significant variability in the immune responses among any group of individuals. Although antibodies are selected on the basis of their ability to form complexes with an antigen, this does not imply that such antibodies may only bind to this antigen. Cross reactivity often permits antibodies to bind substances structurally similar to their cognate antigen [7–10]. While to some extent it is possible to predict the antigenicity of proteins with a known structure [11], the considerable variation between healthy individuals in the reactivity of antibodies [12] makes it essentially impossible to predict if antibodies to antigens, e.g., in formulations involving nanomaterials, may have been preformed. Fortunately, several tests are now possible to broadly investigate if antibody reactivity would allow for the binding of Ig to chosen materials [12].

Secreted antibody to non-proteinous antigens such as lipids or carbohydrates can also be produced, but this process involves T cells only in a limited way and the response is usually weaker than that found for protein antigens. This process depends on the ability macromolecules with a repeated structural motif to cluster or cross-link several B cell receptors in the cell membrane. In addition, immunoglobulins are also produced in a way that appears to not be driven by antigen recognition or T cell involvement. Based on studies in mice, it appears that these so-called natural antibodies are produced by a specialized subset of B lymphocytes [13]. Insight into the biology of natural antibodies in man is lacking. The exact mode of antigen recognition by these antibodies remains enigmatic, but their binding profile suggests promiscuous interactions with many protein and non-protein ligands. In the context of nanotechnology and biocompatibility, it is important to note that the choice of coatings for nanoparticles and other nanostructured devices often are biopolymers, which are targets for T cell-independent antibody formation, mainly because these biopolymers are of a non-proteineous nature.

10.2.2 Antibody Effector Mechanisms and the Activation of the Complement System

The binding of antibodies to antigens triggers several functions of the immune system, usually referred to as "effector mechanisms," which depends on the isotype of the antibody. These mechanisms comprise the ability to (1) neutralize function of intruding microorganisms or other foreign bodies, (2) facilitate the uptake of foreign bodies through receptors on the surface leukocytes that bind antibodies, or (3) activation of the complement system as discussed below in this section.

Antibodies are able to neutralize functions of infectious microbial organisms by simple binding to key molecules of these organisms. Several studies have demonstrated that nanoparticle formulations of various antigens enhance the immune response, i.e., antibody synthesis, compared with the response of the naked antigen [14–16]. It is unclear, however, if nanomaterials enhance the immune response compared with particulate formulations with larger particles, which routinely are used as adjuvants in vaccines. While the particle-enhanced immune response may serve certain purposes in vaccine formulations, it is likely that the strong response could generate antibodies that would interfere with other functions of nanoparticles, e.g., the targeting to specific tissues and drug release. Similarly, binding of antibodies to these or other types of nanomaterials may also be speculated to alter chemical properties of surfaces with regard to hydrophilicity, surface roughness, and the presentation of cues for cell adhesion. Since the function of many nanomaterials critically depends on these properties, such antibody "biofouling" could potentially incapacitate the function of the material [17]. However, the current insight into such processes is limited.

A significant effector mechanism of antibodies involves a processes referred to as "opsonization" derived from an ancient Greek word meaning "preparing for food." A group of leukocytes that

includes monocytes, macrophages, dendritic cells, and neutrophil granulocytes is capable of phagocytosis (literally meaning "eating") of particulate material. The same process also plays a role in the interaction between these cells and solid materials where phagocytes may enable restructuring or degradation of the material. Binding of antibodies to particles greatly facilitates the uptake of these particles by phagocytes and stimulates the production of cytokines. Following the contact between the phagocyte and the antibody-coated particle, receptors for the Fc part of antibodies mediate the uptake of the particles in membrane-clad vesicles into phagocyte cytoplasm. Here, the vesicles are fused with lipid vesicles with enzymes, typically esterases, which may degrade not only protein species but also other polymers. In processes where phagocytes interact with surfaces or objects vastly larger than the cell itself, the cells show signs of incomplete, or frustrated, phagocytosis, which releases enzymes and oxygen radicals to the extracellular environment [18, 19]. The enzymes may eventually affect the successful integration of the nanomaterial in the body.

A third effector mechanism of antibody binding is comprised by the activation of the complement system [20, 21]. The complement system consists of approximately 30 soluble components in human plasma and receptors expressed on the cell surface. Following antibody binding to target surfaces, the C1 complexes bind the antibodies and through its enzymatic components activate complement factors C2 and C4 through cleavage of these proteins into the fragments C2a and C2b as well as C4a and C4b. The C2a and C4b fragments form an enzyme that cleaves C3 into C3a and C3b. Since C3b together with the b fragment of complement factor B (Bb) also is an enzyme that may cleave C3, a positive amplification loop is established, which rapidly covers a target surface with C3b fragments. The C3 and C4 proteins are structurally similar and both of these proteins forms a covalent adduct with hydroxyl or amine groups on the activating surface. The process is controlled by Factor I that inactivates the C3bBb complex by cleavage of C3b into iC3b. Both the C3b and iC3b fragments are facilitators of receptor-mediated phagocytosis and appropriate receptors are expressed on all phagocytes. C3a, the small fragment of C3 following cleavage during activation, together with other small fragments of complement factors (usually referred to as anaphylatoxins), is a potent mediator of inflammation, notably with an influence on the endothelial barrier. Strong activation of the

complement system may consequently cause a breakdown in the function of vascular system leading to a rapid and life-threatening drop in blood pressure (shock) and disseminated intravascular coagulation.

While the above-mentioned activation pathway with antibody as the initiating event is referred to as the "classical" pathway, other antibody independent pathways of complement activation also exist. These include the "alternative pathway" where a spontaneous deposition of autoactivated C3 on surfaces catalyzes further deposition of C3b through formation of the C3bBb convertase. On host cell, such deposition is avoided by cell surface-expressed molecules that catalyzes the proteolytic degradation of C3. During the past 20 years of research, it has become evident that certain lectins, i.e., carbohydrate-binding proteins that are not antibodies, also may contribute to the activation of the complement system through the "lectin pathway" in plasma [22]. Mannan-binding lectin (MBL) binds glycans with terminal mannose, *N*-acetylglucose, or glucose residues. These are typically exposed on the surfaces of viruses, bacteria, and fungi and the opsonization of these microorganisms via complement deposition is clearly important to avoid infections. MBL mediates complement deposition through the associated MBL-associated serine proteases (MASP), notably through the activation of C4 and C2 by MASP-2. More recently, the group of ficolins has also attracted attention [23]. While ficolins also associate with MASP-2, their ligands are not primarily carbohydrates but acetylated compounds, including acetylated sugars, e.g., *N*-acetylglucosamine.

10.2.3 Cell-Bound Receptors

In addition to the soluble factors mentioned above, a large number of receptors expressed on the cell surface of leukocytes are also relevant in the immune response to nanomaterials. Several of these are involved in uptake of particulate material. These receptors can be classified as mainly part of the innate immune system. Unlike the genes encoding antibodies, the proteins are encoded by germ-line genes that are not subject to any somatic recombination or mutation. The ligand-binding potential of these receptors is unaltered throughout life and is conserved in the human population.

On the surface of several phagocytes, notably macrophages and dendritic cells, several lectins are expressed [24, 25]. Many of these share structural characteristics of the ligand-binding domain with MBL although they serve roles not involving the complement system. Their major functions appear to pertain to antigen uptake through recognition of microbial carbohydrates. However, a role as "scavenger receptors," i.e., receptors that serve to remove decayed molecular species from circulation, has also been suggested [26]. One specific example is the macrophage mannose receptor (MMR). The receptor consists of eight carbohydrate recognition domains, however, with only two of these contributing to the ability of recognizing carbohydrate moieties. As suggested by the name terminal mannose residues in glycans are ligands together with fucose and *N*-acetylglucosamine residues. MMR is a powerful agent in supporting phagocytic uptake of particles with an appropriate exposure of carbohydrates. It should be noted that lectin-mediated particle uptake is probably not unique to phagocytic cells. This was elegantly demonstrated by Ezekowitz et al. by simple transfection of a mammalian cell line with no or little resemblance to mammalian leukocytes with a construct expressing MMR [27]. At least the initial phases of phagocytosis, i.e., internalization of yeast particles, was completed by these cells suggesting that the ability of phagocytosis is not exclusive to leukocytes but may rather depend on the expression of cell surface receptors that supports the binding to such particles. This is interesting with the broad expression of lectins since it opens the possibility that a large number of cells this way are capable of receptor-mediated particle uptake.

Integrins are also important in both phagocytosis and cellular signaling [28, 29]. These receptors are heterodimers consisting of one alpha chain and one beta chain, both with transmembrane domains and tightly linked to the cytoskeleton. Research carried out over the past decade strongly supports the idea that the ligand binding by integrins is regulated by the conformation of the receptors. In the resting, non-ligand-binding state the receptor is kept in a bent conformation. Upon activation through cellular stimulation, which involves rearrangements of the cytoskeleton, the bent conformation is changed by allosteric signaling to an unbent, or elongated, conformation that supports ligand binding. A total of 17 integrin alpha and 8 beta chains have been identified, and these form a total of 24 known heterodimers that differ considerably in ligand specificity and cellular expression. The function of integrins can largely be divided into three groups, namely (1) cell–extracellular matrix adhesion, (2) cell–cell adhesion, and (3) cell–pathogen adhesion. A large number of receptors, which contain either the β_3 or β_1 chain, bind a motif in proteins consisting of arginine, glycine, and aspartic acid (RGD) [30]. Such motifs are found in many proteins in the extracellular matrix, including collagens and fibronectin as well as proteins of microbial origin. However, it should be noted that the RGD motifs in proteins are so common that it is difficult to imagine that the mere presence of this motif in a protein implies that the protein is a functional significant integrin ligand. A similar aspect has been addressed in analyses of the function of the family of β_2 integrins. This family comprises the four receptors $\alpha_L\beta_2$ (also known as LFA-1 or CD11a/CD18), $\alpha_M\beta_2$ (Mac-1, complement receptor 3, CD11b/CD18), $\alpha_X\beta_2$ (p150,95, complement receptor 4, or CD11c/CD18), and $\alpha_D\beta_2$ (CD11d/CD18), which are exclusively expressed on leukocytes. These receptors support key functions of leukocytes, including diapedesis through the endothelium and migration in the extra cellular matrix. The function of integrin $\alpha_L\beta_2$ is well established and pertains mainly to binding to intercellular adhesion molecule (ICAM)-1 during diapedesis and formation of contact with antigen presenting cells. $\alpha_L\beta_2$ binds a relatively limited number of ligands that also include ICAM-2 and ICAM-3, which are structurally very similar to ICAM-1 [31]. By contrast, the integrins $\alpha_M\beta_2$ and $\alpha_X\beta_2$ have been reported to bind a large number of ligands with no structural similarity and these include several proteins, endogenous and microbial carbohydrate oligomers, and lipopolysaccaharide [32]. Furthermore, both in the case of $\alpha_M\beta_2$ and $\alpha_X\beta_2$, procedures for destroying higher-order protein structure appear to enhance binding to the unfolded protein [33–35]. A rational for explaining these findings was derived from studies of $\alpha_X\beta_2$ where it appeared that the receptor ligand-binding domain (the I domain) binds strongly to the side chain of glutamic acid residues as well as to several other acid compounds, including carboxylated alkyl chains [34]. In particular, polyanions such as polyglutamic acid and heparin are strong ligands for $\alpha_X\beta_2$ [34, 36]. Interestingly, while $\alpha_M\beta_2$ and $\alpha_X\beta_2$ apparently share many ligands, polyanions are not strong ligands for $\alpha_M\beta_2$. By contrast, it appears that peptides carrying positively charged side chains bind $\alpha_M\beta_2$ well, while this is not the case for $\alpha_X\beta_2$ [37]. It is tempting to speculate that the shared ability to recognize structurally decayed macromolecular species but opposing requirements with regard to the electrostatic charge of bound polymers reflects the need of leukocytes to both bind naturally occurring anionic and cationic polymers. Such properties of ligand recognition by the receptors are also of direct relevance for the interaction between leukocytes and nanomaterials, which are often functionalized with charged groups, e.g., carboxyl and amine groups.

10.3 Nanomaterials and the Immune System

With the introduction above to functions of the immune system, it is possible to outline a number of important principles that regulate the immune response to nanomaterials. Below, emphasis is given to how the chemical composition of materials may trigger or avert the immune response. Many composites of nanomaterials are biopolymers, meaning that these materials are equivalent to or derived from biological materials. However, while such properties often ensure that materials are chemically compatible with the body through low or no toxicity and by permitting degradation, their composition resembles that of many microbial biopolymers. In consequence, the immune system produces a strong response to the introduction of these materials in the body, which may cause a number of undesirable effects ranging from neutralization of the function to shock in the host receiving treatment with nanomaterials. Emerging literature suggests that ultrastructural properties of materials also may play a significant role in regulating the immune response. Specifically, it appears that materials with relevant dimensions on the nanometer scale may interfere with molecular functions of the immune system by manipulating the ultrastructure of proteins.

10.3.1 Biopolymers and the Immune Response

While many biopolymers were chosen as coatings for nanomaterials due to their low metabolic toxicity and degradability, it is now clear that at least some of these represent a special challenge with regard to the immune response they elicit.

One example is the application of dextran to cover or embed ultrasmall superparamagnetic iron oxide (USPIO) particles used clinically as contrast agent in magnetic resonance imaging. Dextran, a branched high-oligomer of glucose, is well tolerated in most patients when administered in formulations of plasma volume expanders following blood loss [38]. It should be noted, however, that most, if not all, individuals produce antibodies of all isotypes to dextran [39]. Formulations of dextran-coated particles used for parenteral administration of iron suggest a more mixed outcome with regard to tolerance compared with soluble dextran. Intolerance to iron dextran complexes has been reported with an incidence of approximately 0.6% of life-threatening anaphylactic reactions [40]. One explanation for the stronger reaction to the particle formulation may relate to the generation of neo-epitopes on the particle surfaces [41]. As discussed in more detail below, another aspect may pertain to the molecular geometry of the interaction of antibodies with dextran epitopes on the surface of a particle. While the anaphylactic reaction presents a safety issue in the treatment with such particles, surprisingly, the antibody-mediated opsonization may also serve an important role in the function of these particles. Evidence suggests that the application of USPIO particles as a contrast agent in magnetic resonance imaging depends on the phagocytic uptake of these particles. If so, the deposition of antibodies on the particles acts to facilitate their function, which — both in imaging of the tumors and in the case of neural imaging — to a large extent appears to rely on the labeling of macrophages in zones of inflammation [42, 43]. This is situation is, of course, not necessarily to be encountered in all settings where bioimaging or other applications of nanoparticles are desired, and care must therefore be taken in evaluating the pharmaceutical potentials of such particles.

A second frequently used biopolymer for making nanoparticles is chitosan. Chitosan is made by de-acetylating chitin, mainly consisting of *N*-acetyl-D-glucosamine, and derived from crustaceans, in particular shrimp. Chitosan is composed of repeating units of D-glucosamine, together with residual *N*-acetyl-D-glucosamine units. Because of the charge of proteonated amine groups, chitosan polymers carry a high positive charge, which is used for making relatively stable complexes with nucleic acid polymers such as plasmidic expression vectors and small interfering RNAs. From several animal studies, it is well documented that chitosan particles are an excellent vehicle for the transport of nucleic acid into several cell types [44]. Chitosan easily triggers complement activation, probably in consequence of pre-formed antibodies as well as the ability of MBL and ficolins to bind *N*-acetyl glucosamine carbohydrate residues in the polymer [45]. As in the case of dextran the ability of the immune system to respond to chitosan is likely to derive from the presence of chitin in microbial organisms that the immune system functions to keep at check. Chitin is part of the cell wall of certain fungi and recent literature has demonstrated that several pattern recognition molecules of the immune system promote the immune recognition of chitosan in blood and on mucosal surfaces [46]. It is uncertain how these recognition mechanisms may interfere with the function of chitosan particles. As in the case of dextran-coated particles, chitosan particles were successfully applied for the modulation of the function of phagocytic cells [47]. Therefore, the success of these strategies is likely to involve the efficient opsonization of the particles. However, in settings not targeting phagocytic cells, the same processes are likely to present obstacles to efficient drug delivery.

DNA has proven to be a remarkably versatile polymer for the formation of nanomaterials with nearly any conceivable structure [48, 49]. The well-characterized and stable structure of the DNA double helix provides sufficient rigidity to support the structure of objects with a size of several nanometers. These structural properties suggest a potential function of DNA-built structures as vehicles for drug delivery and controlled release [50]. However, in spite of several suggestions for applications of such nanomaterials *in vivo*, surprisingly little effort has been spent on considering the physiologic response to the injection of DNA with a complex engineered structure. In the body, DNA is rarely found in the naked state in healthy individuals but is usually in complex with proteins, in particular histones. Apparently the DNA-protein complexes may serve important anti-inflammatory roles [51]. Leukocytes carry receptors, notably those belonging to the family of Toll-like receptors that bind DNA and trigger an inflammatory response [52]. The GC-rich DNA of bacteria is a strong stimulant of the inflammatory response and may act as an adjuvant in the immune response to microbial antigens. In cystic fibrosis patients, DNA massively accumulates in the lung fluid, and there is evidence that the DNA acts as proinflammatory agent [53]. This suggests, of course, that the application of DNA-built nanomaterials could induce a similar response. A further concern over the immune response to injected DNA comes from the observation that 40–60% of patients suffering from systemic lupus erythematosus (SLE) carry antibodies to double-stranded DNA [54]. SLE is a serious chronic autoimmune disorder, which is fatal in some cases. The formed "anti-self" antibodies, including the antibodies to

DNA, attack cells of the cardiovascular system, leading to the decay of the blood vessels in critical organs such as the kidneys. In this way, SLE is a classic demonstration of the dangerous inflammation mediated by autoantibodies. Plasmid DNA has routinely been administered to both animals and humans in gene therapy and gene vaccination trials apparently without significant induction of allergic responses. An often-cited report by Madaio [55] also found that the injection of DNA seemed to induce no significant antibody response. However, an important point also made in this report was the observation that the structure of the DNA molecules affected the immunogenicity such that poly(dG):poly(dC), poly(dT-dG):poly(dC-dA), and left-handed Z-DNA were more able than B-DNA to induce an immune response [55]. This clearly raises a question concerning the consequences of administering a large amount of DNA with a complex structure to the body.

An important source of biopolymers used in nanotechnology is constituted by charged lipids applied for the formation of lipid vesicles or liposomes. Through relatively simple procedures such as the extrusion of lipid suspensions, it is possible to create liposomes with well-defined sizes and the ability to perform targeted transport of drugs, typically by conjugating the liposomes with antibodies to cell surface markers on target cells [56]. In the case of cancer therapy, liposomes have also been conjugated with RGD peptides to facilitate the uptake by β_1 and β_3 integrin-expressing cells. Many animal models have shown the efficacy of such strategies with regard to the suppression of inflammation and slowing of cancer cell growth [57]. A less studied area is leukocyte activation by artificial liposomes. Both microbial organisms and the immune cells produce a large number of vesicular structures. In the case of bacteria, these structures may well contribute to immune evasion by acting as a decoy target for antibodies or other proteins binding to microbial surface structures [58]. Leukocytes liberate a large number of vesicles in the process of migration in the tissue [59]. The homeostasis of lipids is maintained by number of specialized receptors expressed on many cell types, including macrophages, which ingest lipid particles in blood. The uptake by leukocytes is interesting as lipids play a major role in leukocyte signaling and resolution of inflammation [60]. Therefore, it is not surprising that reports have found several immunomodulatory effects of the administration of lipids. Also, it is well established that the inclusion of, in particular, cationic lipids may serve as an adjuvant in enhancing the immune response to several antigens [61]. These properties certainly call for investigations addressing whether lipid formulations applied for making drug-carrying liposome may influence the function of the immune system.

Several coatings that suppress or reduce the immune response have been developed. Notably polyethylene glycol (PEG) is efficient in increasing the circulation time of nanoparticles apparently due to significant reduction of these particles in activating the complement system [43, 62, 63]. Even so, a recent report points to that certain mechanisms involving ficolins and complement factors of the lectin pathway may activate complement by ficolin binding to PEG [64, 65]. Furthermore, antibodies may also recognize PEG pointing to the importance of repeated injection of PEG in experimental animal models to evaluate antibody formation.

10.3.2 Size, Shape, and the Immune Response

The size of nanoparticles and other nanomaterials is a factor in determining the immune response. This is not surprising when considering that particles with diameters of 20–200 nm take dimensions similar to many viruses and debris from the growth of larger microorganisms such as yeasts and bacteria. The immune system comprises many mechanisms for handling such material, which complicates evasion.

The physiological importance of the size of nanomaterials, e.g., nanoparticles, has mainly been emphasized in relation to the penetration of particles into the tissue through leaky vessels or in cellular uptake [66]. Receptor-mediated uptake of particulate material by macrophages is possible for particles larger than approximately 50 nm. Smaller particles are also found intracellularly, but the uptake is likely to depend on spontaneous mechanisms such as pinocytosis. The distinction between receptor-mediated particle uptake and other routes of uptake is significant since the ligation of receptors on the leukocyte cell surface, e.g., β_2 integrins, supports the synthesis of cytokines such as TNF-α. Consequently, as demonstrated by several studies in the area of environmental medicine, particle size may have a role in determining the immune response [67] although a simple relation between particle size and immune response is not likely to exist. As discussed by others [68], particle size is not necessarily a well-defined property due to the ability of certain types of particles to aggregate in the presence of biomacromolecules, e.g., albumin. These problems can be dodged by appropriate modifications of the particle surface. Using a layer of PEG, Larsen et al. recently demonstrated that smaller rather than larger USPIO accumulated tumors in an experimental model. The accumulation involves macrophages in the tumor tissue. As expected, smaller particles with a diameter of 20 nm were less efficiently phagocytosed than larger particles with a diameter of 40 nm [43].

While the influence of particle size on phagocytosis is well established, a surprising role of particle shape was uncovered by Champion and Mitragoti [69]. The comparisons were made with particles with distinct geometric shapes, including spheres, oblate ellipsoids, prolate ellipsoids, elliptical disks, rectangular disks, and "UFOs" with appropriate variation in sizes, thickness and aspect ratios. All particles were opsonized by an IgG-coating. Obloid objects were more readily phagocytosed than spherical or UFO-like objects. By contrast, the volume of the particles did not seem to affect the phagocytosis as prominently as shape. Supported by microscopical analyses, Champion and Mitragoti suggested that actin polymerization in the phagocyte play a role in the shape dependence of phagocytosis [69]. Interestingly, there is evidence that phagocytosis of naturally occurring targets for the immune system such as certain bacteria also is a process where oblate bacteria cells are ingested in a non-random fashion with regard to the ultrastructure of the uptake [69]. Although the biology of this phenomenon is poorly understood, it encourages a speculation that the shape sensitivity of phagocytosis serves some purpose in elimination of bacteria.

The regulation of the immune response by target surface topology is not restricted to processes involving phagocytosis. Pedersen et al. recently reported that complement activation by dextran-coated nanoparticles depended on the diameter of the particles in such a way that larger particles (with a diameter of 600 nm) failed activation, while smaller particles (with a diameter of 250 nm) strongly activated complement [70]. The activation was initiated by the classical pathway and comparison of the responses from donors identified IgM antibodies to dextran as playing a major role in the complement activation. In solution, IgM is a planar molecule [4]. It was previously suggested that this conformation does not permit binding of the C1 complex and hence complement activation, while the surface-bound molecule in a "staple"-like conformation exposes binding sites for C1 [4, 71]. Comparison between the established structure of IgM, specifically the conformation suggested to permit binding of the C1 complex and hence activate complement, and the dimensions of the particles suggested that binding of IgM only to the ~100 nm to ~250 nm particles, but not the 600 nm particles, would support the "staple"-like conformation (Figure 10.1). The critical feature was suggested to be the curvature of the particles [70], which also in other cases appears as a topological feature that may distort or change the ultrastructure of surface-bound proteins [72]. The report by Pedersen et al. may consequently be an example of how nanostructured features can manipulate protein structure and function. In the case of the immune response, such induced changes in protein structure may be critical as an increasing number of examples show how the function of proteins in the immune system is regulated by their conformation.

10.3.3 Structural Decay of Adsorbed Proteins and the Immune Response

All nanomaterials introduced into the human body are exposed to proteins and other biomacromolecules that may potentially coat solvent-exposed surfaces of the material. The physisorption of the molecules is referred to as "biofouling" and will often dramatically change the properties of nanoparticles with regard to colloidal stability and *in vivo* circulation time. Non-colloidal nanomaterials such as implants may also be affected with regard to tissue integration or other functionality. Some of these changes are attributable to simple alterations in the physico-chemical properties of the nanomaterials, including changes in the surface electrostatic potential and hydrophobicity, usually making such contributions as the aggregation of the particles. However, the biofouling may also contribute to unwanted immunological reactions. Many investigations suggest that nanostructuring of surfaces acts to control properties of cellular adhesion or cellular uptake by manipulating protein structure of the adsorbed proteins, including membrane-bound receptors. However, a contribution from the spontaneous adsorption of proteins is difficult to prevent. It is a well-established property of protein adsorption of protein onto materials such as polystyrene that the adsorption may not only change the conformation of the protein but also denature the protein, thereby losing its structure [34, 73]. Interestingly, recent research points to that certain receptors in the leukocyte cell membrane may specifically recognize structurally decayed proteins, while their structurally intact counterparts are significantly weaker ligands [34]. Integrins, in particular those recognizing RGD motifs, are sensitive to the structure of their target ligands since structural changes may expose novel RGD motifs otherwise non-accessible for binding. The mechanisms of ligand recognition by integrins $\alpha_M\beta_2$ and $\alpha_X\beta_2$ (described above) was demonstrated to be strongly influenced by structural integrity of the protein when adsorbed onto surfaces [34, 37]. The denaturation of albumin enhanced its binding to both of these receptors [33]. Surface-induced denaturation of this protein also enhanced the production of the pro-inflammatory TNF-α by adhering leukocyte-like cells, probably through the stronger binding to the integrins that support signaling [74]. The surface-induced denaturation of proteins is not only affected by qualitative properties of the surfaces, e.g., hydrophobicity or electrostatic charge, but also by the amount of protein deposited on the surface [34]. High amounts of deposited protein protect against denaturation by limiting the contact of each molecule with the surface, while, by contrast, coatings with low amounts of protein destroys the structure of the adsorbed proteins. It has been shown in several studies that nanostructuring of surfaces indeed regulates the amount of protein adsorbed to the surface [75]. Thus, leukocyte adhesion and cytokine production are likely to play an important role in the response nanostructured materials that is either engineered directly to manipulate or by accident challenge the structure of adsorbed proteins.

10.4 Conclusions

The successful application of artificial materials in the body is dependent not only on metabolic compatibility with the human organism but also on an absent or limited response from the immune system. Many non-toxic molecules have been identified for the manufacture of biocompatible materials. However, as outlined above, while their biological origin may support a low metabolic toxicity, the resemblance to molecules also found on the surface of microbes induces a strong response from the immune system upon application to the body. This is a particularly important phenomenon in nanomedicine as the structural features manipulated in the engineering of nanomaterials are on nanometer scale and thus comparable to structures on the microbes. In conclusion, when designing such materials, careful evaluation of their immunogenicity is required to achieve safety and functionality in medical treatment.

References

1. Murphy, K., P. Travers, and M. Walport (2008) *Janeway's Immunobiology*, 7th Ed. (Garland Science, USA).
2. Abbas, A.K., and A. H. Lichtman (2009) *Basic Immunology*, 3rd Ed. (Saunders Elsevier, USA).
3. King, L. B., and R. B. Corley (1989) Characterization of a presecretory phase in B-cell differentiation, *Proc. Natl. Acad. Sci. U S A*, ***86***, pp. 2814–2818.
4. Perkins, S. J., A. S. Nealis, B. J. Sutton, and A. Feinstein (1991) Solution structure of human and mouse immunoglobulin M by synchrotron X-ray scattering and molecular graphics modelling. A possible mechanism for complement activation, *J. Mol. Biol.*, ***221***, pp. 1345–1366.
5. Cerutti, A. (2008) The regulation of IgA class switching, *Nat. Rev. Immunol.*, ***8***, pp. 421–434.
6. McHeyzer-Williams, L. J., and M. G. McHeyzer-Williams (2005) Antigen-specific memory B cell development, *Annu. Rev. Immunol.*, ***23***, pp. 487–513.
7. Debler, E. W., G. F. Kaufmann, R. N. Kirchdoerfer, J. M. Mee, K. D. Janda, and I. A. Wilson (2007) Crystal structures of a quorum-quenching antibody, *J. Mol. Biol.*, ***368***, pp. 1392-1402.
8. Stanfield, R. L., M. K. Gorny, S. Zolla-Pazner, and I. A. Wilson (2006) Crystal structures of human immunodeficiency virus type 1 (HIV-1) neutralizing antibody 2219 in complex with three different V3 peptides reveal a new binding mode for HIV-1 cross-reactivity, *J. Virol.*, ***80***, pp. 6093–6105.
9. Fouraux, M. A., A. van der Heijden, W. J. van Venrooij, and G. J. Pruijn (2002) Cross-reactivity of the anti-La monoclonal antibody SW5 with early endosome antigen 2, *Immunology*, ***106***, pp. 336–342.
10. Chitarra, V., P. M. Alzari, G. A. Bentley, T. N. Bhat, J. L. Eisele, A. Houdusse, J. Lescar, H. Souchon, and R. J. Poljak (1993) Three-dimensional structure of a heteroclitic antigen–antibody cross-reaction complex, *Proc. Natl. Acad. Sci. U S A*, ***90***, pp. 7711–7715.

11. Peters, B., and A. Sette (2007) Integrating epitope data into the emerging web of biomedical knowledge resources, *Nat. Rev. Immunol.*, ***7***, pp. 485–490.

12. Legutki, J. B., D. M. Magee, P. Stafford, and S. A. Johnston (2010) A general method for characterization of humoral immunity induced by a vaccine or infection, *Vaccine*, ***28***, pp. 4529–4537.

13. Manz, R. A., A. E. Hauser, F. Hiepe, and A. Radbruch (2005) Maintenance of serum antibody levels, *Annu. Rev. Immunol.*, ***23***, pp. 367–386.

14. Huang, M. H., S. C. Lin, C. H. Hsiao, H. J. Chao, H. R. Yang, C. C. Liao, P. W. Chuang, H. P. Wu, C. Y. Huang, C. H. Leng, S. J. Liu, H. W. Chen, A. H. Chou, A. Y. Hu, and P. Chong (2010) Emulsified nanoparticles containing inactivated influenza virus and CpG oligodeoxynucleotides critically influences the host immune responses in mice, *PLoS One*, ***5***, pp. e12279.

15. Slutter, B., S. Bal, C. Keijzer, R. Mallants, N. Hagenaars, I. Que, E. Kaijzel, W. van Eden, P. Augustijns, C. Lowik, J. Bouwstra, F. Broere, and W. Jiskoot (2010) Nasal vaccination with *N*-trimethyl chitosan and PLGA based nanoparticles: nanoparticle characteristics determine quality and strength of the antibody response in mice against the encapsulated antigen, *Vaccine*, ***28***, pp. 6282–6291.

16. Rice-Ficht, A. C., A. M. Arenas-Gamboa, M. M. Kahl-McDonagh, and T. A. Ficht Polymeric particles in vaccine delivery, *Curr. Opin. Microbiol.*, 13, pp. 106–112.

17. Yeh, P. Y., J. N. Kizhakkedathu, J. D. Madden, and M. Chiao (2007) Electric field and vibration-assisted nanomolecule desorption and anti-biofouling for biosensor applications, *Colloids Surf. B Biointerfaces*, ***59***, pp. 67–73.

18. Dorger, M., S. Munzing, A. M. Allmeling, and F. Krombach (2000) Comparison of the phagocytic response of rat and hamster alveolar macrophages to man-made vitreous fibers in vitro, *Hum. Exp. Toxicol.*, ***19***, pp. 635–640.

19. Wettero, J., T. Bengtsson, and P. Tengvall (2000) Complement activation on immunoglobulin G-coated hydrophobic surfaces enhances the release of oxygen radicals from neutrophils through an actin-dependent mechanism, *J. Biomed. Mater. Res.*, ***51***, pp. 742–751.

20. Walport, M. J. (2001) Complement. First of two parts, *N. Engl. J. Med.*, ***344***, pp. 1058–1066.

21. Walport, M. J. (2001) Complement. Second of two parts, *N. Engl. J. Med.*, ***344***, pp. 1140–1144.

22. Holmskov, U., S. Thiel, and J. C. Jensenius (2003) Collections and ficolins: humoral lectins of the innate immune defense, *Annu. Rev. Immunol.*, ***21***, pp. 547–578.

23. Fujita, T. (2002) Evolution of the lectin-complement pathway and its role in innate immunity, *Nat. Rev. Immunol.*, ***2***, pp. 346–353.

24. Mukhopadhyay, S., A. Pluddemann, and S. Gordon (2009) Macrophage pattern recognition receptors in immunity, homeostasis and self tolerance, *Adv. Exp. Med. Biol.*, ***653***, pp. 1–14.

25. van Kooyk, Y. (2008) C-type lectins on dendritic cells: key modulators for the induction of immune responses, *Biochem. Soc. Trans.*, ***36***, pp. 1478–1481.

26. Gordon, S. (2002) Pattern recognition receptors: doubling up for the innate immune response, *Cell*, ***111***, pp. 927–930.

27. Ezekowitz, R. A., D. J. Williams, H. Koziel, M. Y. Armstrong, A. Warner, F. F. Richards, and R. M. Rose (1991) Uptake of *Pneumocystis carinii* mediated by the macrophage mannose receptor, *Nature*, ***351***, pp. 155–158.

28. Hynes, R. O. (2002) Integrins: bidirectional, allosteric signaling machines, *Cell*, ***110***, pp. 673–687.

29. Springer, T. A. (1994) Traffic signals for lymphocyte recirculation and leukocyte emigration: the multistep paradigm, *Cell*, ***76***, pp. 301–314.

30. Ruoslahti, E. (1996) RGD and other recognition sequences for integrins, *Annu. Rev. Cell. Dev. Biol.*, ***12***, pp. 697–715.

31. Shimaoka, M., J. Takagi, and T. A. Springer (2002) Conformational regulation of integrin structure and function, *Annu. Rev. Biophys. Biomol. Struct.*, ***31***, pp. 485–516.

32. Plow, E. F., T. A. Haas, L. Zhang, J. Loftus, and J. W. Smith (2000) Ligand binding to integrins, *J. Biol. Chem.*, ***275***, pp. 21785–21788.

33. Davis, G. E. (1992) The Mac-1 and p150,95 beta 2 integrins bind denatured proteins to mediate leukocyte cell-substrate adhesion, *Exp. Cell Res.*, ***200***, pp. 242–252.

34. Vorup-Jensen, T., C. V. Carman, M. Shimaoka, P. Schuck, J. Svitel, and T. A. Springer (2005) Exposure of acidic residues as a danger signal for recognition of fibrinogen and other macromolecules by integrin alphaXbeta2, *Proc. Natl. Acad. Sci. U S A*, ***102***, pp. 1614–1619.

35. Yalamanchili, P., C. Lu, C. Oxvig, and T. A. Springer (2000) Folding and function of I domain-deleted Mac-1 and lymphocyte function-associated antigen-1, *J. Biol. Chem.*, ***275***, pp. 21877–21882.

36. Vorup-Jensen, T., L. Chi, L. C. Gjelstrup, U. B. Jensen, C. A. Jewett, C. Xie, M. Shimaoka, R. J. Linhardt, and T. A. Springer (2007) Binding between the integrin alphaXbeta2 (CD11c/CD18) and heparin, *J. Biol. Chem.*, ***282***, pp. 30869–30877.

37. Stapulionis, R., C. L. Oliveira, M. C. Gjelstrup, J. S. Pedersen, M. E. Hokland, S. V. Hoffmann, K. Poulsen, C. Jacobsen, and T. Vorup-Jensen (2008) Structural insight into the function of myelin basic protein as a ligand for integrin alpha M beta 2, *J. Immunol.*, ***180***, pp. 3946–3956.

38. Roberts, J. S., and S. L. Bratton (1998) Colloid volume expanders. Problems, pitfalls and possibilities, Drugs, 55, pp. 621–630.

39. Pinegin, B. V., A. V. Kulakov, E. A. Makarov, P. W. Ledger, and R. M. Khaitov (1995) The occurrence of natural antibodies to minimal component of bacterial cell wall (*N*-acetylglucosaminyl-*N*-acetylmuramyl dipeptide) in sera from healthy humans, *Immunol. Lett.*, **47**, pp. 33–37.

40. Michael, B., D. W. Coyne, S. Fishbane, V. Folkert, R. Lynn, A. R. Nissenson, R. Agarwal, J. W. Eschbach, S. Z. Fadem, J. R. Trout, J. Strobos, and D. G. Warnock (2002) Sodium ferric gluconate complex in hemodialysis patients: adverse reactions compared to placebo and iron dextran, *Kidney Int.*, ***61***, pp. 1830–1839.

41. Lynch, I., K. A. Dawson, and S. Linse (2006) Detecting cryptic epitopes created by nanoparticles, *Sci. STKE*, ***2006***, pp. pe14.

42. Desestret, V., J. C. Brisset, S. Moucharrafie, E. Devillard, S. Nataf, J. Honnorat, N. Nighoghossian, Y. Berthezene, and M. Wiart (2009) Early-stage investigations of ultrasmall superparamagnetic iron oxide-induced signal change after permanent middle cerebral artery occlusion in mice, *Stroke*, ***40***, pp. 1834–1841.

43. Larsen, E. K., T. Nielsen, T. Wittenborn, H. Birkedal, T. Vorup-Jensen, M. H. Jakobsen, L. Ostergaard, M. R. Horsman, F. Besenbacher, K. A. Howard, and J. Kjems (2009) Size-dependent accumulation of PEGylated silane-coated magnetic iron oxide nanoparticles in murine tumors, *ACS Nano*, ***3***, pp. 1947–1951.

44. Andersen, M. O., K. A. Howard, and J. Kjems (2009) RNAi using a chitosan/siRNA nanoparticle system: *in vitro* and *in vivo* applications, *Methods Mol. Biol.*, ***555***, pp. 77–86.

45. Bertholon, I., C. Vauthier, and D. Labarre (2006) Complement activation by core-shell poly(isobutylcyanoacrylate)-polysaccharide nanoparticles: influences of surface morphology, length, and type of polysaccharide, *Pharm. Res.*, ***23***, pp. 1313–1323.

46. Sorrell, T. C., and S. C. Chen (2009) Fungal-derived immune modulating molecules, *Adv. Exp. Med. Biol.*, ***666***, pp. 108–120.

47. Howard, K. A., S. R. Paludan, M. A. Behlke, F. Besenbacher, B. Deleuran, and J. Kjems (2009) Chitosan/siRNA nanoparticle-mediated TNF-alpha knockdown in peritoneal macrophages for anti-inflammatory treatment in a murine arthritis model, *Mol. Ther.*, ***17***, pp. 162–168.

48. Chhabra, R., J. Sharma, Y. Liu, S. Rinker, and H. Yan (2010) DNA self-assembly for nanomedicine, *Adv. Drug Deliv. Rev.*, ***62***, pp. 617–625.

49. Seeman, N. C. Nanomaterials based on DNA, *Annu. Rev. Biochem.*, ***79***, pp. 65–87.

50. Andersen, E. S., M. Dong, M. M. Nielsen, K. Jahn, R. Subramani, W. Mamdouh, M. M. Golas, B. Sander, H. Stark, C. L. Oliveira, J. S. Pedersen, V. Birkedal, F. Besenbacher, K. V. Gothelf, and J. Kjems (2009) Self-assembly of a nanoscale DNA box with a controllable lid, *Nature*, ***459***, pp. 73–76.

51. Gorgani, N. N., and A. N. Theofilopoulos (2007) Contribution of histidine-rich glycoprotein in clearance of immune complexes and apoptotic cells: implications for ameliorating autoimmune diseases, *Autoimmunity*, ***40***, pp. 260–266.

52. Lenert, P. (2010) Nucleic acid sensing receptors in systemic lupus erythematosus: development of novel DNA- and/or RNA-like analogues for treating lupus, *Clin. Exp. Immunol.*, ***161***, pp. 208–222.

53. Pressler, T. (2008) Review of recombinant human deoxyribonuclease (rhDNase) in the management of patients with cystic fibrosis, *Biologics*, ***2***, pp. 611–617.

54. Pisetsky, D. S., and I. A. Vrabie (2009) Antibodies to DNA: infection or genetics?, *Lupus*, ***18***, pp. 1176–1180.

55. Madaio, M. P., S. Hodder, R. S. Schwartz, and B. D. Stollar (1984) Responsiveness of autoimmune and normal mice to nucleic acid antigens, *J. Immunol.*, ***132***, pp. 872–876.

56. Peer, D. (2010) Induction of therapeutic gene silencing in leukocyte-implicated diseases by targeted and stabilized nanoparticles: a mini-review, *J. Control. Release* ***148***, pp. 63–68.

57. Garanger, E., D. Boturyn, and P. Dumy (2007) Tumor targeting with RGD peptide ligands-design of new molecular conjugates for imaging and therapy of cancers, *Anticancer Agents Med. Chem.*, ***7***, pp. 552–558.

58. Ellis, T. N., and M. J. Kuehn (2010) Virulence and immunomodulatory roles of bacterial outer membrane vesicles, *Microbiol. Mol. Biol. Rev.*, ***74***, pp. 81–94.

59. Distler, J. H., D. S. Pisetsky, L. C. Huber, J. R. Kalden, S. Gay, and O. Distler (2005) Microparticles as regulators of inflammation: novel players of cellular crosstalk in the rheumatic diseases, *Arthritis Rheum.*, ***52***, pp. 3337–3348.

60. Serhan, C. N. (2010) Novel lipid mediators and resolution mechanisms in acute inflammation. To resolve or not?, *Am. J. Pathol.*, ***177***, pp. 1576–1591.

61. Perrie, Y., A. R. Mohammed, D. J. Kirby, S. E. McNeil, and V. W. Bramwell (2008) Vaccine adjuvant systems: enhancing the efficacy of sub-unit protein antigens, *Int. J. Pharm.*, ***364***, pp. 272–280.

62. Paillard, A., C. Passirani, P. Saulnier, M. Kroubi, E. Garcion, J. P. Benoit, and D. Betbeder (2010) Positively-charged, porous, polysaccharide nanoparticles loaded with anionic molecules behave as 'stealth' cationic nanocarriers, *Pharm. Res.*, ***27***, pp. 126–133.

63. Morille, M., T. Montier, P. Legras, N. Carmoy, P. Brodin, B. Pitard, J. P. Benoit, and C. Passirani (2010) Long-circulating DNA lipid nanocapsules as new vector for passive tumor targeting, *Biomaterials*, ***31***, pp. 321–329.

64. Moghimi, S. M., A. J., Andersen, S. H. Hashemi, B. Lettiero, D. Ahmadvand, A. C. Hunter, T. L. Andresen, I. Hamad, and J. Szebeni (2010) Complement activation cascade triggered by PEG-PL engineered nanomedicines and carbon nanotubes: the challenges ahead, *J. Control. Release*, ***146***, pp. 175–181.

65. Hamad, I., A. C. Hunter, J. Szebeni, and S. M. Moghimi (2008) Poly(ethylene glycol)s generate complement activation products in human serum through increased alternative pathway turnover and a MASP-2-dependent process, *Mol. Immunol.*, ***46***, pp. 225–232.

66. Moghimi, S. M., A. C. Hunter, and J. C. Murray (2005) Nanomedicine: current status and future prospects, *FASEB J.*, ***19***, pp. 311–330.

67. Oberdorster, G. (1996) Significance of particle parameters in the evaluation of exposure-dose-response relationships of inhaled particles, *Inhal. Toxicol.*, ***8*** Suppl, pp. 73–89.

68. Ruenraroengsak, P., J. M. Cook, and A. T. Florence (2010) Nanosystem drug targeting: facing up to complex realities, *J. Control. Release*, 141, pp. 265–276.

69. Champion, J. A., and S. Mitragotri (2006) Role of target geometry in phagocytosis, *Proc. Natl. Acad. Sci. U S A*, ***103***, pp. 4930–4934.

70. Pedersen, M. B., X. Zhou, E. K. Larsen, U. S. Sorensen, J. Kjems, J. V. Nygaard, J. R. Nyengaard, R. L. Meyer, T. Boesen, and T. Vorup-Jensen (2010) Curvature of synthetic and natural surfaces is an important target feature in classical pathway complement activation, *J. Immunol.*, ***184***, pp. 1931–1945.

71. Roux, K. H. (1999) Immunoglobulin structure and function as revealed by electron microscopy, *Int. Arch. Allergy Immunol.*, ***120***, pp. 85–99.

72. Mandal, H. S., and H. B. Kraatz (2007) Effect of the surface curvature on the secondary structure of peptides adsorbed on nanoparticles, *J. Am. Chem. Soc.*, ***129***, pp. 6356–6357.

73. Moskowitz, K. A., B. Kudryk, and B. S. Coller (1998) Fibrinogen coating density affects the conformation of immobilized fibrinogen: implications for platelet adhesion and spreading, *Thromb. Haemost.*, ***79***, pp. 824–831.

74. Brevig, T., B. Holst, Z. Ademovic, N. Rozlosnik, J. H. Rohrmann, N. B. Larsen, O. C. Hansen, and P. Kingshott (2005) The recognition of adsorbed and denatured proteins of different topographies by beta2 integrins and effects on leukocyte adhesion and activation, *Biomaterials*, ***26***, pp. 3039–3053.

75. Vallet-Regi, M. Nanostructured mesoporous silica matrices in nanomedicine, *J. Intern. Med.*, ***267***, pp. 22–43.

Chapter 11

Complement Activation, Immunogenicity, and Immune Suppression as Potential Side Effects of Liposomes

Janos Szebeni[a] and Yechezkel (Chezy) Barenholz[b]
[a] *Nanomedicine Research and Education Center,*
Semmelweis University and Bay Zoltan Foundation for Applied Research,
Budapest, and Faculty of Health Sciences, Miskolc University, Miskolc, Hungary
[b] *Laboratory of Membrane and liposome Research, Institute of Medical Research Israel Canada (IMRIC), The Hebrew University-Hadassah Medical School,*
Jerusalem, Israel
Jszebeni2@gmail.com, yb@cc.huji.ac.il, chezyb@gmail.com

Some therapeutically relevant liposomes are recognized by the immune system as foreign, and the resulting innate or specific immune response can be adverse to the host. The innate response can involve the activation of the complement (C) system, which, via liberation of anaphylatoxins (C5a, C3a), underlies an acute hypersensitivity syndrome called C activation-related pseudoallergy (CARPA). CARPA represents a potential barrier to the clinical use of reactogenic liposomes in cardiac patients, as a main manifestation of C activation in the body may be cardiopulmory distress. The adverse immune

Handbook of Harnessing Biomaterials in Nanomedicine: Preparation, Toxicity, and Applications
Edited by Dan Peer

ISBN 978-981-4316-46-0 (Hardback), 978-981-4364-27-0 (eBook)
www.panstanford.com

response to liposomes involving specific immunity is exemplified by PEGylated nanoliposome-induced transient IgM production, which causes accelerated blood clearance (ABC). Immunosuppression occurs mostly with anticancer and antifungal liposomes. This chapter updates the information on CARPA, accelerated blood clearance (ABC phenomenon), and immunosuppression; highlights their common and specific causes; and discusses their mechanisms.

11.1 Introduction

Today, 46 years after the discovery of liposomes [10, 25], 34 years after their first injection in man against Gaucher's disease [12] and with more than 10 liposomal drugs in clinical use [63, 92, 93], the adverse effects of liposomes on the immune system represent a relatively poorly explored territory within "liposomology."

This, however, will likely change in the near future as the rising number of advanced liposome-based drugs reach *in vivo* testing. These advanced nano-liposomes include targeting ligands and/or proteins or nucleic acids as the active ingredient, making the particles more complex than the currently approved liposomal drugs. Therefore, they may carry increased risk of recognition by the immune system as foreign. Unless we understand the cellular and molecular processes underlying the ensuing protective/defensive response, the absence of adverse effects — a unique asset of simple liposomes — will probably become the exception rather than the rule. The immunological effects of liposomes will extend its present focus, from the use of liposomes as vaccines, to mapping an uncharted network of hypersensitivity and immunogenicity reaction pathways. As the safety of medicinal nanoparticles comes more to the fore, reactogenicity and immunogenicity testing may join the list of toxicity and QC assays required by regulatory agencies. A deeper insight into the fine immunomodulatory effects of such complex nano-particles may also lead to a need to revise our views on immune suppression, not as a side effect but as contributor to therapeutic benefit. This seems to be the case with Doxil, the first nano-drug approved by the US FDA, which is the subject of Chapter 12.

It looks like future nano-particle based drugs will have a less smooth path of safety clearance compared with what we used to have so far, a toll we may need to pay for nursing small-molecular-weight conventional drugs into the nano dimension, which is surveyed by the immune system with "eager eyes" (Figure 11.1).

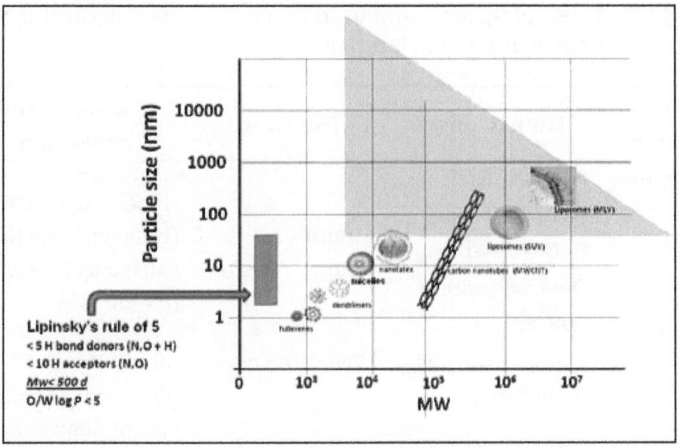

Figure 11.1 Immune recognition of nanoparticles. Map of different nanoparticles on a diameter vs. Mw chart; blue shaded area is the region of immune recognition. Liposomes and carbon nanotubes, with their length, fall into the "sight" of the immune system, while smaller nanoparticles (fullerenes, dendrimers, micelles and complex polymeric particles (e.g., nanolatex) are, in theory, below the size and Mw thresholds of immune recognition. The green "Lipinsky box" shows the position of traditional small-molecular weight drugs [62]. See also Color Insert.

11.2 Types and Features of Immune Responses to Liposomes

The immune effects of liposomes can be stimulatory or inhibitory, weak, moderate or severe, all with a broad individual variation in the time of onset and duration (Table 11.1). In additions to the above time-related differences, the immune effects of liposomes also differ in the part of the immune system primarily affected, i.e., whether the nonspecific, innate, or the specific, adaptive arm of immunity undergoes stimulation or suppression. The term *reactogenicity* is used to imply a broad activation process that involves the innate as well as the adaptive arm of the immune system, while *immunogenicity* usually refers to specific antibody induction with the involvement of B and T cells. Of note, *antigenicity*, i.e., the capability of liposomes to expose antigens, does not necessarily mean reactogenicity or immunogenicity, as antigens may remain unrecognized or can induce immune suppression (tolerance).

Table 11.1 Types of liposome-induced immune changes according to the time of onset and duration

Type of change	Time of onset	Duration	Example and reference
Stimulation	Immediate (within seconds to minutes) Delayed (within hours)	Minutes to hours	Hypersensitivity (infusion) reactions caused by liposomes [84–86, 89]
	Late (within days to months)	Weeks to years	Immunity to liposomal antigens, e.g. influenza or hepatitis B [2, 13]
Inhibition	Short term	Hours to days	Liposomal alendronate [21]
	Long term	Days to months	Doxil-induced immunosuppression [1, 37, 79]

To date, two aspects of the impact of liposomes on the immune system were explored: first, in the 1970s, the late-onset, long-lasting immunogenic properties of phospholipid bilayers were recognized and utilized as antigen carriers and adjuvants. Since then, numerous vaccine candidates have reached advanced clinical trials, and two products, an influenza (Inflexal® V) and a hepatitis A vaccine (Epaxal®) have reached the market; both are based on influenza virus-like liposomes ("immune-potentiating reconstituted influenza virosomes"). Another proteoliposome-based hepatitis-B vaccine in current testing worldwide is based on yeast derived or mammalian recombinant, 22 nm-hepatitis B surface antigen particles carried by multilamellar liposomes [26, 27].

The second "bad" aspect of immune stimulation by liposomes, i.e., the rise of immune responses with adverse consequences, emerged only some 20 years later, after clinical studies started with liposome-based antifungal and anticancer drugs (Ambisome and Doxil) [11, 18, 34, 36, 66, 77]. The rest of the chapter focuses only on the latter, adverse immune responses to liposomes. It was our goal to highlight the common grounds of immune stimulation, to provide examples of reactogenicity, immunogenicity and immune suppression, and to outline recent theories about the mechanism of these phenomena.

11.3 General Causes Behind Immune Recognition of Liposomes

Among many structural features, two stand out as fundamental reasons for immune recognition of liposomes: (1) the diameter of vesicles, roughly in the 50–200 nm range and (2) absence on the liposomal bilayer surface of those membrane proteins or other structures that are present on blood cells and endothelial cells, which normally prevent these cells from C attack. As for the size factor, Table 11.2 shows that there is a remarkable overlap between the size range of many clinically used liposomes and pathogenic human viruses belonging to different viral families. This overlap, however, may not be simple coincidence, but rather the consequence of those common physicochemical rules and forces that force bilayer membranes to form vesicles in live systems and in test tubes; in fact, liposomes are considered as the archetype bilayer vesicles that predated cellular evolution over millions of years [9, 23, 24].

As a remarkable example of common natural forces involved in the formation of viruses and liposomes, Figure 11.2 shows that the visual appearance of Doxil (a) is almost indistinguishable from that of HIV-1 (b). Figure 11.2c also illustrates that most globular viruses under the electron microscope look very much like large unilamellar vesicles (LUV), while paramyxoviruses look like typical multilamellar vesicles (MLV). Of note, hepatitis B surface antigen particles are almost indistinguishable from small unilammelar vesicles (SUV) [26].

In addition to viruses, liposomes also resemble ectosomes, i.e., membrane vesicles detached from cells, as well as most other ecto-organelles and cellular debris that form upon cell death. Nanobacteria, the smallest self-replicating pathogens, are also in the liposome size range (100–200 nm) [19]. In essence, liposomes mimic the size and shape of pathogenic microbes and some subcellular structures against which nature developed strong eliminatory mechanisms via humoral and cellular immune responses.

Table 11.2 Size ranges of clinically applied liposomes and human viruses

Liposomal drug	*Size (d, nm)		Virus family	*Size (d, nm)	
	Low end	High end		Low end	High end
Ambisome	45	80	Adeno	70	90
Amphotec Amphocyl	115	115	Arena	50	300
DaunoXome	45	45	Calici	35	40
Doxil (Caelyx)	80	95	Corona	120	160
Epaxal	100	200	Flavi	40	60
Inflexal V	100	200	Hepadna	42	42
			Herpes	100	120
			Orthomyxo	80	55
			Papova	45	250
			Paramyxo	120	300
			Pox	250	75
			Reo	75	120
			Retro	80	180
			Rhabdo	75	70

*Low and high ends are the minimal and maximal values in the size range obtained from microbiology textbooks (viruses), and drug information (liposomes) or other internet sources. Of note, the sizes of many other FDA-approved liposomes (e.g., Abelcet, Visudyne, DepoCyt, Extrasorb, DepoDur) are different from those listed in the table, or were not found in the literature.

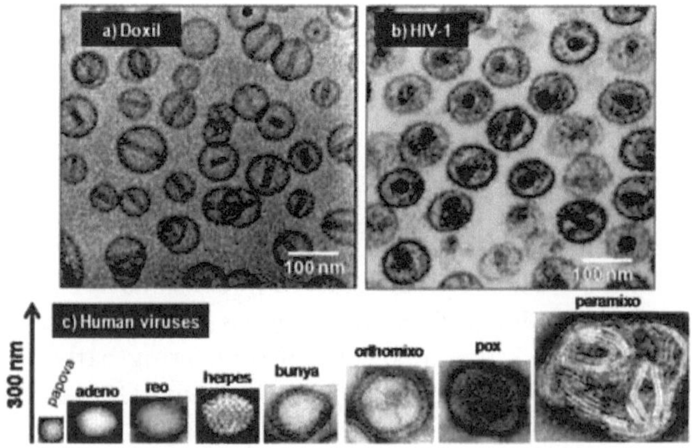

Figure 11.2 Electron microscopic images of Doxil (a), HIV-1 (b), and other common human viruses (c) scaled to each other in the nanometer region, illustrating the morphological similarity of liposomes and viruses.

The second major cause underlying the immune recognition of liposomes is the lack of self-discriminating molecules on the bilayer membrane. Figure 11.3 shows those that are engaged in protecting cells from attack by the C system, referred to as C control proteins (CCPs). These include C receptor type 1 (CR1), decay accelerating factor (DAF), membrane cofactor protein (MCP) and CD59.

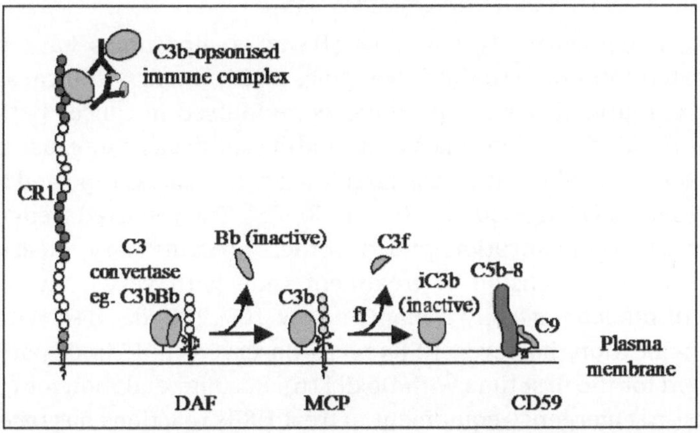

Figure 11.3 Complement control proteins on blood cells, endothelial and other cells that normally prevent host damage by C attack. They are not present on current liposomes (reproduced from [44] with permission).

Figure 11.3 also illustrates the activities of these proteins [44]: CR1 binds C3b and C4b and promotes their physical dissociation (decay accelerating activity). Furthermore, CR1 also enhances the catalytic lysis of C3 convertases by the plasma serine protease, factor I (fI) (cofactor activity). Furthermore, CR1 binds C3b-opsonised particles and immune complexes, extracting them from the activation cascade and carrying them to -among others, to cells of the RES. DAF binds C3 convertase and accelerates its decay to subunits; MCP displays fI-cofactor activity, while CD59, as the last defense line against C damage, interferes with C9 unfolding and polymerizing to form the membrane attack complex (MAC) [44]. In the absence of the above membrane proteins, which normally prevent host damage by C attack, the mistake of the immune system to recognize beneficial liposomal medicines becomes irreversible "friendly fire." The ensuing inflammatory reaction causes harm to both the body and the liposomal drug.

11.4 Consequences of Immune Recognition of Liposomes

11.4.1 Acute Hypersensitivity Reactions

11.4.1.1 Symptoms and occurrence

Acute hypersensitivity reactions (HSRs) to liposomes have been reported from time to time, ever since 1986, the first clinical study wherein large doses of liposomes were infused in cancer patients [76]. All kinds of liposomes and lipid-based drugs can cause such reactions, as follows from the large variety of vesicles reported to be reactogenic [15, 22, 30, 32, 38–41, 70, 75]. The reported frequency following premedication and/or other precautionary measures, such as the extension of treatment time with very slow initial rate of infusion, usually remains below 10% [28, 82, 84]. Without premedication, however, HSRs were observed in 45% of patients treated for the first time with Doxil [16]. Recommendation for ready access to emergency equipment to treat HSRs reactions has recently become part of the box insert of Doxil [28].

Table 11.3 categorizes the symptoms of HSRs according to organ systems involved [80–84]. The wide range of symptoms reflects complex and highly individual pathomechanism. Of note, death, whenever it occurs, is mostly due to cardiac anaphylaxis, as a result of massive anaphylatoxin (C3a, C5a) release and their impact on the heart [84, 86].

Table 11.3 Symptoms of acute hypersensitivity (infusion) reactions*

Cardio-vascular	Broncho-pulmonary	Muco-cutaneous	Neuro-psychosomatic	Autonomic
arrhythmia	apnea	cyanosis	back pain	chills
carcinogenic shock	bronchospasm	erythema	chest pain	diaphoresis
edema	coughing	flushing	chest tightness	diarrhea
hypertension	dyspnea	rash	headache	dizziness
hypotension	hyperventilation	rhinitis	feeling of imminent death	fever
hypoxia	laryngospasm	swelling	fright	nausea

Cardio-vascular	Broncho-pulmonary	Muco-cutaneous	Neuro-psychosomatic	Autonomic
myocardial infarction	pulmonary infiltration	urticaria	panic	sweating
tachycardia	respiratory distress		rigors	vomiting
ventricular fibrillation	shortness of breath		tightness of chest, throat	wheezing

*Compilation of symptoms was based on the adverse events reports in the box labels of liposomes and other reactogenic nanomedicines.

11.4.1.2 Complement activation by liposomes as an underlying mechanism of hypersensitivity reactions

Features of C activation and CARPA. Since the recognition of C activation by liposomes in 1968/69 [4, 47, 48, 56], numerous studies analyzed this phenomenon *in vitro* and *in vivo* under various conditions. As reviewed previously [80–84], the outcomes of these experiments were highly variable as a consequence of the substantial differences in vesicles studied, animal models, serum sources and experimental conditions. Nevertheless, numerous common and basic features of the phenomenon have been uncovered both *in vitro* [8, 14, 17, 20, 33, 42, 43, 45, 47, 56, 64, 67, 69, 71, 72, 74, 80, 81, 83, 84, 90] and *in vivo* [85–89], summarized in Tables 11.4 and 11.5, respectively.

Mechanisms involved in C activation and CARPA. In commenting on the mechanisms of some of the effects listed in Table 11.4, surface charge is perhaps the best known enhancer of C activation induced by nanoparticles and liposomes. A closer scrutiny of the phenomenon at atomic level revealed that the oxygen moiety of the mPEG-phospholipid is responsible for enhanced C activation, at least for the case of mPEGylated dipalmitoylphosphatidylcholine (DPPC) liposomes [68]. The evidence included the lack of activation by non-PEGylated vesicles and the inhibition of C activation by methylation of the oxygen moiety on mPEG-DPPE phosphate [68]. In other studies it was further shown that the C activating negative charge needs to be part of conventional anionic phospholipids, as carboxylic acid-modified vesicles having the same surface charge and electrophoretic mobility failed to induce significant C activation [78]. These observations suggest that C activation is specific to the structure of acidic groups, and negative surface or zeta potential *per se*, may not necessarily imply C activating potency.

Table 11.4 Observations on C activation by liposomes *in vitro*

- All types of liposomes can activate C, with neutral small unilamellar vesicles (SUV) being the least reactogenic.[1]
- The sensitivity of human serum for C activation by different liposomes shows substantial individual (human to human) variation.
- A serum sensitive to a certain liposome is not necessarily sensitive to other liposomes: the individual (human to human) sensitivity variation is large and formulation specific.
- C activation may proceed on both the classical and the alternative pathways.
- Activation triggers include the binding to the vesicles of IgG, IgM, CRP[2], C1q, C3, and potentially, MBL[3] and ficolin.
- C activation is enhanced by
    - positive or negative surface charge
    - increasing liposome size in the 70–300 nm range
    - inhomogeneity
    - endotoxin contamination
    - presence of aggregates
    - presence of doxorubicin or similar drugs in the extraliposome medium that can bind to liposomes and induce aggregation and/or surface modification
    - presence of high amounts of cholesterol in the bilayer membrane (e.g., 71 mole %)
    - PEGylation of liposomes by insertion of the negatively charged PEG-PE, but not with insertion of the neutral PEG-DS[4]
- C activation can be inhibited by known C inhibitors.[5]

[1] Egg PC SUV were injected in 10 humans (6 weekly injections) each at a dose up to 300 mg/kg without indication of C activation (Shmeeda, Barenholz, and Chaiejceck, unpublished).

[2] CRP, C reactive protein.

[3] MBL, mannose binding lectin.

[4] DS, 3-polyethyleneglycol-methoxy polyethylene glycol-oxycarbonyl-3-amino-1,2- propandiol distearoyl ester.

[5] For example, by soluble C receptor type I (sCR1) [89, 90].

In keeping with the above conclusions, liposomes in which the negatively charged PEG-DSPE was replaced with near-neutral PEG-DS showed lack of (or minimal) cardiopulmonary reactivity in pigs [87].

Regarding the impact of doxorubicin or similar drugs that can bind to and aggregate liposomes or lipids, it seems important to consider that the number of liposomes introduced in the circulation upon each treatment (in the order of 10^{13} Doxil liposomes) represents substantial phospholipid bilayer surface (in the order of $\sim$10–30 cm^2). Thus, small changes in liposome surface can translate to large changes in overall surface, which may have a major biological impact. In the case of Doxil, the presence of low curvature oval, elongated (coffee-bean-like), or irregular liposomes and aggregates in commercial vials [87], may have a significant impact on the surface area of vesicles exposed to blood. This suggestion, taken together with a recent report on the significant influence of minor differences in liposome surface curvature on C activation via the classical pathway (via IgM binding) [73] raises the possibility that doxorubicin could indirectly contribute to C activation via modifying the surface of liposomes.

11.4.2 Mechanism of Liposome Reactions and Its Individual Variation

Among the symptoms of HSRs (Table 11.3), there is no single, or unique, symptom that would be liposome-specific. Like many micellar and particulate drugs, radiocontrast agents, monoclonal antibodies, and enzyme therapeutics, liposomes are "only" triggers of a complex chain of events that involves (1) C activation, (2) binding of anaphylatoxins to their specific receptors on mast cells, basophils, and other anaphylatoxin-receptor-positive cells (macrophages), (3) activation of the latter cells to release a host of vasoactive mediators, including histamine, tryptase, PAF, LTB_2, LTB_4, LTC_4, LTD_4, LTE_4, TXA_2, PGD_2 and TXD_4 [57] (Figure 11.4). Some of these mediators (e.g., PAF, histamine, tryptase and TXA_2) are preformed and liberated from the cells immediately upon activation, while others are *de novo* synthesized and, hence, are liberated slower [57]. This differential, multistep release of allergomedins from anaphylatoxin-responsive cells may explain the individual variation in the start of clinical symptoms. Specifically, the activation of H1 receptors leads to vasoconstriction and vascular leakage and is responsible for the cardiovascular and cutaneous symptoms of anaphylaxis. H2 receptors, in turn, increase cellular cAMP levels and cause vasodilation, increased heart rate and pulse pressure. Another potentially important factor in individual variation of HSR symptoms is the relative abundance of reactive cells in different organs of response, i.e., in the skin, lung, heart, bowel, etc. [57, 60, 61, 84].

Table 11.5 Observations on C activation-related pseudoallergy caused by liposomes

- All types of liposomes can cause CARPA in animals and man, with neutral SUV being the least reactogenic (see Table 11.4).
- The sensitivity of different animals to different liposomes shows substantial variation.
- The sensitivity of different species to liposomal CARPA decreases roughly in the following order: pig> dog> human (hypersensitive) > rabbit> sheep > rat> mouse.
- The minimum effective reactogenic dose of liposomes in rats is 10–100 times higher than that in pigs or dogs.
- The individual variation of the cardiopulmonary changes associated with porcine liposome-induced CARPA is lower than that of dogs.
- In pigs, pulmonary hypertension, while in dogs, systemic hypotension are the dominant cardiopulmonary symptoms of CARPA.
- Both in pigs and dogs, the cardiopulmonary changes can decrease or entirely disappear after the second or third dosing, a reflection of tachyphylaxis (tolerance induction, unpublished observations).
- The latter phenomenon allows the development of desensitization protocols using empty (placebo) liposomes (unpublished observations).
- Both in pigs and dogs, leukopenia followed by leukocytosis and thrombocytopenia are varying hematological abnormalities associated with CARPA.
- The rise of plasma thromboxane A2 (measured as TXB2) closely parallels the hemodynamic changes in pigs, indicating that TXA2 is a rate limiting mediator. TXB2 also rises in other species during CARPA.
- CARPA can be inhibited in pigs with C inhibitors (e.g., sCR1, anti-porcine C5 antibody and indomethacin).
- Based on the minimal effective reactogenic dose, porcine and canine CARPA may represent a model of human CARPA in hypersensitive individuals

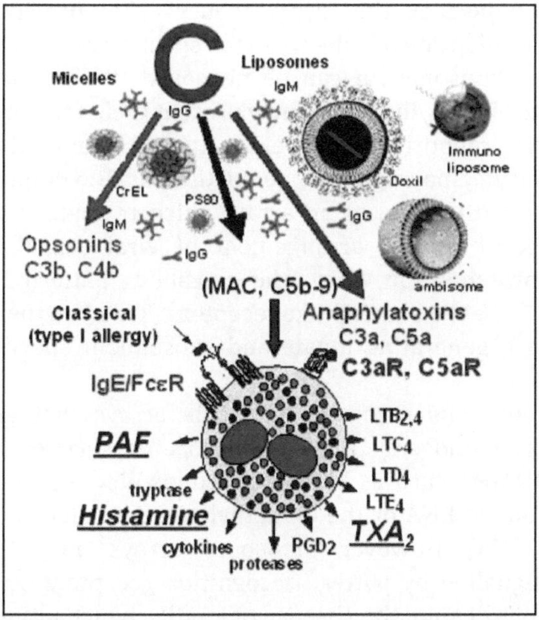

Figure 11.4 Mechanism of complement activation-related pseudoallergy (CARPA) caused by liposomes and micelles. Crel-Cremophor EL, PS80-polysorbate 80, R-receptor. See also Color Insert.

11.5 Immunogenicity of Liposomes

Being built from natural, or natural-like (regarding stereochemistry and composition), synthetic or semisynthetic phospholipids, liposomes are generally not immunogenic. This statement is in apparent conflict with the intense ongoing R&D of liposomal vaccines; however, it should not be forgotten that these vaccines include protein, carbohydrate, or lipid antigens and adjuvants as well as other mediators, such as lipid A, muramyl dipeptide and its derivatives, interleukin-1 and interleukin-2 in addition to the phospholipid bilayer, which also acts as an adjuvant in its own right [3]. When adjuvants are used, specific antibodies are induced against all liposome components, including structural (phospho)lipids, cholesterol and even squalene, a cholesterol precursor triterpene [5–7, 65].

As for the underlying cause of the intrinsic adjuvant capability of phospholipid bilayers, promoting specific immune response to liposomal antigens and non-antigenic lipid components (without additional adjuvant), the "array theory" [91] provides a likely explanation. Adapting this theory to the special case of immunogenic non-vaccine liposomes, it can be proposed that because of their similarity to viruses, liposomes may present their surface conjugates or protruding repetitive surface elements to APC and other immune cells (monocyte/macrophages, dendritic cells, B lypmphocytes and mast cells) in the form of an array, which resembles the regular and symmetric spatial arrangement of viral capsid glycolipids and glycoproteins, for which the so-called "pattern recognition receptors" (e.g., LPS and Toll-like receptors (TLRs) on the above cells readily react, generating innate and subsequent specific immune responses.

Originally TLRs recognize molecule arrays that are broadly shared by pathogens (called pathogen-associated molecular patterns, PAMPs, such as LPS, lipoproteins, lipopeptides, flagellin, double-stranded RNA or the unmethylated CpG islands of bacterial and viral DNA). However, "liposomal arrays" may also trigger "danger" signaling by pattern recognition receptors on the above immune cells despite the absence of PAMPs, which ultimately leads to antibody production against the "pseudo-PAMPs" on liposomes and their phospholipid support. The resultant immune response may or may not differ from a standard immune response to vaccines, depending on the pathway of immune activation.

An example of non-standard, partial immunogenicity is the so-called "ABC phenomenon", i.e., accelerated blood clearance of PEGylated liposomes, a phenomenon that has great clinical relevance. As shown by Ishida and colleagues [49–55, 58, 59], repeated injection of PEGylated liposomes in mice and rats causes rapid clearance of liposomes from the bloodstream, due to the formation of anti-PEG IgM in the spleen. Importantly, the phenomenon is absent with PEGylated liposomes encapsulating doxorubicin, which is consistent with the lack of ABC in cancer patients treated with Doxil. On the other hand, free doxorubicin given in doses that correspond to the amount given in Doxil, restores ABC. These data indicate that immune cells responsible for the ABC phenomenon might be selectively affected by doxorubicin encapsulated in PEGylated liposomes, as detailed in the section on liposome-induced immune suppression below. Since the ABC phenomenon was also observed in BALB/c nu/nu mice, but not in BALB/c SCID mice, it was suggested that antibody production represents a T cell-independent, B cell response, and that PEGylated liposomes might be recognized by B cells as a thymus-independent type 2 antigen [58]. Based on the array theory, as delineated above, it can be hypothesized that PEGylated liposomes trigger B cells via some of their TLRs, for PEG looks to B cells like viral spikes. The ABC phenomenon is illustrated in Figure 11.5.

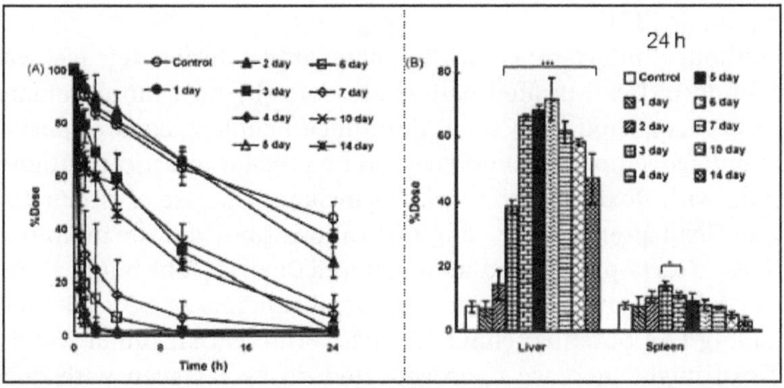

Figure 11.5 Blood clearance rate of PEgylated liposomes in rats (A) and tissue accumulation 24 hours after administration. The figure, reproduced from [51] (with permission), illustrates the acceleration of liposome clearance after repeated injection (on days 2 to 14), of liposomes with paralleling increase in liver and spleen deposition.

11.6 Immune Suppression by Liposomes

It is well known that liposomes are taken up mainly by cells of the reticuloendothelial system (RES) in the liver, spleen, bone marrow and elsewhere, which cells are also part of the nonspecific, innate immune system. Therefore, it has been asked for a long time whether macrophage saturation by liposomes, leading to immune suppression, could be an issue, a potential risk for infection. There is ample evidence that clinically applied doses of non-cytotoxic liposomes generally do not cause immune suppression, at least not major, clinically important blockage of macrophage function. However, the situation is different with anticancer liposomes loaded with cytotoxic drugs, which may cause different levels of immunosuppression.

Administration of Doxil in mice, for example, was shown to interfere with the clearance of bacteria from blood, which was explained by macrophage suppression [79]. Further evidence, in mice, of partial RES blockage by liposomal doxorubicin was the dose-dependent pharmacokinetics of Doxil, resulting in slower clearance and disproportional increase of tumor uptake at higher doses (in the 2.5 to 20 mg/kg range) [37]. The clearance slow-down effect was not seen with free doxorubicin administration at a similar dose or after doxorubicin-free liposomes were co-administered with free doxorubicin [37].

Although interference with innate antibacterial defense was not found in Doxil-treated patients to date (by now more humans have been injected with Doxil than mice), clinical signs of partial macrophage suppression do seem to be present in cancer patients treated with Doxil. Evidence for this includes the rise of circulation $T_{1/2}$ of Doxil after repeated administrations [35], and the inhibition of HSRs to carboplatin by co-administered Doxil [1]. The implications of partial immune suppression by Doxil remains to be evaluated, including two potential clinical benefits. One is that tumor uptake of Doxil might increase upon repeated doses (as seen with dose escalation in mice [37]), resulting in increased therapeutic efficacy by the same dose, or allowing dose reduction without loss of efficacy. The second is that Doxil may provide therapeutic advantage over paclitaxel or gemcitabine in combination chemotherapies with carboplatin, as HSRs to carboplatin have become dose-limiting during treatment of platinum sensitive recurrent cancer [1].

11.7 Conclusions and Outlook

Immunosafety may become a key issue in current and future R&D of liposomes and other nanomedicines. Its significance is emphasized by examples of postmarketing drug recalls, industry guidelines on immunotoxicity testing and recent calls for collaborative research in the fields of nanotoxicology and immunogenicity [29, 31, 46]. Clearly, the currently used immunotoxicology endpoints (e.g. lymphoid organ weight and histology, lymphocyte proliferation, cytotoxicity and antibody production tests, cytokine assays, skin irritation test) have little, or no predictive value in assessing the risk of HSRs, nor do they predict the immunogenicity of complex liposomes or other nano-bio-hybrid drugs. An almost insurmountable difficulty in this regard is the high complexity and species and individual variability of the immune processes involved in the latter phenomena.

As for assessing the risk of HSRs mediated by C, to our knowledge, the only direct approaches are the *in vitro* C activation measurements in normal human sera (NHS), the *in vivo* porcine and canine CARPA tests and the basophil leukocyte activation-based allergenicity assays, provided mostly as services by a few contract research organizations (CROs). A combination of these tests can predict in a rough, semiquantitative way the likely presence, severity and frequency of CARPA caused by a certain drug in most people, and also in individual patients. The unique benefit of the large animal (pig and dog) model of CARPA is that the endpoints, i.e., cardiopulmonary and hematological changes, when they occur, not only reveal the potential reactogenicity of the drug, but also model the physiological changes occurring in hypersensitive individuals. As mentioned in the text above (Table 11.5), liposome-induced CARPA in pigs and dogs provides a model of the infusion reactions seen in hypersensitive individuals. Focusing on liposomes, the C and CARPA tests are useful in assessing their risk of causing HSRs, enabling early abandonment of highly reactogenic formulations. For lack of a valid animal model for assessing the immunogenicity of human or humanized protein containing liposomes, securing of immune safety of these products seems to be an even greater challenge than solving the HSR problem.

What gives hope in this challenging "terra nova" is that interest will never cease in improving the therapeutic efficacy of available drugs, or creating new drugs whose molecular buildup gets increasingly complex. Hopefully it is not too far in the future that we can equip liposomes and other drug carrier nano-systems with immune evasive capabilities, and/or "teach" the immune system to distinguish these nanotech marvels from harmful viruses or other nano-organisms.

Acknowledgments

The authors gratefully acknowledge the financial support by the Barenholz Fund and the National Office for Research and Technology (NKTH), Budapest (CARPA777,NANOMEDI and TÁMOP-4.2.1.B-09/1/KMR-2010-0001 and 4.1.2.B-10/2/KONV-2010-0001, with support by the European Union, co-financed by the European Social Fund).

References

1. Alberts, D. S., Liu, P. Y., Wilczynski, S. P., Clouser, M. C., Lopez, M. A., Michelin, D. P., Lanzotti, V. J., and Markman, M. (2008). Randomized trial of pegylated liposomal doxorubicin (PLD) plus carboplatin versus carboplatin in platinum-sensitive (PS) patients with recurrent ovarian or peritoneal carcinoma after failure of initial platinum-based chemotherapy (South West Oncology group protocol S0200). *Gynecol. Oncol.* 108, pp. 90–94.
2. Altina, J. G., and Parish, C. R. (2006). Liposomal vaccines — targeting the delivery of antigen. *Methods* 40, pp. 39–52.
3. Alving, C. R. (1991). Liposomes as carriers of antigens and adjuvants. *J. Immunol. Methods* 140, pp. 1–13.
4. Alving, C. R., Kinsky, S. C., Haxby, J. A., and Kinsky, C. B. (1969). Antibody binding and complement fixation by a liposomal model membrane. *Biochemistry* 8, pp. 1582–1587.
5. Alving, C. R., Koulchin, V., Glenn, G. M., and Rao, M. (1995). Liposomes as carriers of peptide antigens: induction of antibodies and cytotoxic T lymphocytes to conjugated and unconjugated peptides. *Immunol. Rev.* 145, pp. 5–31.
6. Alving, C. R., and Swartz, G. M. (1991). Antibodies to cholesterol, cholesterol conjugates, and liposomes: implications for atherosclerosis and autoimmunity. *Crit. Rev. Immunol.* 10, pp. 441–453.
7. Alving, C. R., Swartz, G. M. J., Wassef, N. M., Ribas, J. L., Herderick, E. E., Virmani, R., Kolodgie, F. D., Matyas, G. R., and Cornhill, J. F. (1996). Immunization with cholesterol-rich liposomes induces anti-cholesterol antibodies and reduces diet-induced hypercholesterolemia and plaque formation. *J. Lab. Clin. Med.* 127, pp. 40–49.
8. Alving, C. R., Urban, K. A., and Richards, R. L. (1980). Influence of temperature on complement-dependent immune damage to liposomes. *Biochim. Biophys. Acta* 600, pp. 117–125.
9. Bangham, A. D. (1993). Liposomes: the Babraham connection. *Chem. Phys. Lipids* 64, pp. 275–285.
10. Bangham, A. D., and Horne, R. W. (1964). Negative staining of phospholipids and their structural modification by surface active agents as observed in the electron microscope. *J. Mol. Biol.* 8, pp. 660–668.
11. Barenholz, Y. (2006). Amphipathic weak base loading into preformed liposomes having a transmembrane ammonium ion gradient: from the bench to approved DOXIL, In *Liposome Technology Vol 2* (G. Gregoriadis, ed.), pp. 1–26. Informa Healthcare, New York, NY.

12. Belchetz, P. E., Crawley, J. C., Braidman, I. P., and Gregoriadis, G. (1977). Treatment of Gaucher's disease with liposome-entrapped glucocerebroside: beta-glucosidase. *Lancet* 8029, pp. 116–117.

13. Bergers, J. J., Otter, W. D., and Crommelin, J. A. (1996). Liposome-based cancer vaccines. *J. Liposome Res.* 6, pp. 339–355.

14. Bonte, F., and Juliano, R. L. (1986). Interactions of liposomes with serum proteins. *Chem. Phys. Lipids* 40, pp. 359–372.

15. Cabriales, S., Bresnahan, J., Testa, D., Espina, B. M., Scadden, D. T., Ross, M., and Gill, P. S. (1998). Extravasation of liposomal daunorubicin in patients with AIDS-associated Kaposi's sarcoma: a report of four cases *Oncol. Nurs. Forum* 25, pp. 67–70.

16. Chanan-Khan, A., Szebeni, J., Savay, S., Liebes, L., Rafique, N. M., Alving, C. R., and Muggia, F. M. (2003). Complement activation following first exposure to pegylated liposomal doxorubicin (Doxil): possible role in hypersensitivity reactions. *Ann. Oncol.* 14, pp. 1430–1437.

17. Chonn, A., Cullis, P. R., and Devine, D. V. (1991). The role of surface charge in the activation of the classical and alternative pathways of complement by liposomes. *J. Immunol.* 146, pp. 4234–4241.

18. Chopra, R., Blair, S., Strang, J., Cervi, P., Patterson, K. G., and Goldstone, A. H. (1991). Liposomal amphotericin B (AmBisome) in the treatment of fungal infections in neutropenic patients. *J. Antimicrob. Chemother.* 28 Suppl B, pp. 93–104.

19. Ciftcioglu, N., McKay, D. S., Mathew, G., and Kajander, E. O. (2006). Nanobacteria: fact or fiction? Characteristics, detection, and medical importance of novel self-replicating, calcifying nanoparticles. *J. Investig. Med.* 54, pp. 385–394.

20. Cunningham, C. M., Kingzette, M., Richards, R. L., Alving, C. R., Lint, T. F., and Gewurz, H. (1979). Activation of human complement by liposomes: a model for membrane activation of the alternative pathway. *J. Immunol.* 122, pp. 1237–1242.

21. Danenberg, H. D., Golomb, G., Groothuis, A., Gao, J., Epstein, H., Swaminathan, R. V. P., Seifert, P., and Edelman, E. R. (2003). Liposomal alendronate inhibits systemic innate immunity and reduces in-stent neointimal hyperplasia in rabbits. *Circulation* 108, pp. 2798–2804.

22. de Marie, S. (1996). Liposomal and lipid-based formulations of amphotericin B. *Leukemia* 10, Suppl. 2., pp. S93–S96.

23. Deamer, D. (2009). On the origin of systems. Systems biology, synthetic biology and the origin of life. *EMBO Rep.* 10, Suppl 1, pp. S1–4.

24. Deamer, D. W. (2008). Origins of life: how leaky were primitive cells? *Nature* 454 (7200), pp. 37–38.

25. Deamer, D. W. (2010). From "banghasomes" to liposomes: a memoir of Alec Bangham, 1921–2010. *FASEB J.* 24, pp. 1308–1310.

26. Diminsky, D., Moav, N., Gorecki, M., and Barenholz, Y. (1999). Physical, chemical and immunological stability of CHO derived hepatitis B surface antigen (HBsAg) particles. *Vaccine* 18, pp. 3–17.

27. Diminsky, D., Schirmbeck, R., Reimann, J., and Barenholz, Y. (1997). Comparison between hepatitis B surface antigen (HBsAg) particles derived from mammalian cells (CHO) and yeast cells (Hansenula polymorpha): composition, structure and immunogenicity. *Vaccine* 15, pp. 637–647.

28. Doxil. (2010). Package insert. www.Doxil.com 2010 November.

29. Dujmovic, I. H. (2005). Comparison of two guidelines on immunotoxicology testing of medicinal products. *Arh. Hig. Rada. Toksikol.* 56, pp. 265–268.

30. Eckardt, J. R., Campbell, E., Burris, H. A., Weiss, G. R., Rodriguez, G. I., Fields, S. M., Thurman, A. M., Peacock, N. W., Cobb, P., Rothenberg, M. L., et al. (1994). A phase II trial of DaunoXome, liposome-encapsulated daunorubicin, in patients with metastatic adenocarcinoma of the colon. *Am. J. Clin. Oncol.* 17, pp. 498–501.

31. EMEA. (2000). Note for guidance on repeated dose toxicity. CPMP/SWP/1042/99.

32. Fossa, S. D., Aass, N., and Paro, G. (1998). A phase II study of DaunoXome in advanced urothelial transitional cell carcinoma. *Eur. J. Cancer* 34, pp. 1131–1132.

33. Funato, K., Yoda, R., and Kiwada, H. (1992). Contribution of complement system on destabilization of liposomes composed of hydrogenated egg phosphatidylcholine in rat fresh plasma. *Biochim. Biophys. Acta* 1103, pp. 198–204.

34. Gabizon, A., Catane, R., Uziely, B., Kaufman, B., Safra, T., Cohen, R., Martin, F., Huang, A., and Barenholz, Y. (1994). Prolonged circulation time and enhanced accumulation in malignant exudates of doxorubicin encapsulated in polyethylene-glycol coated liposomes. *Cancer Res.* 54, pp. 987–992.

35. Gabizon, A., Isacson, R., Rosengarten, O., Tzemach, D., Shmeeda, H., and Sapir, R. (2007). An open-label study to evaluate dose and cycle dependence of the pharmacokinetics of pegylated liposomal doxorubicin. *Cancer Chemother. Pharmacol.* 61, pp. 695–702.

36. Gabizon, A., Shmeeda, H., and Barenholz, Y. (2003). Pharmacokinetics of pegylated liposomal Doxorubicin: review of animal and human studies. *Clin. Pharmacokinet.* 42, pp. 419–436.

37. Gabizon, A., Tzemach, D., Mak, L., Bronstein, M., and Horowitz, A. T. (2002). Dose dependency of pharmacokinetics and therapeutic efficacy of pegylated liposomal Doxorubicin (DOXIL) in murine models. *J. Drug Targeting* 10, pp. 539–548.

38. Gill, P. S., Espina, B. M., Muggia, F., Cabriales, S., Tulpule, A., Esplin, J. A., Liebman, H. A., Forssen, E., Ross, M. E., and Levine, A. M. (1995). Phase I/II clinical and pharmacokinetic evaluation of liposomal daunorubicin. *J. Clin. Oncol.* 13, pp. 996–1003.

39. Gill, P. S., Wernz, J., Scadden, D. T., Cohen, P., Mukwaya, G. M., von Roenn, J. H., Jacobs, M., Kempin, S., Silverberg, I., Gonzales, G., Rarick, M. U., Myers, A. M., Shepherd, F., Sawka, C., Pike, M. C., and Ross, M. E. (1996). Randomized phase III trial of liposomal daunorubicin versus doxorubicin, bleomycin, and vincristine in AIDS-related Kaposi's sarcoma. *J. Clin. Oncol.* 14, pp. 2353–2364.

40. Girard, P. M., Bouchaud, O., Goetschel, A., Mukwaya, G., Eestermans, G., Ross, M., Rozenbaum, W., and Saimot, A. G. (1996). Phase II study of liposomal encapsulated daunorubicin in the treatment of AIDS-associated mucocutaneous Kaposi's sarcoma. *AIDS* 10, pp. 753–757.

41. Guaglianone, P., Chan, K., DelaFlor-Weiss, E., Hanisch, R., Jeffers, S., Sharma, D., and Muggia, F. (1994). Phase I and pharmacologic study of liposomal daunorubicin (DaunoXome). *Invest. New Drugs* 12, pp. 103–110.

42. Hamad, I., Al-Hanbali, O., Hunter, A. C., Rutt , K. J., Andresen, T. L., and Moghimi, S. M. (2010). Distinct polymer architecture mediates switching of complement activation pathways at the nanosphere-serum interface: implications for stealth nanoparticle engineering. *ACS Nano* 4, pp. 6629–6638.

43. Harashima, H., Sakata, K., Funato, K., and Kiwada, H. (1994). Enhanced hepatic uptake of liposomes through complement activation depending on the size of liposomes. *Pharm. Res.* 11, pp. 402–406.

44. Harris, C. L., and Morgan, B. P. (2004). The many faces of the membrane regulators of complement, In *The Complement System: Novel Roles in Health and Disease* (J. Szebeni, ed.). Kluwer, Boston.

45. Hashimoto, Y., Sugawara, M., and Endoh, H. (1983). Coating of liposomes with subunits of monoclonal IgM antibody and targeting of the liposomes. *J. Immunol. Methods* 62, pp. 155–162.

46. Hastings, K., L,. (2002). Implications of the new FDA/CDER immunotoxicology guidance for drugs. *Int. Immunopharmacol.* 11, pp. 1613–1618.

47. Haxby, J. A., Gotze, O., Muller-Eberhard, H. J., and Kinsky, S. C. (1969). Release of trapped marker from liposomes by the action of purified complement components. *Proc. Natl. Acad. Sci. U.S.A.* 64, pp. 290–295.

48. Haxby, J. A., Kinsky, C. B., and Kinsky, S. C. (1968). Immune response of a liposomal model membrane. *Proc. Natl. Acad. Sci. U.S.A.* 61, pp. 300–307.

49. Ishida, T., Harada, M., Wang, X. Y., Ichihara, M., Irimura, K., and Kiwada, H. (2005). Accelerated blood clearance of PEGylated liposomes following preceding liposome injection: effects of lipid dose and PEG surface-density and chain length of the first-dose liposomes. *J. Control. Release* 105, pp. 305–317.

50. Ishida, T., Ichihara, M., Wang, X., and Kiwada, H. (2006). Spleen plays an important role in the induction of accelerated blood clearance of PEGylated liposomes. *J. Control. Release* 115, pp. 243–250.

51. Ishida, T., Ichihara, M., Wang, X., Yamamoto, K., Kimura, J., Majima, E., and Kiwada, H. (2006). Injection of PEGylated liposomes in rats elicits PEG-specific IgM, which is responsible for rapid elimination of a second dose of PEGylated liposomes. *J. Control. Release* 112, pp. 15–25.

52. Ishida, T., Ichikawa, T., Ichihara, M., Sadzuka, Y., and Kiwada, H. (2004). Effect of the physicochemical properties of initially injected liposomes on the clearance of subsequently injected PEGylated liposomes in mice. *J. Control. Release* 95, pp. 403–412.

53. Ishida, T., Maeda, R., Ichihara, M., Irimura, K., and Kiwada, H. (2003). Accelerated clearance of PEGylated liposomes in rats after repeated injections. *J. Control. Release* 88, pp. 35–42.

54. Ishida, T., Masuda, K., Ichikawa, T., Ichihara, M., Irimura, K., and Kiwada, H. (2003). Accelerated clearance of a second injection of PEGylated liposomes in mice. *Int. J. Pharm.* 255, pp. 167–174.

55. Ishihara, T., Takeda, M., Sakamoto, H., Kimoto, A., Kobayashi, C., Takasaki, N., Yuki, K., Tanaka, K., Takenaga, M., Igarashi, R., Maeda, T., Yamakawa, N., Okamoto, Y., Otsuka, M., Ishida, T., Kiwada, H., Mizushima, Y., and Mizushima, T. (2009). Accelerated blood clearance phenomenon upon repeated injection of PEG-modified PLA-nanoparticles. *Pharm. Res.* 10, pp. 2270–2279.

56. Kinsky, S. C., Haxby, J. A., Zopf, D. A., Alving, C. R., and Kinsky, C. B. (1969). Complement-dependent damage to liposomes prepared from pure lipids and Forssman hapten. *Biochemistry* 8, pp. 4149–4158.

57. Knol, E. F., Mul, F. P., Lie, W. J., Verhoeven, A. J., and Roos, D. (1996). The role of basophils in allergic disease. *Eur. Respir. J. Suppl.* 22, pp. 126s.

58. Koide, H., Asai, T., Hatanaka, K., Akai S, Ishii T, Kenjo, E., Ishida, T., Kiwada, H., Tsukada, H., and Oku, N. (2010). T cell-independent B cell response is responsible for ABC phenomenon induced by repeated injection of PEGylated liposomes. *Int. J. Pharm.* 392, pp. 218–223.

59. Koide, H., Asai, T., Hatanaka, K., Urakami, T., Ishii, T., Kenjo, E., Nishihara, M., Yokoyama, M., Ishida, T., Kiwada, H., and Oku, N. (2008). Particle size-dependent triggering of accelerated blood clearance phenomenon. *Int. J. Pharm.* 362, pp. 197–200.

60. Lieberman, P. (1989). The use of antihistamines in the prevention and treatment of anaphylaxis and anaphylactoid reactions. *Singapore Med. J.* 30, pp. 290–293.

61. Lieberman, P. (1991). Anaphylactoid reactions to radiocontrast material. *Clin. Rev. Allergy* 9, pp. 319–338.

62. Lipinski, C. A., Lombardo, F., Dominy, B. W., and Feeney, P. J. (1997). Experimental and computational approaches to estimate solubility and permeability in drug discovery and development settings. *Adv. Drug Deliv. Rev.* 23, pp. 3–25.

63. Marcato, P. D., and Duran, N. (2008). New aspects of nanopharmaceutical delivery systems. *J. Nanoscience Nanotechnol.* 8, pp. 1–14.

64. Masaki, T., Okada, N., Yasuda, R., and Okada, H. (1989). Assay of complement activity in human serum using large unilamellar liposomes. *J. Immunol. Methods* 123, pp. 19–24.

65. Matyas, G. R., Wassef, N. M., Rao, M., and Alving, C. R. (2000). Induction and detection of antibodies to squalene. *J. Immunol. Methods* 245, pp. 1–14.

66. Meunier, F., Prentice, H. G., and Ringdén, O. (1991). Liposomal amphotericin B (AmBisome): safety data from a phase II/III clinical trial. *J. Antimicrob. Chemother.* 28 Suppl B, pp. 83–91.

67. Moghimi, S. M., Andersen, A. J., Hashem, S. H., Lettiero, B., Ahmadvand, D., Hunter, A. C., Andresen, T. L., Hamad, I., and Szebeni, J. (2010). Complement activation cascade triggered by PEG-PL engineered nanomedicines and carbon nanotubes: the challenges ahead. *J. Control. Release* 146, pp. 175–181.

68. Moghimi, S. M., Hamad, I., Andresen, T. L., Jörgensen, K., and Szebeni, J. (2006). Methylation of the phosphate oxygen moiety of phospholipid-methoxy(polyethylene glycol) conjugate prevents PEGylated liposome-mediated complement activation and anaphylatoxin production. *FASEB J.* 20, pp. 2591–2593.

69. Mold, C., and Gewurz, H. (1980). Activation of human complement by liposomes: serum factor requirement for alternative pathway activation. *J. Immunol.* 125, pp. 696–700.

70. Money-Kyrle, J. F., Bates, F., Ready, J., Gazzard, B. G., Phillips, R. H., and Boag, F. C. (1993). Liposomal daunorubicin in advanced Kaposi's sarcoma: a phase II study. *Clin. Oncol. (R. Coll. Radiol.)* 5, pp. 367–371.

71. Okada, N., Yasuda, T., Tsumita, T., and Okada, H. (1983). Membrane sialoglycolipids regulate the activation of alternative complement pathway by liposomes containing trinitrophenylaminocaproyldipalmitoylphosphatidylethaolamine. *Immunology* 48, pp. 129–140.
72. Ozato, K., Ziegler, H. K., and Henney, C. S. (1978). Liposomes as model membrane systems for immune attack. II. The interaction of complement and K cell populations with immobilized liposomes. *J. Immunol.* 121, pp. 1383–1388.
73. Pedersen, M. B., Zhou, X., Larsen, E. K. U., Sorensen, U. S., Kjems, J., Nygaard, J. V., Nyengaard, J. R., Meyer, R. L., Boesen, T., and Vorup-Jensen, T. (2010). Curvature of synthetic and natural surfaces is an important target feature in classical pathway complement activation. *J. Immunol.* 184, pp. 1931–1945.
74. Richards, R. L., Habbersett, R. C., Scher, I., Janoff, A. S., Schieren, H. P., Mayer, L. D., Cullis, P. R., and Alving, C. R. (1986). Influence of vesicle size on complement-dependent immune damage to liposomes. *Biochim. Biophys. Acta* 855, pp. 223–230.
75. Richardson, D. S., Kelsey, S. M., Johnson, S. A., Tighe, M., Cavenagh, J. D., and Newland, A. C. (1997). Early evaluation of liposomal daunorubicin (DaunoXome, Nexstar) in the treatment of relapsed and refractory lymphoma. *Invest. New Drugs* 15, pp. 247–253.
76. Sculier, J. P., Coune, A., Brassinne, C., Laduron, C., Atassi, G., Ruysschaert, J. M., and Fruhling, J. (1986). Intravenous infusion of high doses of liposomes containing NSC 251635, a water-insoluble cytostatic agent. A pilot study with pharmacokinetic data. *J. Clin. Oncol.* 4, pp. 789–797.
77. Solomon, R., and Gabizon, A. (2008). Clinical pharmacology of liposomal anthracyclines: Focus on pegylated liposomal doxorubicin. *Clin. Lymphoma Myeloma* 8, pp. 21–32.
78. Sou, K., and Tsuchida, E. (2008). Electrostatic interactions and complement activation on the surface of phospholipid vesicle containing acidic lipids: effect of the structure of acidic groups. *Biochim. Biophys. Acta* 1778, pp. 1035–1041.
79. Storm, G., ten Kate, M. T., Working, P. K., and Bakker-Woudenberg, A. (1998). Doxorubicin entrapped in sterically stabilized liposomes: effects on bacterial blood clearance capacity of the mononuclear phagocyte system. *Clin. Cancer Res.* 4, pp. 111–115.
80. Szebeni, J. (1998). The interaction of liposomes with the complement system. *Crit. Rev. Ther. Drug Carrier Syst.* 15, pp. 57–88.

81. Szebeni, J. (2001). Complement activation-related pseudoallergy caused by liposomes, micellar carriers of intravenous drugs and radiocontrast agents. *Crit. Rev. Ther. Drug Carr. Syst.* 18, pp. 567–606.

82. Szebeni, J. (2004). Complement activation-related pseudoallergy: mechanism of anaphylactoid reactions to drug carriers and radiocontrast agents, In *The Complement System: Novel Roles in Health and Disease* (J. Szebeni, ed.), pp. 399–440. Kluwer, Boston.

83. Szebeni, J. Baranyi, L. Savay, S. Milosevits, J. Bodo, M. Bunger, R. Alving, C. R. The interaction of liposomes with the complement system: *in vitro* and *in vivo* assays. *Methods Enzymol.* 373, pp. 136–154.

84. Szebeni, J. (2005). Complement activation-related pseudoallergy: a new class of drug-induced immune toxicity. *Toxicology* 216, pp. 106–121.

85. Szebeni, J., Baranyi, B., Savay, S., Bodo, M., Morse, D. S., Basta, M., Stahl, G. L., Bunger, R., and Alving, C. R. (2000). Liposome-induced pulmonary hypertension: properties and mechanism of a complement-mediated pseudoallergic reaction. *Am. J. Physiol.* 279, pp. H1319–H1328.

86. Szebeni, J., Baranyi, L., Sávay, S., Bodó, M., Milosevits, J., Alving, C. R., and Bünger, R. (2006). Complement activation-related cardiac anaphylaxis in pigs: role of C5a anaphylatoxin and adenosine in liposome-induced abnormalities in ECG and heart function. *Am. J. Physiol.* 290, pp. H1050–H1058.

87. Szebeni, J., Bedőcs, P., Rozsnyay, Z., Weiszhár, Z., Rosivall, L., Cohen, R., Garbuzenko, O., Báthori, G., Tóth, M., Bünger, R., and Barenholz, Y. (2011). Liposome-induced complement activation and related cardiopulmonary distress in pigs: factors promoting reactogenicity of Doxil and Ambisome. *Nanomed. Nanotechnol. Biol. Med.* In press.

88. Szebeni, J., Bunger, R., Baranyi, L., Bedocs, P., Toth, M., Rosivall, L., Barenholz, Y., and Alving, C. R. (2007). Animal models of complement-mediated hypersensitivity reactions to liposomes and other lipid-based nanoparticles. *J. Liposome Res.* 17, pp. 107–117.

89. Szebeni, J., Fontana, J. L., Wassef, N. M., Mongan, P. D., Morse, D. S., Dobbins, D. E., Stahl, G. L., Bünger, R., and Alving, C. R. (1999). Hemodynamic changes induced by liposomes and liposome-encapsulated hemoglobin in pigs: a model for pseudo-allergic cardiopulmonary reactions to liposomes. Role of complement and inhibition by soluble CR1 and anti-C5a antibody. *Circulation* 99, pp. 2302–2309.

90. Szebeni, J., Wassef, N. M., Hartman, K. R., Rudolph, A. S., and Alving, C. R. (1997). Complement activation *in vitro* by the red blood cell substitute, liposome-encapsulated hemoglobin: Mechanism of activation and

inhibition by soluble complement receptor type 1. *Transfusion* 37, pp. 150–159.

91. van de Wert, M., and Moller, E. H. (2008). Immunogenicity of biopharmaceuticals: causes, methods to reduce immunogenicity, and biosimilars, In *Immunogenicity of Biopharmaceuticals*" (M. van de Wert and E. H. Moller, eds.), pp. 97–111. Springer, AAPS Press.
92. Venkatraman, S. S., Ma, L. L., Natarajan, J. V., and Chattopadhyay, S. (2010). Polymer- and liposome-based nanoparticles in targeted drug delivery. *Front. Biosci. (Schol. Ed.)* 2, pp. 801–814.
93. Wagner, V., Dullaart, A., Bock, A.-K., and Zweck, A. (2006). The emerging nanomedicine landscape. *Nature Biotechnol.* 24, pp. 1211–1217.

Chapter 12

Doxil® — The First FDA-Approved Nano-Drug: From an Idea to a Product

Yechezkel (Chezy) Barenholz
Laboratory of Membrane and Liposome Research,
Institute of Medical Research Israel Canada (IMRIC),
The Hebrew University-Hadassah Medical School, Jerusalem 91120, Israel
yb@cc.huji.ac.il, chezyb@gmail.com

Doxorubicin in liposomes (abbreviated and registered as Doxil) is an anticancer nano-drug. Doxil is based on three unrelated principles: (i) using sterically stabilized liposomes, steric stabilization being achieved by the presence of pegylated distearoyl phosphatidylethanolamine (2000Da PEG-DSPE), which results in long blood circulation time of the liposomes; (ii) high and stable remote loading of doxorubicin driven by a transmembrane ammonium sulfate gradient, which also allows for drug release at the tumor; and (iii) having the liposome lipid bilayer in the "liquid ordered" phase based on the high-T_m (53°C) hydrogenated soy phosphatidylcholine, and on cholesterol. In order to take advantage of the enhanced permeability and retention (EPR) effect and to achieve passive targeting of the liposomes into the tumor, the liposomes are nano-scale. This chapter describes the downs and ups of pre-Doxil and Doxil formulations, and how the lessons learned from the failure of pre-Doxil liposomal doxorubicin formulations were turned into the

Handbook of Harnessing Biomaterials in Nanomedicine: Preparation, Toxicity, and Applications
Edited by Dan Peer

ISBN 978-981-4316-46-0 (Hardback), 978-981-4364-27-0 (eBook)
www.panstanford.com

Doxil success. It demonstrates that such a development requires a multidisciplinary approach and is highly dependent on understanding and optimal use of physicochemical and nano-technology principles. Doxil, which is considered today the gold standard in liposome-based drug delivery systems, has opened the road to the development of other anticancer and anti-inflammatory nano-drugs that make used of the EPR effect and remote drug loading.

12.1 Historical Perspectives

I will never forget the cool, early morning (01:00 AM) in November 1995 when most of the Liposome Technology Inc. (LTI) employees and I were waiting in the big, noisy storage area of LTI at 1050 Hamilton Court, Menlo Park, CA, with a lot of food, drinks, and many discussions waiting nervously to see online the FDA's Oncologic Drug Advisory Committee (ODAC) meeting in Washington, DC, at which a recommendation to the FDA to approve or disapprove **Doxil®** for Kaposi's sarcoma indication should be given. ODAC's session started at 08:00 AM Eastern time (05:00 CA time). The happy end of that morning was that Doxil's approval was recommended. Doxil is actually an abbreviation of the words "**DOX**orubicin **In** **L**iposomes."

Doxil vials ((Figure 12.1) were distributed for clinical use by Sequus Pharmaceuticals (previously LTI) as early as 1996.

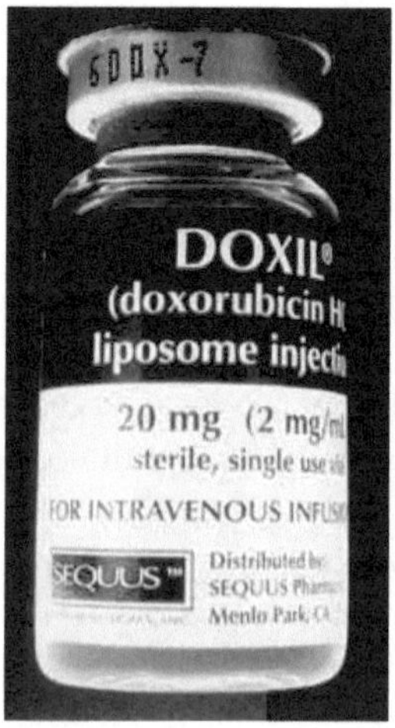

Figure 12.1 Doxil vial as sold by Sequus Pharmaceuticals (1996). See also Color Insert.

Direct work on Doxil development was initiated in Israel and the USA 7.5 years earlier; however, the history of Doxil goes back to 1979, when Alberto Gabizon and I started collaborating on the development of liposomes as a drug delivery system of cytotoxic drugs for the treatment of cancer. This idea stems from Paul Ehrlich's (1906) classical "magic bullet" working hypothesis that by targeting the desired drug to the diseased tissue, the "therapeutic index" (ratio) and "the protective ratio" of the drug (for definitions see Wikipedia) should be significantly increased by either improving therapeutic efficacy or lowering toxicity, and preferably by combination of both. The overall effect is the improvement of drug therapeutic effects.

Liposomes were proposed as a good option for a drug delivery system (DDS) by Alec Bangham already in the 1960s, soon after he described liposomes as an excellent model system for biological membranes in 1964 (for historical perspectives, see Barenholz, 1992; Bangham, 1993; Lasic, 1996).

However, in 1979, 15 years after liposomes' first description by Bangham (rev. in Bangham, 1993), the use of liposomes as a drug delivery system was still in its infancy. When, on January 4, 2011, I searched in Delphion, which covers all patents and patent applications (granted and pending), I found that until January 1979, mention of liposomes anywhere in the text of the patents (including background) was only 170 times, whereas in the claims (protected), liposomes were referred to only 33 times. Today the situation is much different. Anywhere in the patents' text (including background), liposomes are mentioned 224,836 times and in the patents' claims (protected), liposomes are referred to 19,210 times.

Similar differences exist regarding scientific publications, comparing less than 1200 publications that involved liposomes in January 1979, while today more than 0.1% of all scientific papers published in life and health sciences involve liposomes. As of this writing (April 4, 2011), Doxil has more than 171,000 Google citations.

Despite the poor and minimal information available on liposomes as a DDS in 1979, Gabizon and I selected liposomes as our preferred DDS. Our decision was based on the common knowledge at that time, which can be summarized as follows:

- Liposomes can act as a reservoir of both hydrophilic and amphipathic low- and high-molecular-weight drugs/agents.

- The drugs/agents are "encapsulated" as is, namely, in their native form without the need of covalent binding or other chemical modification;
- For hydrophilic and amphipathic drugs/agents, encapsulation is "passive" in nature, which means it is done during the process of liposome fabrication. For amphipathic drugs/agents, encapsulation is determined mainly by the interaction of the drug/agent with the liposomal membrane (Barenholz, 2003; Kedar et al., 1994a, 1994b; Joseph et al., 2006; Even-Or et al., 2010). For water-soluble drugs, the encapsulation is determined by two main parameters: drug/agent degree of solubility in the lipid hydration medium and the liposome trapped aqueous volume (Barenholz, 2001, 2003, Grant et al., 2001). This means that for most applications of water-soluble drugs that require nano-liposomes, the passive loading approaches are a poor option (especially for drugs/agents having poor aqueous solubility) as the product will have a drug-to-lipid ratio that is too low for achieving therapeutic drug concentration for human use. For example the therapeutic dose of doxorubicin is ~ 50 mg/m^2 (~100 mg per each administration);
- The pharmacokinetics (PK) and biodistribution (BD) of the drug/agent encapsulated are modified to a large extent by being encapsulated in liposomes, especially to achieve high accumulation in the RES and to avoid many other tissues (e.g., heart). This can be controlled to some extent by the physicochemical properties of the liposomes [size distribution, electrical charge, and level of rigidity (fluidity)];
- The physicochemical properties can be controlled by liposome lipid composition and method of liposome preparation;
- Phospholipids, glycolipids, and sterols, which are the main building blocks of liposomes, are of natural sources, or are semi-synthetic or fully synthetic, having natural stereochemistry, and therefore believed to be biocompatible.

In the 1980s, the overall expectation of liposomes as a broad spectrum drug delivery system was low. This was summarized in an almost "lethal" (to the medical application of liposomes) *Cancer Research* paper by Poste et al. (1982). This 1982 important paper claimed the following:

> Functional and ultrastructural studies of liposomes injected i.v. into inbred C57BL/6N mice were performed **to determine whether free liposomes can traverse capillaries**. In the liver and spleen, organs with discontinuous (sinusoidal) capillaries, ultrastructural and cell fractionation studies revealed that small (300 to 800 Å diameter), sonicated, unilamellar liposomes were more efficient in penetrating liver sinusoids to interact with hepatocytes than were large (0.5 to 10 μm) multilamellar liposomes. Ultrastructural studies of the behavior of liposomes in the continuous capillaries of the lungs revealed that circulating phagocytic cells engulf the liposomes in the capillaries. **Transcapillary migration of free liposomes was not observed. We conclude that free liposomes are unable to extravasate to reach the alveoli for subsequent engulfment by alveolar macrophages. Instead, liposomes in the lung capillaries are engulfed by circulating blood phagocytes, which subsequently migrate to the alveoli to become alveolar macrophages**. Experiments on the recruitment of blood monocytes into the lungs subjected to whole- or partial-body X-radiation confirmed that transfer of i.v.-injected liposomes to the alveolar compartment was mediated by blood monocytes. **The inability of liposomes to escape from continuous capillaries and their rapid uptake by circulating and fixed phagocytic cells calls into question the feasibility of using liposomes to "target" drugs to cells in extravascular tissues.**

This and Poste's 1983 publication were "catastrophic" to the medical application of liposomes as it led the scientific community as well as the major grant agencies, the pharma industry, and the venture capital community to lose interest in this field. It took 10 more years for the field to recover and gain back some trust that enabled the development of more than 10 FDA-approved liposomal drugs from 1995 to the present.

The above Poste et al. papers were published at the stage when we were in the middle of the development of our liposomal doxorubicin formulation and set the conditions for our selection of liver tumors as the preferred tumor choice. Only very little help from very few published papers was available to us in 1979. Very few relevant papers were published till then, exemplified by Gregoriadis et al. (1974) and Richardson et al. (1979). A few other groups all over the world that were "fed" by the same available scientific information were working in parallel to us on the development of similar systems (see below).

As described above, the 1980s were problematic for the field of liposome medical applications. Nevertheless, it was an exciting time for the development of liposomal drugs as three startup companies were founded in the United States alone, Vestar at Pasadena, CA, The Liposome Company (TLC) at Princeton, NJ, and Liposome Technology Inc. (LTI) at Menlo Park, CA; none of them survived. Although support money was short, these companies succeeded to initiate, and later in the 1990s, when money became more available, to develop most of the FDA-approved liposomal drugs. Interestingly, all three companies selected and had different intellectual property (I.P.) on liposomal anthracyclines as one of their leading products [Doxil® of LTI (now sold by Johnson & Johnson, DaunoXome of Vestar (now sold by Diatos), and Myocet of TLC (now sold by Zenous Pharma Sopherion Therapeutics)]. This clearly demonstrates that these three leading (at that time) startup companies worked along similar lines of thought.

12.2 First-Generation Liposomal Doxorubicin — Liver-Directed Liposomal Doxorubicin

12.2.1 Background

The common knowledge available in 1980 on liposomes as drug carriers (see above) suggests that liposomes should be mainly useful to treat diseases that are localized at RES organs, which are enriched with MPS activities. Therefore, we selected liver hepato-cellular carcinoma as the tumor target of choice. This tumor type, although not a major disease in the Western world, is the most abundant tumor in Japan and a very common one in China. Our idea was that the liposomes loaded with the drug will be cleared fast from the circulation by the RES system and will be taken up efficiently by the phagocytic cells, mainly in the liver. There the liposomes were expected to reach and be processed at the phagosomes and endosomes, followed by drug release to the cytoplasm. From there, it can be further released to the circulation and become available and kill the cancer cells that reside in the liver in proximity to the

RES cells. The optimal chemical stability at low endosome/lysosome pH and the fact that the doxorubicin is an amphipathic weak base is supportive of the MPS cells acting as a doxorubicin depot. In effect, the liposomes deliver the drug to the MPS cells, which serve as a drug depot for liver tumor treatment.

A high dose of doxorubicin (50 mg/m^2) is needed to achieve therapeutic efficacy. The physicochemical properties and especially the low doxorubicin solubility are unfavorable to achieve sufficient passive loading into a 100-nm liposome's intraliposome aqueous phase. Therefore larger liposomes have to be used.

At that time, we (Gabizon and Barenholz) were not the only group that selected doxorubicin (or anthracyclines) as the anticancer drug of choice for the development of liposome-based cancer treatment. Other scientists in academia worked along similar considerations, which were based on the same common knowledge (Rahman et al., 1980, 1985, 1986a, 1986b; Forssen and Tokes, 1979, 1981, 1983; Olson et al., 1982; Van Hossel et al., 1984; Mayhew et al., 1983, 1985, 1987; Strom et al, 1987, and others).

Most liposomal doxorubicin formulations developed during the 1980s took advantage of doxorubicin's being an amphipathic weak base that can associate efficiently with negatively charged membrane lipids. Doxorubicin's mannose amine-derived positive charge allows for association with negatively charged phospholipids (such as PS, PA, PG, and DPG), while its amphipathicity supports doxorubicin partition to the liposome lipid bilayer (Forssen and Tokes, 1979, 1981; Mayhew et al., 1983a, 1983b; Rahman et al., 1985; Storm et al., 1987). The working hypothesis behind all these studies called for the use of liposomes that are larger than the nano-scale, as they can better and faster be taken up by the RES system and be processed there to release the drug. Not less important is that liposomes of such size may have high enough drug levels associated with them to reach therapeutic levels for human treatment.

We selected doxorubicin as our drug of choice on the basis of medical, scientific, and practical considerations. Doxorubicin, like many other anthracyclines, is produced by one of the *Streptomyces* bacteria, (*Streptomyces peucetius* var. caesius). It was discovered in the 1960s near the Adriatic Sea, which explains the source of the brand name Adriamycin. It showed significant anticancer activity (Blum and Carter, 1974; McKelvey et al., 1976; Gundersen et al., 1986). Doxorubicin acts on the nucleic acids of dividing cells by two main mechanisms of action. First, it inhibits DNA and RNA synthesis by intercalating between base pairs of the DNA/RNA strands, thus preventing the replication of rapidly growing cancer cells. This mechanism is based on the chemistry and physics of the doxorubicin molecule (its positively charged mannose amine, which binds efficiently to negatively charged nucleic acid phosphate diester groups, and the excellent fit of the drug anthroquinone planar ring structure for intercalation into the double stranded DNA). All together, these structural features lead to high affinity of the drug to double stranded nucleic acids in a way that is not metabolism dependent. Second, doxorubicin inhibits topoisomerase II enzyme, preventing the relaxing of super-coiled DNA and thus blocking DNA transcription and replication. Its third major biological effect is that it forms iron-mediated free radicals that cause oxidative changes to DNA, proteins, and cell membrane lipids. Especially sensitive are the mitochondrial membranes due to their high level of the negatively charged phospholipid cardiolipin, for which doxorubicin has high affinity. This property was the basis of Rahman and coworkers' (1980, 1985, 1986a, 1986b) selection of cardiolipin as their formulation's negatively charged lipid. This oxidative induced damaging effect is now considered one of the main reasons for doxorubicin's toxicities and side effects. The fact that heart muscle is enriched in mitochondria explains in part the drug's cardiotoxicity. Routine treatment by doxorubicin is given intravenously using a relatively high drug dose, in the range of 10 to 50 mg/m^2 (rev. in Weiss, 1992; Skeel, 1999; Minotti et al., 2004; Takimoto and Calvo, 2008; Kenyon, 2008).

Doxorubicin is considered one of the most effective anticancer drugs ever developed, and therefore it became one of the main "first line" anticancer drugs almost from its discovery. It is effective against more types of cancer (including leukemias, lymphomas, and breast, uterine, ovarian, and lung cancers) than any other class of chemotherapy agents (Skeel, 1999; Weiss, 1992, Minotti et al., 2004).

However, like most other chemotherapeutic drugs, doxorubicin has toxicities and side effects attached to its use. Its most dangerous toxicity is the cumulative dose-dependent cardiotoxicity (irreversible congestive heart failure), which considerably limits its usefulness (upper accumulative dose of 550 mg/m^2). Its other side effects include severe myelosuppression, nausea and vomiting, mucocutaneous effects [(stomatitis, alopecia, severe local tissue damage, and hyperpigmentation of skin overlying veins used for drug injection) (Skeel, 1999; Peng et al., 2005; Takimoto and Calvo, 2005; Kenyon, 2008)].

It is the combination of doxorubicin's clinical use for such a broad spectrum of tumor types and the very large number of patients treated with it, combined with its major deficiencies of dose-limiting and accumulating-dose-limiting toxicities, that made it very appealing and attractive to us (and others) and was the major driving force for selecting doxorubicin as the drug of choice for delivery by liposomes. The scientific supportive reasons that were available in 1980 were that the drug's stability (Beijnen et al., 1985), chemistry, and physicochemical properties were well established and drug ADME (**a**bsorption, **d**istribution, **m**etabolism, and **e**xcretion) was common knowledge (Andrews et al., 1980).

Our practical reasons that supported and encouraged work with doxorubicin were its distinct spectral properties, which allow easy quantification of doxorubicin level, its chemical degradation, and even state of aggregation, as well as changes in its local environment (pH and level of hydrophobicity). Doxorubicin's reasonably high molar extinction at 486 nm (12,500 OD/M) allows for its easy quantification by a spectrophotometer, especially when combined with HPLC. Another major practical advantage of doxorubicin is its long wavelength (>550 nm) and high quantum yield fluorescence emission. The use of fluorescence detection increases the limit of detection by more than 100-fold. The fluorescence excitation and emission spectra are distinguished from each other, and both are sensitive to the environment. Doxorubicin's excitation and emission fluorescence spectra are both sensitive to the absorbance variables described above, but at much higher (>300-fold) sensitivity. This enables one to follow doxorubicin PK and BD for long periods of time (Barenholz and Amselem, 1993, 1993b; Haran et al., 1993; Barenolz et al., 1993, 1993a; Amselem et al., 1993a, 1993b; Bandak et al., 1999; Gabizon et al., 1994, 2003).

12.2.2 Liposomal Doxorubicin (First Generation): From Design to Formulation, Characterization, and Stability

We designed, studied, and compared a few liposomal formulations, all having three lipid components: (1) a phosphatidylcholine (PC) as the "liposome-forming lipid"; (2) cholesterol, which is needed to eliminate phase transitions and to increase physical stability in biological fluids; (3) a negatively charged phospholipid as a source of the negative charge needed to increase and stabilize doxorubicin association (partition) to the liposomes' membranes. During eight years (1980–1988), we studied the fabrication and the physicochemical properties of many liposomal compositions loaded with doxorubicin. For these, we compared small unilamellar, large unilamellar, large oligolamellar, and large multilamellar liposomes, referred to as SUV, LUV, OLV, and MLV, respectively. In all of the above, most doxorubicin was associated with the liposomes' bilayer(s). We also studied short- and long-term physical stability (defined by changes in size distribution and drug-to-lipid mole ratio), and chemical stability of the lipids and the doxorubicin of the formulation. In our *in vivo* studies in mice, we studied pharmacokinetics (PK) and biodistribution (BD) in normal and tumor-bearing mice, as well as toxicity and tolerability in rodents, and finally their therapeutic efficacy in tumor-bearing mice (several models). The specific *in vitro* screening parameters included efficiency of drug capture (encapsulation = association), preservation of *in vitro* cytotoxicity (on tumor cells in culture), and the stability of drug–liposome association in body fluids. The *in vivo* screening parameters included *in vivo* tissue distribution with special focus on levels in the heart, and anticancer activity. Representative tumor models relevant to liver tumor were used. Toxicological evaluation included general toxicology and cardiotoxicity. The technical screening included critical analysis of the factors involved in the pharmaceutical development with focus on shelf life, wet versus lyophilized formulations, quality control tests, etc. Our studies on this system are described in many publications (Gabizon et al., 1982; Gabizon et al., 1983; Gabizon et al., 1985; Gabizon et al., 1986a, 1986b; Gabizon et al., 1988a, 1988b; Gabizon et al., 1989a, 1989b; Druckman et al., 1989; Goren et al., 1990; Goren D. (Ph.D. thesis, 1990); Amselem et al., 1993]. Our studies clearly demonstrated that the negatively charged lipids (at physiological pH) in the formulation were essential to meet the needs of high efficiency of doxorubicin encapsulation. The fact that the level of drug loading (capture) is ~50-fold higher than the trapped aqueous volume determined by ^{3}H-inulin (Amslem et al., 1990; Haran et al., 1993) indicated that most of the captured drug is not in the intraliposome aqueous phase but rather associated with the negatively charged liposomal membranes. Diphosphatidyl glycerol (cardiolipin, DPG), phosphatidyl glycerol (PG), and phosphatidylserine (PS) were all active in improving the encapsulation, with DPG encapsulation being the best in terms of drug association, in agreement with the highest association constant of DPG doxorubicin of 1.6×10^{-6}, compared with 1.8×10^{-4} for PS and ~0.0 for PC (Goormarghitigh and Ruysschaert, 1984). Exposure to serum (without large dilution!) did not cause significant doxorubicin release. For practical reasons such as DPG availability and cost (at that time), as well as potential immunogenicity, we excluded the DPG from our studies.

Another important aspect of this research was that unilamellar vesicles (either SUV < 100 nm or LUV > 100 nm in diameter) capture much less drug and lose their drug content faster than vesicles of the same lipid composition in larger sizes and lamellarity (Goren et al., 1990; Goren, 1990) including either large (>100 nm) oligolamellar (OLV) or multilamellar large vesicles (MLV). Large and small are functional definitions that describe vesicles in which the external two leaflets of the external lipid bilayer have different (SUV) or almost the same (OLV and MLV) curvature (Lichtenberg and Barenholz, 1988). This was another warning signal that could predict a failure in humans, which we did not understand in the early 1980s.

Finally, we found that formulations composed of saturated lipids have significantly lower drug capture than the formulations that are based on phospholipids of the identical headgroups but having unsaturated hydrocarbon chains. Namely, unsaturated phospholipids seemed to be superior to saturated phospholipids. This may be explained by the larger free volume in the membrane composed of unsaturated lipids, which leaves more space for the drug.

With both PS- and PG-containing OLV (as the negatively charged lipid), we achieved a similar drug to lipid ratio over the broad range of 0.05–0.26 (depending on fine tuning, Amselem et al., 1990, 1992), but as PS is less chemically stable and more expensive, PG became our negatively charged lipid of choice. The formulation was optimized for various variables, of which level of PG (demonstrated in Figure 12.2) was a main one.

The result of all these optimization processes was our preferred formulation for OLV-DOX, a liposome 300–500 nm in diameter. It was composed of egg PC : egg PG : cholesterol (7 : 3 : 4 mole ratio) and was fabricated by extrusion (Amselem et al., 1989–90, 1990, 1992). Due to the use of egg-derived unsaturated phospholipids

(PC and PG), acyl chains were composed of ~50 mole% unsaturated fatty acids [C18:1 (30.2%) > C18:2 (16.3%) > C20:4 (3.5%) > C22: 5 (0.9%) > C22:6 (0.7%)] (Barenholz and Amselem, 1993). We had to deal with two types of chemical stability issues: acyl ester hydrolysis and lipid auto/peroxidation (Lichtenberg and Barenholz, 1988). Major efforts were dedicated to solve these stability issues. The best protection against oxidative damage was obtained by inclusion in the lipid mixture of 1.5 mole% D-α-tocopherol succinate (TCS). This by itself was not sufficient, and therefore the fabrication and storage of the formulation was done in the presence of the highly efficient iron ion chelator Desferal (deferoxamine mesylate) using the aqueous medium of 0.15 M NaCl (saline) containing 200 mM Desferal, at pH range of pH 5.7–6.8 at 4°C (Barenholz and Gabizon, 1990, 1991; Amselem et al., 1990; Barenholz and Amselem, 1993; Barenholz et al., 1993). Under such conditions, doxorubicin degradation was minimal (<5%), lipid hydrolysis was low (<5%), cholesterol degradation was below detection limit, and lipid oxidation was minimal even after 19 months storage at 4°C (Barenholz and Amselem, 1993). TCS acts as a pro-antioxidant slowly hydrolyzing and continuously supplying α-tocopherol as an active antioxidant, while Desferal is one the most potent iron chelating agents, which effectively neutralizes iron ions that are highly potent inducers of lipid and doxorubicin auto/peroxidation (Lichtenberg and Barenholz, 1988, Barenholz and Amselem, 1993).

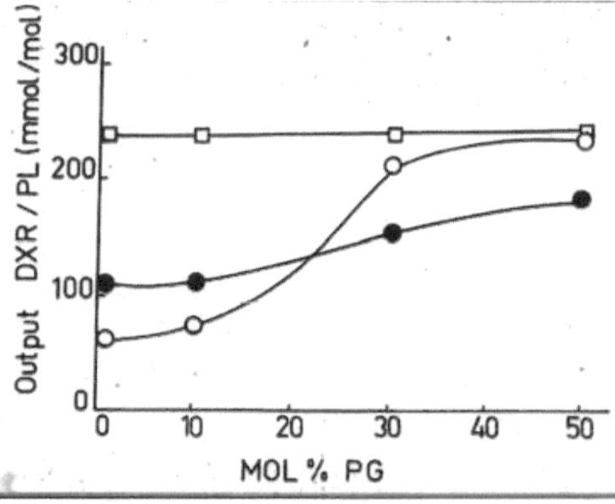

Figure 12.2 Optimization of OLV-DOX to the mole percent PG. Effect on doxorubicin (DXR) association with the liposomes (Amselem et al., 1990). The white square equals input DXR:PL ratio; White circle equals DXR loading method I; Black circle equals DXR loading method II.

The optimal doxorubicin-loaded egg (E)-derived phospholipids and cholesterol (EPC/EPG/Cholesterol/TCS 7:3:4:0.2) OLV-DOX formulation showed reasonable shelf life and good physical stability in plasma (<5% release in 1 h at 37°C). However, today, we know that this way of testing was misleading, as the dilution of the OLV-DOX used was small.

12.2.3 Cytotoxicity to Cells in Culture (*in vitro*)

In vitro testing of this formulation (OLV-DOX) indicated that the drug encapsulation in the OLV has almost no effect on the IC_{50} (compare 1.1×10^{-8M} for the liposomal drug with 1.8×10^{-8M} for the free drug) in the two cell lines studied [J-6456 lymphoma and P388 leukemia, (Gabizon and Barenholz, 1988)]. At the time the experiment was performed, we did not understand that this should be a warning signal of the "viability" of this formulation as it suggested unwanted relatively fast dilution-dependent major drug leakage from the liposomes to the cell growth medium. At a later stage, when we evaluated why this formulation failed in humans (see below), we found that no growth inhibition of the cells (no cytotoxicity) was observed in the presence of the cation exchanger Dowex-50 [which selectively and efficiently binds the positively charged free doxorubicin, but not liposome-associated drug (Druckmann et al., 1989; Amselem et al., 1990)]. The same removal of drug cytotoxicity by the cation exchanger was obtained for free doxorubicin (F-DOX), indicating that in both cases, drug enters the cells in its free (nonliposomal) form.

12.2.4 Pharmacokinetics and Biodistribution Studies in Mice

Preclinical PK and BD studies of the above optimal OLV-DOX in normal and tumor-bearing mice met all of our objectives and expectations. Biodistribution studies showed that the encapsulation of DOX into these OLV increased liver (the target organ) and spleen DOX uptake concomitantly with reducing DOX levels in the heart, kidneys, and small intestine, as well as reducing organ and plasma clearance of the drug (Gabizon et al., 1982, 1983). In mice bearing liver metastasis, the DOX level after i.v. injection of OLV-DOX reached a level severalfold higher than after injection of an equal amount of

F-DOX. This was paralleled by a large reduction in the viability of tumor cells isolated from the liver of tumor-bearing mice (by Percoll density gradient) after injection of OLV-DOX, which was achieved only after administration of OLV-DOX and not of F-DOX.

12.2.5 Toxicity

We studied the toxicity of a few liposomal doxorubicin formulations of different lipid compositions in small rodents as a part of the selection process of the optimal formulation. Here we will summarize our comparison of the leading formulation of EPC/EPG/Cholesterol/TCS 7:3:4:0.2 OLV-DOX with free drug (F-DOX). The comparison included a few studies that included single-dose and multi-dose experiments (Gabizon et al., 1986b). We demonstrated that OLV-DOX is much less toxic than F-DOX; LD_{50} value of OLV-DOX is twofold higher than the LD_{50} value of F-DOX. The lower toxicity of OLV-DOX was also demonstrated by higher, close to normal, body weight and organ weights and almost no histopathological damage to the kidney and myocardium. The low level of cardiotoxicity observed was fully reversible. It is also very important that despite the fact that i.v. administration of OLV-DOX resulted in high accumulation of doxorubicin in the liver, hepatotoxicity was minimal and limited to some megalonucleosis, with slight changes in liver function observed at the end of a six-month-long experiment in rodents. The much lower toxicity of OLV-DOX than of F-DOX is related first to the fact the encapsulation in the OLV affected dramatically the drug biodistribution, with much less drug reaching the heart and the kidneys (Gabizon et al., 1982, 1983). However, this is not the only effect of the encapsulation. Not less important is the effect on subcellular distribution, which results in the diminishing interaction of the intracellular doxorubicin with the mitochondria. The latter may explain part of the chronic free drug toxicity (related to the high affinity of the drug to the mitochondrial lipid DPG. The bottom line of the toxicity studies is that our OLV-DOX is significantly less toxic than F-DOX.

12.2.6 Therapeutic efficacy

For the therapeutic efficacy, we studied two *in vivo* models of tumor-bearing mice with major involvement of RES organs, the J-6456 lymphoma with predominant dissemination to the liver (Gabizon et al., 1982, 1983, 1985) and the BCL1 leukemia, which infiltrates mainly the spleen and bone marrow (Gabizon et al., 1986a). In both models, OLV -DOX was much superior to F-DOX at equal drug dose and, as higher doses of OLV-DOX can be administered due to its superior LD_{50}, the therapeutic efficacy of OLV-DOX is much higher than that of F-DOX. Levels of the drug after administration OLV-DOX i.v. administration at the J-6456 lymphoma cells isolated from the liver of tumor-bearing mice (by Percoll density gradient) were more than three-fold higher than after injection of an equal dose of F-DOX for at least the first 64 h post drug administration (i.e., compare 195 ng and 25 ng of drug per 10^7 isolated lymphoma cells for DOX-OLV and F-DOX, respectively, at 24 h post injection). Table 12.1 is one of many examples that clearly show that the therapeutic efficacy of DOX-OLV in mice bearing J-6456 metastatic lymphoma was also much superior to an equal dose of F-DOX.

One explanation for the fact that we did not get a cure or many long-term (>100 days) mice survivors is that the result of the presence of metastatic lymphoma cells in tissues other than liver and spleen, to which OLV-DOX does not deliver high drug levels.

This is an important lesson to learn about our OLV-DOX performance.

Table 12.1 Superior anti-tumor activity of OLV-DOX over F-DOX based on survival time (days)[a]

Exp	No. of Mice	Mean ± s.e.	Median (range) p^a
Untreated	7	19.3 + 0.5	18.5 (18–21) <0.01
F-DOX	8	40.5 + 2.3	40.0 (28–50) <0.01
OLV-DOX (PG:PC:Chol)	8	71.1 + 12.9	53.0 (41–148)

Note: For more details, see Gabizon et al. (1985).

[a]BALB/c mice inoculated with 10^6 J-6456 cells and treated i.v. with 8 mg kg^{-1} doxorubicin in either free or liposome-entrapped form.

[b]Wilcoxon test: F-DOX analyzed versus Untreated; OLV-DOX analyzed versus F-DOX.

Overall, the above results suggest that our treatment modality with OLV-DOX may meet the expectation of being superior to F-DOX in treatment of liver tumors including liver metastasis in humans.

In 1985, based on the above formulation design and characterization, combined with acceptable toxicology (significantly better than F-DOX), superior PK, BD, and therapeutic efficacy in small rodents (compared with F-DOX), we started to plan and apply for a phase I clinical trial approval at the Hadassah University Hospital. IND application was submitted and was approved in 1985 by the Hadassah University Hospital Helsinki Committee and the Israel Ministry of Health (MOH).

12.2.7 Scale-Up

The preparation for the clinical trials required fabrication of the OLV-DOX at liter-scale batches, concomitantly with the development of quality control assays (Barenholz et al., 1989; Gabizon et al., 1989b; Amselem et al., 1989–90, 1990, 1992, 1993a, 1993b; Gabizon et al., 1991; Barenholz and Amselem, 1993; Barenholz and Crommelin, 1994).

12.3 OLV-DOX Clinical Trials

12.3.1 What Was Known in 1985 on "First in Man" Studies and the Clinical Use of Liposomes as Carriers of Drugs and Imaging Agents?

The first clinical use of liposomes dates back to 1974, when the fate of radiolabeled liposomes was examined in three cancer patients (Gregoriadis et al., 1974). This was followed by Gregoriadis and coworkers' use of liposomes as a carrier for the enzyme glucocerebroside (a beta-glucosidase) for enzyme replacement therapy for Gaucher's disease treatment (Belchetz et al., 1977). More extensive studies in humans with radiolabeled "fluid"-phase sonicated liposomes indicated that the major tissues of liposome uptake are the liver and spleen (Richardson et al., 1979). A similar study in which the distribution of technetium-99m-labeled MLV in patients with Hodgkin's disease was performed by Perez-Soler et al. (1985). The earliest report in the literature on the therapeutic use of liposomes as drug carriers given systemically to a sizable group of patients described the experience gained after administration of amphotericin-B in liposomes. It showed clear beneficial antifungal activity without apparent toxicity at doses in which serious toxic effects of the free drug occurs (Lopez-Berestein et al., 1985). A similar study with another (sonicated) liposomal amphotericin-B formulation was performed later in cancer patients with fungal infections by Sculier and coworkers (1988). A pilot human study with the water-insoluble cytotoxic drug NSC 251635 was also performed (Sculier et al., 1986).

One early clinical "first in man" study was performed with a liposomal doxorubicin formulation by Kumai et al. (1985). They reported on a treatment of liver cancer by local (hepatic intra-arterial) injection of small doses of liposomal doxorubicin, up to 15 mg/m^2, in 10 cancer patients with liver metastasis. The main side effect found was fever, which could be explained by a small contamination of the liposomal formulation with endotoxin. Our main take-home lesson from all the above "first in man" trials was that the preparation of liposomal formulations for clinical use is feasible. These early experiments were very helpful in convincing the ethical committee and Israel MOH to grant permission for our "first in man" and phase I clinical trials of OLV-DOX.

12.3.2 Phase I Clinical Trials of Liposomal Doxorubicin (OLV-DOX)

EPC/EPG/Cholesterol/TCS 7:3:4:0.2 OLV-DOX having a doxorubicin (membrane associated) to phospholipid mole ratio of 0.056 and a size distribution of 300–500 nm were used in our clinical trials.

In our first study (Gabizon et al., 1989a, 1989b), 32 patients, most of them with primary or metastatic liver cancer refractory to conventional therapy, were treated. A total of 69 courses of therapy was administered by intravenous infusion of a suspension of OLV-DOX (0.5–2.0 mg DOX/mL) in physiologic saline containing 200 mM Desferal (pH 6.2) at an approximate infusion rate of 2 mL/min given on a 3-week intermittent schedule.

OLV-DOX and phospholipid doses were escalated from 20 mg/m^2 and 0.3 g/m^2 to 120 mg/m^2 and 3.2 g/m^2 for DOX and phospholipids, respectively. Treatment was generally well tolerated, and acute toxic effects such as nausea and vomiting were mild and infrequent. Chills and fever (>38°C) were observed on infusion. Median WBC nadir counts were 2700, 2300, and 700/ml at 85, 100, and 120 mg/m^2, respectively. All three patients receiving 120 mg/m^2 developed grade

4 leukopenia and fever requiring intravenous antibiotics, and, in two of them, severe stomatitis (grades 3 and 4) was observed. Significant hair loss was apparent in all patients receiving doses higher than 50 mg/m^2. This also should have been a warning signal (which we did not understood then) of the possibility of fast drug release from the OLV upon infusion. The maximal tolerated dose (MTD) of OLV-DOX appears to be 120 mg/m^2 , with leukopenia and stomatitis being the dose-limiting factors. While the sub-acute toxicity of OLV-DOX appeared to be qualitatively similar to that of F-DOX, its tolerance was better, as it exceeded the recommended dose of free drug (75 mg/mL) in the standard 3-weekly schedule.

This clinical study with OLV-DOX shows that administration of this formulation to humans is feasible even at higher than conventional dose levels of free drug (60–75 mg/m^2), and it appears to be well tolerated. Based on this phase I study, the recommended starting dose for phase II studies would be 100 mg/m^2. It should be noted that most of the patients in this study suffered from heavy neoplastic involvement of the liver, and most of them had been previously treated with various cytotoxic agents including doxorubicin. There is suggestive evidence that doxorubicin-induced myelosuppression is more severe when the tumor shows a major liver involvement (McKelvey et al., 1976; Gundersen et al., 1986) , This may lead to increase in liposome localization in the bone marrow (Perez-Soler et al., 1985). Therefore it seems that patient populations that have heavy neoplastic involvement of the liver are not suitable for being treated with a high dose of OLV-DOX. However, higher doses could be administered to other patient populations with acceptable toxicity. Regarding acute toxicity, nausea and vomiting appear to be substantially attenuated when compared with the common clinical experience with free DOX at standard 3-weekly doses (Blum and Carter, 1974). Fever, a rather uncommon side effect of free DOX therapy, was observed in a relatively high percentage of cases. Although the immediate reaction may still be attributable to a low amount of endotoxin, undetectable in the rabbit test, the delayed reaction appears to be a specific feature of DOX-OLV. One possible explanation is that this treatment induces interleukin-l secretion by doxorubicin-activated macrophages (Mace et al., 1988) following DOX-OLV localization in tissue macrophages and breakdown of endocytosed liposomes. The sub-acute toxicity of OLV-DOX appears to be qualitatively similar to that of free DOX, with leucopenia and stomatitis being the most significant dose-limiting factors. These data should be another warning signal (that we ignored) that the drug is released fast from the liposomes into the blood circulation. A similar finding has been obtained in a another clinical study (Treat et al., 1989), with DOX encapsulated in liposomes composed of cardiolipin, PC, stearylamine, and cholesterol, although the MTD and recommended dose for Phase II studies reported (90 and 75 mg/m^2, respectively) are lower than in our study. Drug causing myelosuppression may reach the bone marrow in several ways. The ability of liposomes to localize in the bone marrow, a tissue rich in sinusoidal capillaries, has been demonstrated in animals (Gregoriadis and Senior, 1986) and in humans (Perez-Soler et al., 1985). Today our interpretation of these results is that all these formulations that share that doxorubicin is a liposome membrane component, also share a fast dilution-induced drug leakage (release) from the liposomes in the blood circulation, which may explain the myelosuppressive effect of the liposomal formulations. Another possible explanation is that drug that was released from the liver and spleen macrophages reached the circulation after the liposomes were endocytosed and processed. Although human pharmacokinetic studies with liposomal doxorubicin have been previously reported (Gabizon et al., 1989; Rahman et al., 1989), they did not enable discrimination between the various explanations, as the measurements done at that time did not provide separation between plasma free drug and liposome-associated drug in the plasma. These two forms of doxorubicin can now be resolved by the methodology of using the cation exchanger Dowex-50, described by Druckmann et al. (1989).

The bottom line of our first in man clinical trial indicated that while the administration of DOX-OLV to humans is feasible and even up-shifts MTD the major side effects were similar to those of the free drug. This was disappointing and not in agreement with our expectations, which were based on our mice results. There the DOX-OLV was superior in all aspects [PK, BD, tolerability, and efficacy (see above)]. In order to benefit from the disappointing human trial results, we decided to put major efforts into the understanding of the differences observed between the failed human study (Gabizon et al., 1989b) and the successful mice studies (rev. in Gabizon and Barenholz, 1988). For this, we decided to study pharmacokinetics and liposome localization by imaging studies in patients.

12.3.3 OLV-DOX Pharmacokinetics, Biodistribution, and *in vivo* Imaging in Humans

The PK and BD study in humans (Gabizon et al., 1991) included 19 patients receiving OLV-DOX. It was carried out within the framework of a Phase I clinical trial (Gabizon et al., 1989a, 1989b; Barenholz et al., 1990). The formulation of DOX-OLV tested consisted of the DOX-OLV described above. Plasma clearance of total drug extracted from the plasma after DOX-OLV infusion followed a bi-exponential decay curve with a pattern and PK parameters similar to that reported (and confirmed by us) for free DOX. The plasma concentration of drug circulating in liposome-associated form was also determined using the method described by Druckmann et al. (1989), which is based on separation of free and liposome-associated drug by the cation exchanger Dowex-50 (which selectively binds the free drug). These special studies were performed in seven patients. Liposome-associated drug was found to be rapidly cleared from plasma; its ratio to nonliposome-associated drug appeared to correlate with liver reserve, with highest ratios in patients with normal liver function. Liposomes' clearance was measured after free drug and protein-associated drug were removed by Dowex-50 cation-exchange resin (Druckmann et al., 1989). The remaining plasma that contained the OLV-DOX was thereafter processed for HPLC drug analysis as detailed elsewhere (Gabizon et al., 1991a). Measurements of total and liposome-associated plasma doxorubicin were obtained. The levels of free and protein-bound drugs were inferred by subtracting the concentration of liposome-associated drug from that of total doxorubicin. In three of these patients, we also measured the concentration of PG in plasma to follow the clearance of liposomes (Gabizon et al., 1991a; Amselem et al., 1993a). PG was selected as a liposome marker because of its very low concentration in human plasma (less than 5 nmoles/mL) relative to the concentration of total phospholipids (2,000–4,000 nmoles/mL). Phosphatidylethanolamine (PE) was chosen as an internal standard due to its absence in the DOX-OLV formulation and its being in a concentration range of similar order of magnitude to the phospholipids infused as OLV-DOX. Plasma samples were extracted after a complete trinitrophenylation of the plasma aminolipids (PE and phosphatidylserine) and of DOX by trinitrobenzene sulfonate (TNBS). The step of trinitrophenylation was essential to optimize the chromatographic separation. The different phospholipids were quantified using low-phosphorus silica gel thin layer plates. The reduction in PG plasma concentration with time was used to calculate liposome plasma clearance, while the change of ratio of DOX to PG in the plasma was used to calculate rate of DOX release from DOX-OLV in the patients' plasma.

The results obtained in these three patients indicate that liposome-associated doxorubicin has fast clearance, which resembles that of F-DOX. In addition, their ratio of DOX/PG is reduced fast (Figure 12.3, inset) suggesting that liposomes lose most of their drug payload during circulation.

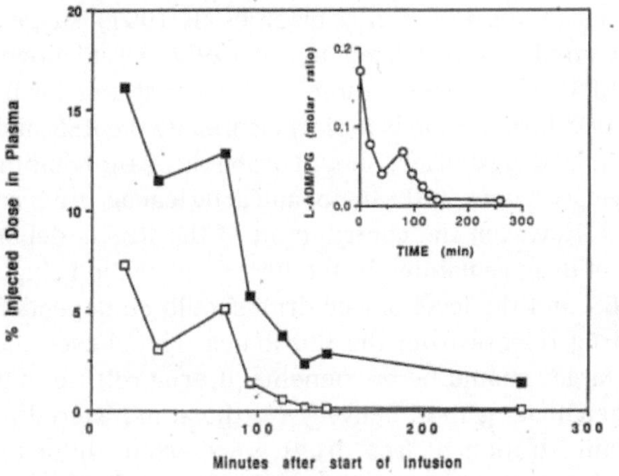

Figure 12.3 Plasma clearance of liposomal doxorubicin (white squares) and PG (black squares). Due to dilution-induced release in plasma, the liposomes reached the liver almost drug free. Adriamycin (ADM) = doxorubicin (DOX). (Gabizon et al., 1991a; Amselem et al., 1993a)

To learn about the liposome organ distribution, imaging studies were carried out with doxorubicin-free ^{111}indium-deferoxamine-labeled liposomes of the same composition and size distribution as the OLV-DOX. These ^{111}In-OLV were prepared by hydration of the lipids in a medium containing 200 mM of the chelating agent deferoxamine mesylate (DF) dissolved in physiological saline. Un-encapsulated DF was removed by passage through a Dowex-50 cation-exchange resin. Liposomes were labeled with ^{111}In by incubation with an ^{111}In-oxine (Amersham) complex at room temperature for about 30 min. Free (unloaded ^{111}In-oxine was removed by gel permeation chromatography. Approximately 90% of the label became liposome-associated. Patients were imaged using a dose of ~700 mCi of ^{111}In and 300 mg phospholipid given by i.v. bolus. Whole body anterior and posterior images were obtained immediately after injection, 2 h and 24 h later, using a Gamma camera (Apex 415 Elscint, Haifa, Israel). For details see Gabizon et al., 1991). The results show clearly that the ^{111}In-OLV were cleared predominantly by liver and spleen and to a lesser extent by bone marrow in seven out of nine patients. In two patients with active hepatitis and severe liver dysfunction, there was minimal liver uptake and increased spleen and bone marrow uptake. For all patients analyzed except one hepatoma patient, intrahepatic and extrahepatic tumors were not imaged by liposomes (Figures 4, 6–9 in Gabizon et al., 1991), suggesting that liposome uptake is restricted to cells of the reticuloendothelial system (RES). These observations indicate that a major fraction of this OLV-DOX formulation is rapidly cleared by the RES, and that the mechanism of drug delivery should probably be the combined result of slow release from the RES depot and drug leakage from circulating liposomes. However, the contribution of the RES is dependent on the level of drug remaining in the liposomes while being taken up by the RES, and the level of free drug should be dependent on the rate of drug release from the liposomes. The slower the release rate, the larger should be the benefits. If drug release in plasma is fast, no beneficial gain of delivery via the administered liposomes (over administration of free drug) is expected. Unfortunately, in human subjects the latter occurred. As shown in Figure 12.2, the OLV-DOX shows fast release of their doxorubicin payload in plasma, and therefore, the therapeutic benefits expected of these liposomes compared to free doxorubicin should be minimal, if any. Figure 12.4 clearly demonstrates that conventional liposomes (OLV-DOX) do not target liver tumor and behave similarly to ^{99}Tc-colloid.

The same OLV-DOX that failed in humans has been shown to have reduced toxicity and improved antitumor efficacy in experimental animal models (rev. in Gabizon and Barenholz, 1988). Namely, the beneficial effects in mice were not reproduced in our Phase I clinical study (Gabizon et al., 1989a, 1989b). Although the maximal tolerated dose (MTD) of DOX-OLV was increased in relation to the MTD of free drug administered at the conventional 3-weekly schedule; in humans the dose-limiting toxicity (the myelotoxicity) of OLV-DOX is very similar to that of free doxorubicin. Thus, although the toxicities of free DOX and OLV-DOX differ somewhat quantitatively, they are qualitatively very similar.

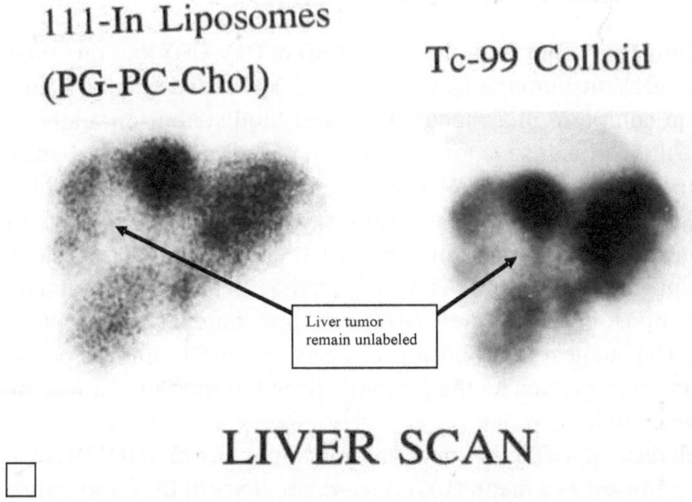

Figure 12.4 Liver scintigraphies 2 h after injection of patient with radiolabeled ^{111}In-OLV or ^{99}Tc-colloid (Gabizon et al., 1991).

The "bottom line" conclusions of our human clinical trials are based on the PK and BD human study in which the results of clearance of drug and the liposomes (DOX and liposome PG) are combined with the results of the radiolabeled ^{111}In-OLV human imaging experiment. The latter clearly indicates that in humans who retain significant liver function, the OLV accumulate in the liver and spleen RES, but without reaching the liver tumor. What is more problematic is that there is a fast dilution-induced drug release of the OLV-DOX in the blood already during the i.v. infusion. This means that in humans, the liposomes reaching the liver are almost drug free, so our basic working hypothesis that the RES will act as a drug depot is not valid for human treatment. Another important conclusion is the confirmation that in humans severe liver dysfunction will have a large effect on RES-directed liposomes; then more liposomes will reach the spleen and the bone marrow, and drug leakage of the circulating liposomes will become the main factor that determines drug fate.

12.3.4 Conclusions of Our Clinical Experience with OLV-DOX as the Basis for the Development of Novel Liposomal DOX for Treatment of Metastatic Tumors

Our study that reports on the PK and BD of OLV-DOX and on imaging of ^{111}In-OLV in humans (Gabizon et al., 1991) is the first study in which a complete pharmacokinetic and biodistribution analysis of a drug-liposome dosage form in human patients was described. The clearance of DOX when delivered as OLV-DOX is a composite of two processes: (i) clearance of liposomes containing DOX by the RES, predominantly liver and spleen and (ii) clearance of DOX released from liposomes in plasma. The analysis that includes PK of total drug (DOX), liposome-associated DOX, and liposome markers (PG and ^{111}In-OLV) suggests that both processes operate in human patients and that factors such as the patient's liver function may affect their relative contribution.

Delivery of DOX in liposome-entrapped form (OLV-DOX) has been proposed as a means to reduce the toxicity of DOX and improve its therapeutic index based on a number of preclinical studies (rev. in Gabizon and Barenholz, 1988).

The PK, BD, and imaging data (Gabizon et al., 1991) suggest that the reduced clinical toxicity of OLV-DOX results from a somewhat lower peak level of free drug and possibly some changes in the tissue distribution of the liposomes, with a partial shift toward OLV and possibly some drug accumulation in the RES at the expense of other tissues. The main limitations of our therapeutic strategy based on OLV-DOX, as revealed by this study, are the significant drug leakage and preferential RES uptake. These shortcomings are probably the result of the basic formulation physicochemical characteristics, such as

(i) Drug entrapment in the liposome bilayer as opposed to encapsulation in liposome aqueous interior. Bilayer-associated drug may be more accessible to be released to the plasma upon dilution and to associate with plasma proteins (Goren et al., 1990; Goren, 1990). This process will be affected by the degree of dilution upon injection, which is also dependent on the mode of administration (greater dilution effect occurs for slow infusion than for bolus injection). The association of doxorubicin with liposomes is related to the drug-liposomes association constant [which determines the liposome/medium (liposome/plasma) partition coefficient (K_p)]. The question is how high K_p has to be in order to prevent a major drug leakage in plasma. This may be a key issue that may explain the difference between our success in rodents and failure in humans (Amselem et al., 1993; Barenholz and Cohen, 1995; Barenholz, 2001, 2003). Plasma volume in mice is ~1.0 mL compared with 3,500 mL in humans. Therefore, upon slow infusion, the liposomes undergo a very large dilution of 3500-fold for each milliliter that reaches the plasma, compared with only a fivefold dilution with the bolus injection of the same liposomes to mice. The fast free drug clearance keeps this huge dilution effect active throughout the time of infusion.

The observation of a sudden burst of drug leakage shortly after injection (Figure 4 in Gabizon et al., 1991) is compatible with the dilution effect.

(ii) The presence of a high mole fraction of PG in the liposome bilayer may accelerate uptake by the RES (Gabizon and Papahadjopoulos, 1988); it may also induce complement activation (Szebeni et al., 2007, and rev. in Szebeni and Barenholz, 2012, this book).

(iii) The liposome size is too large to allow for extravasation in extrahepatic tissues (Hwang, 1987) and to take advantage of the enhanced permeability and retention (EPR) effect that was first described by Matsumura and Maeda (1986) and recently reviewed by Maeda et al. (2009). This effect may allow for selective accumulation of nanoparticles in tumors due to unique micro-anatomy of blood vessels there (but not in normal healthy tissue) being porous and permeable to 100-nm particles. In addition, the tumor tissue is poor in lymphatic drainage, which enables prolonged retention of the nanoparticles there, followed by local (tumor) drug release and/or for the liposomes to be taken up by the tumor cells.

Based on this analysis, the fact that the same dose-limiting bone marrow toxicity was observed with DOX-OLV and with F-DOX is not surprising and can be assigned to a large extent to the fast drug leakage from circulating liposomes.

In view of the OLV-DOX fast plasma drug release and changes in tissue distribution and bioavailability, it is uncertain whether the somewhat increased tolerated dosage of OLV-DOX (over F-DOX) will result in an enhanced antitumor activity. The liposomes used here are cleared quickly by the RES of liver and spleen and to a lesser extent by the bone marrow. Our studies suggest that the mechanism of antitumor activity of OLV-DOX is complex, and presumably results from exposure of tumor cells to drug leaking from circulating liposomes and drug released from the RES. Obviously, drug leakage from circulating liposomes is undesirable since it increases toxicity. Regarding drug release from the RES, the clinical conditions most likely to benefit from this approach are limited. This approach should not work for treatment of solid tumors, as in most solid tumors drug exposure in relation to dosage may be suboptimal. The OLV-DOX will be highly sensitive to factors such as RES/liver function, site of tumor involvement, and proximity of tumor cells to RES cells.

The failure of our OLV-DOX approach in humans has some basic "take home messages" that if used right should lead us to the development of a liposomal doxorubicin formulation that should be less toxic and more efficacious than free DOX in humans. This failure served as the main driving force and as the basis for Doxil® development.

12.4 Doxil® Development

12.4.1 Turning DOX-OLV Failure into Doxil Success

We started our clinical trial of OLV-DOX in 1985. In summer of 1985 after we already had treated two patients, I started my sabbatical at Liposome Technology Inc. (LTI) at Menlo Park. That year LTI also licensed from Yissum two pending patent applications of Barenholz and Gabizon on OLV-DOX (Barenholz and Gabizon, 1990, 1991). One year later, LTI staff became involved in the OLV-DOX clinical trial and expanded it to include, in addition to Israel, also the United Kingdom. The UK studies were led locally by Roger New (Amselem et al., 1992). This trial expansion allowed us to increase patient number. By 1987 it became evident to us that this specific OLV-DOX formulation would not become a viable product and is not good enough for further development. We decided to exploit the results of this study to bring us closer to understand the requirements for a viable product that could overcome all (or at least most) of the deficiencies demonstrated by our OLV-DOX. These included the facts that in this failed formulation, doxorubicin is liposome-membrane-associated and that liposome membrane is composed of two fluid unsaturated phospholipids (having the solid ordered to liquid disordered phase transition much below 37°C): the zwitterionic "fluid" liposome-forming lipid EPC, and the negatively charged "fluid" liposome-forming lipid EPG, and cholesterol. These failed liposomes were oligolamellar, and of size distribution in the range of 200–500 nm. The combination of this size distribution range and lipid composition resulted in fast uptake of the liposomes by the RES; namely, there was no RES avoidance. Not less important are the facts that in the RES the liposomes were not taken up by tumors (Gabizon et al., 1991a, 1991b). These liposomes reached the liver with a very low level of drug (Gabizon et al., 1991a, 1991b Amselem et al., 1993a) due to the fact that most encapsulated drug was membrane-associated (electrostatically) and in humans undergoes fast dilution-induced drug release upon intravenous injection. In addition, such large liposomes could not make use of extravasation typical of nano-particulates (having long circulation time) via the porous blood vessels of the tumor tissue. This unique nano-anatomy can be used as the Achilles' Heel of the cancer tissue for selective accumulation of macromolecules and nanoparticles in the tumor tissue. The latter unique extravasation was described first by Matsumura and Maeda (1986) and referred to as the enhanced permeability and retention (EPR) effect.

The microanatomy of tumor blood vessels and its relevance to tumor therapy was studied extensively by Jain and coworkers (Hashizume et al., 2000), while Bassermann (1986) described the changes in vascular pattern of tumors and surrounding tissues during different phases of metastatic growth. Jain and coworkers also point out the high pressure in tumors (but not in healthy tissues), which reduces drug diffusion from blood vessels into the tumors, thereby reducing the therapeutic efficacy and increasing toxicity of chemotherapy.

After our failed "first in man" clinical trial, we were back at square one, but we were much more educated and more knowledgeable on both the scientific and technological levels of the issues and the need to solve the major problems described above. We were also confident that the development of liposomal doxorubicin is feasible. Therefore we decided to look for an alternative liposomal doxorubicin formulation that can overcome all the above deficiencies and will be able to reach most metastatic solid tumors and will not be limited to liver-residing tumors.

We decided that in order for the liposomes to become an approved anticancer drug, the liposomes should be characterized by the following features:

- They should be at the nano scale (nano-liposomes) so they will be able to take advantage of the EPR effect and extravasate from the blood vessels at the tumor into the tumor tissue.
- In order to be efficacious, the liposomes should reach the tumors loaded with a therapeutically high enough drug level.
- The drug PK and BD should be controlled by the liposomes, with the liposomal drug demonstrating a highly prolonged plasma circulation time to give it the time needed to achieve drug tumor accumulation.
- Drug should be available to tumor cells either by drug release at the tumor site or by the drug loaded nano-liposomes being internalized by the tumor cells.

12.4.2 Requirements to Achieve Therapeutically Efficacious Passively Targeted Drug Loaded Liposomes and Means to Fulfill Them

Table 12.2 summarizes the requirements to achieve therapeutically efficacious passively targeted drug loaded liposomes and means to fulfill them (based on Barenholz, 2007).

Table 12.2 Requirements to achieve therapeutically efficacious passively targeted drug loaded liposomes and means to fulfill them

	Requirements	Solutions
1.	Extended circulation time in intact form in the human plasma	Development of sterically stabilized liposomes (SSL) composed of high T_m lipids, cholesterol, and a lipopolymer such as ^{2000}PEG-DSPE

	Requirements	Solutions
2.	Sufficient levels and stable loading of drug in order for long circulating nano-liposomes to reach disease site with liposomes loaded with drug at a level needed to achieve therapeutic efficacy [$t_{1/2}$ of drug release in blood should be longer than circulation $t_{1/2}$]	Use of pH or ammonium ion gradients for remote (active) loading of amphipathic weak bases or acids into long-circulating nano-liposomes
3.	Extravasation into diseased tissue (tumor)	Using small enough (<120 nm, preferably <100 nm) nano-liposomes in order to efficiently extravasate through the gaps in the tumor vasculature (taking advantage of the EPR effect)
4.	Getting active drug into target cells	Releasing drug from liposomes through selective drug leakage at site due to diseased tissue properties, or using: collapsible ion gradient, or liposomes sensitive to secretory phospholipases, or by applying physical means such as heat (thermosensitive nSSL) or ultrasound or by internalization after active targeting.

Note: For relevant references, see Table 1 in Barenholz (2007).

In order to save time, all four aspects described in Table 12.2 were investigated in parallel at four different locations: LTI laboratories at Menlo Park, CA, by LTI scientists; Papahadjopoulos' Lab at UCSF by Alberto Gabizon; Terry Allen's lab at the University of Alberta in Canada; and Barenholz's lab in Jerusalem.

LTI, Terry Allen, and Alberto Gabizon/Dimitri Papahadjopoulos worked on getting liposomes of extended circulation and RES avoidance, which due to being at the nano-range size can take advantage of the EPR effect [Matsumura and Maeda (1986)]. The EPR effect was expected to result in selective nano-particulate extravasation from the tumor capillaries into the tumor tissue. The liposomes with prolonged circulation time and RES avoidance were termed by Dr. Frank Martin of LTI "Stealth®" liposomes and these unique properties of liposomes were referred to as "Stealthness," which means unseen or unrecognized as particulates by the RES.

At the same time, I and my student Gilad Haran (now a professor at the Weizmann Institute) were working on the development of a remote and stable loading method for doxorubicin, which should enable the formulation to reach sufficient level of drug to achieve therapeutic efficacy in humans under conditions that the drug when reaching the tumor will be bioavailable to the tumor cells (Barenholz and Haran, 1993, 1994; Haran et al., 1993).

12.4.3 Liposomes Having Prolonged Blood Circulation

In 1987 when I came back to Jerusalem after one and a half years of sabbatical at LTI, Alberto Gabizon just started his sabbatical with Dimitri Papahadjopoulos at USCF. Each of us started to work on different aspects related to how to achieve an improved liposomal doxorubicin formulation. Alberto focused his studies on how to prolong blood circulation of liposomes while I focused on how to achieve stable high drug loading into liposomes and nano-liposomes. During his sabbatical, Alberto worked, with LTI support and blessing, on liposome formulations with extended circulation time. Terry Allen at the University of Alberta was the first one to describe such formulations (Allen and Chonn, 1987; Allen, 1989, US patent 4,837,028). In 1986, we, at LTI, decided to support her research on this issue. LTI scientists looked also for long-circulating liposomal formulations of various lipid compositions that differed from those studied by Allen and Gabizon. The latter two scientists added known (but not frequently used) lipids to the liposome lipid composition in order to reach extended circulation time and selective tumor localization with the focus on gangliosides (Allen) or hydrogenated phosphatidylinositol, abbreviated as HPI (Gabizon). LTI scientists tried and studied novel lipids that were not recognized as known natural lipid species (Woodle et al., 1991; Woodle et al., 1990, rev. in Woodle and Lasic, 1992; Woodle, 1993). All these three groups (associated with LTI) worked in parallel on different formulations and all were using small unilamellar liposomes with narrow unimodal size distribution having a mean size of ~100 nm. These nano-liposomes were prepared by medium pressure extrusion using polycarbonate filters with defined pore size (Hunt and Papahadjopoulos, 1985, US patent 4,529,561 licensed by UCSF to LTI). All these three laboratories used different lipid compositions in order to achieve the same goal of extended circulation time, RES avoidance, and intra-tumor accumulation. Terry Allen achieved it by inclusion of sphingomyelin and GM1 ganglioside as liposome-membrane components. Alberto Gabizon was using hydrogenated phosphatidylinositol (HPI) that he included in small liposomes composed of "solid" high-T_m) lipids and cholesterol (Gabizon and Papahadjopoulos, 1988), while LTI scientists started working with DSPE-PEG [(Annie Yau-Yang's idea combined with Carl Redmann's chemical synthesis (Woodle et al., 1991, US patent 5,013,556; Woodle et al., 1990, rev. in Woodle and Lasic, 1992, and in Woodle 1993)]. LTI was not the only group to work with PEG-DSPE: At the same time Volodia Torchilin and Leaf Huang and their teams joined forces and worked on it too (Klivanov et al., 1990), as well as Gregor Cevc's lab in Munich (Blume and Cevc, 1990). A comprehensive review on pegylated liposomes is described in many of the papers of *Stealth Liposomes* (1995), a book edited by Dan Lasic and Frank Martin.

12.4.4 The Lesson Learned from Pegylated Proteins

The inspiration and motivation to start working with pegylated lipids like PEG-DSPE came to Annie Yau-Yang and others at LTI from pioneering research in the 1970s by Frank Davis, Abraham Abuchowski, and colleagues who foresaw the potential of the conjugation of polyethylene glycol (PEG) to proteins (Abuchowski et al., 1977; Abuchowski founded Enzon, Inc., which brought three pegylated drugs to the market. Various length (>350–50,000 Da) chains of PEG polymer are available. Low-molecular-weight drugs were also pegylated. However, the main pegylated products so far are a few proteins and one liposomal formulation — Doxil® (the topic of this review article). For peptides and proteins (including antibody fragments), mainly relatively large PEG polymers of >5000 Da were used. It was found that pegylation helps improve safety and efficacy as well as reduce the immunogenicity of many therapeutics (Veronese and Harries, 2002; Veronese and Pasut, 2005). The suggested mechanism by which pegylation works is that it is a result of the alterations it produces in the physicochemical properties of the molecule to which the PEG residue is covalently attached. These may include changes in level of hydration, conformation, electrostatic binding, and hydrophobicity/hydrophilicity balance. Covalently attached highly flexible and highly hydratedhydrated PEG [three to four molecules of water per 1 ethylene oxide oxygen (Tirosh et al., 1997, 1998)] induce changes in structure and lead to increase in size and bulkiness. All together this results in "steric stabilization," which reduces nonspecific protein–protein interaction and nonspecific protein–cell interactions. These physical and chemical changes increase systemic retention of the therapeutic agent. Also, it can influence the binding affinity of the therapeutic moiety to the cell receptors and can alter the absorption and distribution patterns. PEG polymer has only two reactive OH groups (one at each end of the PEG molecule); in order to prevent the PEG from inducing intra- and inter-cross linkages, one of these hydroxyl groups was methylated.

Pegylation, by increasing the molecular weight of a molecule and its level of hydration, can impart several significant pharmacological advantages over the native unmodified molecule, such as

- Improved agent solubility
- Extended circulating life
- Therefore, reducing dosage frequency, without diminished efficacy with potentially reduced toxicity
- Increased drug stability
- Enhanced protection from proteolytic degradation
- Reduced immunogenicity

In addition, pegylated drugs may have the following commercial advantages:

- Opportunities for new delivery formats and dosing regimens
- Extended patent life of previously approved drugs

This resulted in the development of many pegylated proteins and peptide drugs, (only a few of which made it to the market), so now the clinical value of pegylation is well established. ADAGEN (PEG-bovine adenosine deaminase), manufactured by Enzon Pharmaceuticals, Inc., was the first pegylated protein (approved by the FDA in March 1990) to enter the market. It is used to treat X-chromosome-linked severe combined immunogenicity syndrome, as an alternative to bone marrow transplantation and enzyme replacement by gene therapy. Now a large number of pegylated protein and peptide pharmaceuticals are in clinical use. The most successful examples are

- **PEGASYS:** Pegylated interferon alpha for use in the treatment of chronic hepatitis C and hepatitis B (Hoffmann-La Roche)
- **Pegintron:** Pegylated interferon alpha for use in the treatment of chronic hepatitis C and hepatitis B (Schering-Plough/Enzon)
- **Oncaspar:** Pegylated L-asparaginase for the treatment of acute lymphoblastic leukemia in patients who are hypersensitive to the native unmodified form of L-asparaginase (Enzon). This drug was recently approved as a first-line treatment
- **Neulasta:** Pegylated recombinant methionyl human granulocyte colony-stimulating factor for severe cancer-chemotherapy-induced neutropenia (Amgen)

Many other pegylated peptides and proteins are now in clinical trials or under development.

The success of pegylated proteins was the driving force for the successful development of Doxil® as the first FDA-approved liposomal drug and nano-drug (November 17, 1995). In lipids, PEG chains of >350 to 15,000 were tried (equivalent to 8 to 334 ethylene oxide units) and various considerations, such as the metabolism of the pegylated lipids and the rate of secretion via the kidneys were used in the decision which PEG length to select for lipid pegylation.

12.4.5 Selection of Pegylated Nanoliposomes as the Basis of Doxil

Each of the laboratories working on long circulating liposomes described above has its publications and patents on its unique liposome formulations. In the early 1990s, it became evident that for various scientific and practical reasons (availability, cost, species specificity, etc.) described elsewhere (Woodle, 1993; Allen, 1995), the GM1-ganglioside-based formulation was excluded. At LTI, HPI and PEG-DSPE remained in the race. In order for LTI to decide which of the two lipids will be the one to use in evaluating the novel formulation in human, we performed in 1991 a critical comparative PK experiment in Beagle dogs (Gabizon et al., 1993). Dog is a preferred animal due to its much larger plasma volume (~500 mL), which resembles much better that of human beings in studying the effect of dilution-induced drug release (Gabizon et al., 1991; Amselem et al., 1993a) than small rodents with their very small plasma volume (and therefore almost no dilution).

The Beagle dog doxorubicin PK study clearly demonstrated that although both liposomal formulations were much superior to F-DOX. The PEG-DSPE formulation was better, as it showed much slower plasma clearance than the HPI formulation.

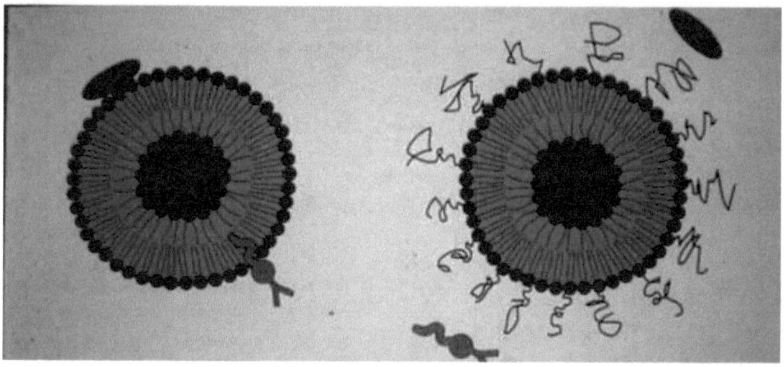

Figure 12.5 A cartoon showing a comparison between conventional and sterically stabilized (pegylated) liposomes (SSL, Stealth liposomes). (Courtesy of the late D. Lasic.) The cartoon shows lack of insertion of opsonins into the membrane of Stealth liposomes. See also Color Insert.

Using mice peritoneal macrophages (obtained from the ascitic fluid of mice treated with thioglycolate), *in vitro*, Doxil showed 40% of the uptake of liposomes of similar size and lipid composition but lacking 5 mole% PEG-DSPE (Emanuel et al., 1996a). This reduction in macrophage uptake is in direct correlation with the increase in plasma circulation time. The increase in mole% of PEG-DSPE can further reduce macrophage uptake and probably increase circulation time (Emanuel et al., 1996a, 1996b). For more details on the effect of PEG-DSPE on nano-liposomes, see Garbuzenko et al. (2005).

12.4.6 Remote Loading of Doxorubicin into Nano Sterically Stabilized Liposomes (nSSL) to Form Doxil

12.4.6.1 The need for remote loading

For liposome formulation designed for metastatic tumor treatment, intravenous (i.v.) administration is the only option, and therefore high loading level and its high stability during storage and blood circulation are required. However, due to the combination of needs for nano-liposomes and high dose of doxorubicin (~50 mg/m^2) to achieve the sufficiently high loading (to be in the range of intra-liposome drug concentration, which is in the range of hundreds of mM) is not an easy task. When the loading is poor, so will be the drug/lipid ratio. This means that either therapeutic levels of drug cannot be reached or therapeutic use of such liposomes will require administering very large amounts of lipids. In addition, when the loading is inefficient there is a great loss of the active agent during the loading and a need to remove unloaded drug. Therefore, the use of liposomes as a vehicle becomes inefficient as well as uneconomical. The major requirements of drug loading into nano-liposomes are (1) to achieve a high level of loading of active agent in the liposome and to make this loading stable during handling and storage, irrespective of the nature of the agent and (2) to fit the release rate of the loaded active agent to specific therapeutic aims of the liposome formulation.

A careful analysis of the currently available loading approaches reveals clearly that the remote loading approach is the best, and in many cases the only, way to achieve the desired intraliposome drug concentration (usually defined as drug to lipid mole ratio) (Barenholz, 2003).

12.4.6.2 Drug classification

In 1985, we looked for a simple way to classify drugs by their physico-chemical features in a way that will enable the formulator to predict which loading approach to use or, specifically, if a drug is suited for a remote loading approach. At that time, with very little available information, we came up with an oversimplified approach and classified all agents into three categories based on their oil/buffer and octanol/buffer partition coefficients (K_p). Category I, molecules having high oil/buffer K_p, are considered lipophilic; these molecules do not fit liposomes as their carrier. Category II, molecules having low oil/buffer partition coefficient and medium to high octanol/buffer K_p, are amphipathic. Category III, molecules of very low values in both partition coefficients, by definition, are defined as being water soluble. For some of the molecules, those which are amphipathic weak acids or bases, the classification between group II and III is pH dependent, which determines the level of ionization of the molecule. (Barenholz and Cohen, 1995; Barenholz, 2001, 2003)).

Although the use of octanol/water partition coefficient to determine suitability of molecules to reside in a lipid bilayer is controversial, it is well established that it is indicative of agent transmembrane diffusion rate (Stein, 1986), and therefore it is relevant to loading efficiency, loading stability, and the drug release profile.

12.4.6.3 Remote loading optimization

Recently, we developed a much more detailed and precise computation means to predict remote loading performance, which is based on more variables than only the partition coefficient (logP and/or logD), including the details on apolar and polar surface areas of the desired molecule (and the ratio between the two surface areas), its pK_a, and logD at different pHs. This enables us to better predict, analyze, and optimize the loading process. In order to have an efficient remote loading, pK_a and logD have to be in a certain range, which means that at least a certain fraction of the loaded molecule has to be uncharged, and in this range of logD, we found the apolar and polar surface areas to be highly informative indicators (Zucker et al., 2009).

That paper describes how applying data-mining algorithms to a data bank based on our laboratory's 15 years of liposome research experience on remote loading of nine different drugs enabled us to build a model that relates drug physicochemical properties and loading conditions to loading efficiency. This model enables choosing candidate molecules for remote loading and optimizing loading conditions according to logical considerations. The model should also help in designing prodrugs suitable for remote loading. This approach is now further improved by including data from over 50 different molecules that were remote loaded in many different laboratories in the world by ion or pH transmembrane gradients (Cern, Goldblum, and Barenholz, in preparation) and are expected to improve and accelerate the development of liposomal formulations for clinical applications.

Only remote (active) drug loading enables transforming pegylated nano-liposomes (nSSL) into an approved efficacious drug. This drug loading approach is based on the strategy of fabricating nano-liposomes that exhibit a transmembrane intraliposome high/extra liposome medium low) ion gradient, which acts as the driving force for the remote loading of amphipathic weak acid or base drugs into these liposomes. Historically, in my laboratory the remote loading approach began from the need to achieve a highly efficient and stable liposomal drug encapsulation that would be stable during storage and after administration during the long circulation time in the blood (up to 100-h half-life; Gabizon et al., 2003). This approach was recently discussed by us in detail for nine different drugs (Zucker et al., 2009). It was applied for remote loading of the amphipathic weak base anticancer drug doxorubicin and was the basis for the first FDA-approved pegylated nano-liposomal anticancer drug Doxil®. Since the approval of Doxil (1995), it was successfully employed for other drugs and agents in our and other laboratories ((Barenholz and Haran, 1993, 1994; Haran et al., 1993, Lasic et al., 1992, 1995; Clerc and Barenholz, 1995, 1998; Bolotin et al., 1994; Barenholz, 2001, 2007, 2010; Grant et al., 2004, Wasserman et al., 2007; Avnir et al., 2008; Zucker et al., 2009).

Overall, from our own experience with nine different drugs (reviewed in Zucker et al., 2009), we concluded that a transmembrane ammonium sulfate gradient is most suitable for stable encapsulation of amphipathic weak bases, while a transmembrane calcium acetate gradient is most suitable for loading amphipathic weak acids.

The basis of these nanochemical loading engines is that liposomes are fabricated to exhibit the desired pH and/or ion gradient by using salts composed of either weak bases (e.g., ammonium) or weak acids (e.g., acetate). The degree of ionization of these compounds is pH dependent. Their ionized species (i.e., ammonium and acetate) have a very low permeability coefficient and octanol-to-buffer partition coefficient and therefore they do not, or only very slowly, permeate the liposome lipid bilayer, while their un-ionized species have high permeability as well as octanol-to-buffer partition coefficient (exemplified by ammonia gas and acetic acid) and therefore can diffuse relatively fast across the lipid bilayer and reach the intraliposome aqueous phase (rev. in Barenholz, 2001, 2007, and Zucker et al., 2009). The magnitude of the intraliposome high/external medium low transmembrane gradient of such ions is the driving force for remote loading, as they can be exchanged with amphipathic drugs (weak acids with acetate and weak bases with ammonium). The counterion of the gradient-forming ion (e.g., sulfate or calcium in the case of ammonium or acetate gradient, respectively) can be selected so that it will control the state of aggregation and precipitation/crystallization of the drug–counterion salt in the intraliposome aqueous phase, thereby contributing to control the efficiency and stability of remote loading, as well as drug release rate at various temperatures (Clerc and Barenholz, 1998; Barenholz et al., 2001; Wasserman et al., 2007).

It is important to note that the successful application of this nano-chemical engine benefits from the very small trapped aqueous volume of nanoliposomes (i.e., 2.21×10^5 nm^3 for a 37.5 nm radius liposome), which supports faster and higher accumulation, as well as intraliposome precipitation of drug–counterion salt in crystalline or noncrystalline forms.

12.4.6.4 Ammonium sulfate transmembrane gradient driven doxorubicin loading into nSSL

For the remote loading of doxorubicin into nSSL we applied the transmembrane ammonium sulfate gradient under conditions that $[(NH_4)_2SO_4]_{lip}$ >> $[(NH_4)_2SO_4)]_{med}$ (lip is the nSSL and med is the extraliposome medium). Figure 12.6 describes the overall mechanism of this loading process. The drug loading is actually a base exchange of the amphipathic weak base drug with the ammonium ions. For doxorubicin >90% drug encapsulation was obtained. Doxorubicin is accumulated in the intraliposome aqueous phase, where it reaches a concentration > 100-fold the drug level in the loading medium (this explains why we refer to it as active loading, as it goes against the drug concentration gradient). Based on various spectral analyses including X-ray diffraction (Barenholz and Haran, 1993; Haran et al., 1993; Lasic et al., 1992, 1995) almost all the encapsulated doxorubicin is in the intra-liposome aqueous phase and most of it is in the form of aggregated (crystalline) $[doxorubicin]_2SO_4$ salt. The loading is dependent on the ammonium ion gradient, while the loading stability is dependent on the liposome lipid composition and on the level of $[doxorubicin]_2SO_4$ precipitation, as well as temperature. The transmembrane ammonium–sulfate-gradient-driven drug loading differs from most other remote loading approaches since it neither requires fabrication of liposomes in acidic pH, nor alkalinization of the extra-liposome aqueous phase.

Doxil is a good example of remote loading by an ammonium sulfate gradient under conditions that $[(NH_4)_2SO_4]_{lip}$ >> $[(NH_4)_2SO_4)]_{med.}$ Figure 12.6 describes the overall mechanism of this loading process.

(For more details see Barenholz and Haran, 1993, 1994; Haran et al., 1993, Bolotin et al., 1994; Lasic et al., 1992; Lasic et al., 1995; Clerc and Barenholz, 1998; Barenholz, 2001; Barenholz, 2007; Zucker et al., 2009).

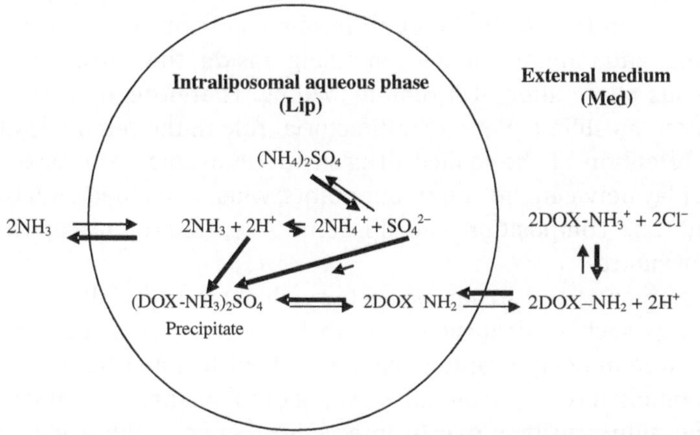

Figure 12.6 doxorubicin remote loading into nSSL exhibiting a transmembrane ammonium ion gradient. The thick arrows represent the processes occurring during drug loading, and the thin arrows represent the processes occurring during drug release.

The efficiency of loading by this method and its stability are dependent on

(1) The large (~10^{12}) difference in permeability coefficient of the neutral ammonia (10^{-1} cm/sec) and the SO_4^{2-} anion (>10^{-12} cm/sec)
(2) The initial pH gradient having the $[H^+]_{lip} >> [H^+]_{med}$
(3) The low solubility of (doxorubicin)$_2$-SO_4 (<2 mM), which also minimizes intraliposomal osmotic pressure and therefore helps keep liposome integrity
(4) The asymmetry in doxorubicin partition coefficient (K_p)
(K_p lip/external med > K_p lip/intra lip med)
(K_p oct/external med > K_p oct/intra lip med)
(Barenhoz and Cohen, 1995; Barenholz, 1998).

K_p is a partition coefficient between the two phases defined in the brackets. Lip = liposome membrane, med = aqueous medium either external or intraliposomal, oct = bulk octanol phase.

This asymmetry means that the K_p of DOX in the extraliposomal medium supports influx in a direction opposite to the ammonium sulfate gradient (namely, into the liposomes), while the K_p of DOX in the intraliposomal aqueous phase acts to reduce partition into the membrane, thereby reducing the desorption rate (k_{off}). The reduction in DOX K_p in the intraliposomal aqueous phase is driven by the ammonium sulfate remaining inside the intraliposomal aqueous phase after DOX remote loading. Therefore, it seems that ammonium sulfate plays a multifactorial role in the remote loading and retention of the loaded drug in the liposomes. For Doxil the interplay between the above four points, when combined with Doxil membrane composition and liposome size, determines liposome performance.

Another issue, so far neglected, which is especially relevant to drugs such as doxorubicin, is their tendency to self-aggregate (reviewed in [21]), forming oligomers of various mer number. This phenomenon results from the stacking of the planar aromatic rings of the anthracyclines due to interaction between the π electrons of the rings. This self-aggregation is facilitated by increasing ionic strength. DOX dimers appear already at 1 μM and larger aggregates at higher DOX concentrations. The effect of such oligomerization on therapeutic efficacy is not yet clear. However, based on simple geometric considerations, it is obvious that nonmonomeric DOX cannot interact with DNA in the same way as monomeric DOX, and the exact location between the two DNA strands should differ [21]. Therefore, the way by which the drug is internalized (monomers versus aggregated form) by the tumor cell may be an important factor in drug efficacy.

The breakthrough in using remote (active) loading driven by the transmembrane ammonium sulfate gradient for the doxorubicin is one of the main reasons that enabled successful clinical use of Doxil and its approval by the regulatory agencies worldwide.

12.4.6 The Role of Drug Release Rate (k_{off})

The results of liposome loading when combined with liposome structure, lipid composition, and site of injection will determine rate of drug release in plasma (Barenholz and Cohen, 1995). For example, for i.v.-administrated liposomal drug formulations, only when the drug release (determined by k_{off}) is slower than the liposome clearance (k_c) will the liposome determine drug pharmacokinetics and biodistribution. When $k_{off} > k_c$, then the ratio k_{off}/k_c is a measure of the rate of drug release *in vivo*. Controlling this ratio is obligatory to achieve controlled drug release in blood or in the tissues reached by the liposomes. Therefore, this ratio also affects therapeutic efficacy of the liposomal drug. For drugs of fast clearance, when $k_{off} >> k_c$ the benefits of use of liposomes for drug delivery will be minimal or none, as the performance of the liposomal drug will be similar to that of the free drug. This is exemplified by our first-generation failed OLV-DOX formulation (see above). An efficient and functional way to test the release rate is a cytotoxicity test measuring doxorubicin IC_{50} in cell culture. As described by Horowitz et al. (1992) Doxil has about a 2-order of magnitude higher IC_{50} (lower cytotoxic activity) than free doxorubicin, while as described in Section 12.2.3, our failed OLV-DOX had similar IC_{50} to free doxorubicin. These differences demonstrate nicely that the large dilution-induced release that basically "killed" the performance of OLV-DOX in humans does not occur in Doxil. To make sure that our interpretation is correct, we studied the effect of nigericin on doxorubicin release and IC_{50}. Nigericin is an ionophore that breaks the pH and ammonium gradient by exchanging the intraliposome proton with potassium ion. The exposure of Doxil to nigericin caused complete drug release, which was paralleled by reducing the IC_{50} to the low level of free doxorubicin, proving that Doxil's excellent drug retention is the reason for its poor IC_{50} (Horowitz et al., 1992).

However, the opposite (very low k_{off}) is as bad. Namely, when k_{off} is too slow and there is no liposome uptake by the target cells, there will be no therapeutic efficacy even if the loaded liposomes will reach the target very efficiently, as the free drug concentration at the target tissue will be too low, as exemplified by sterically stabilized cisplatin liposomes (Lasic et al., 1999; Barenholz, 2001; Peleg-Shulman et al., 2001).

12.4.7 Doxil: Each Part Matters

In Doxil, each part matters and contributes to the optimized performance (Figure 12.7). Doxil is an excellent example to demonstrate the obligatory role of lipid biophysics in the success of liposome-based drugs.

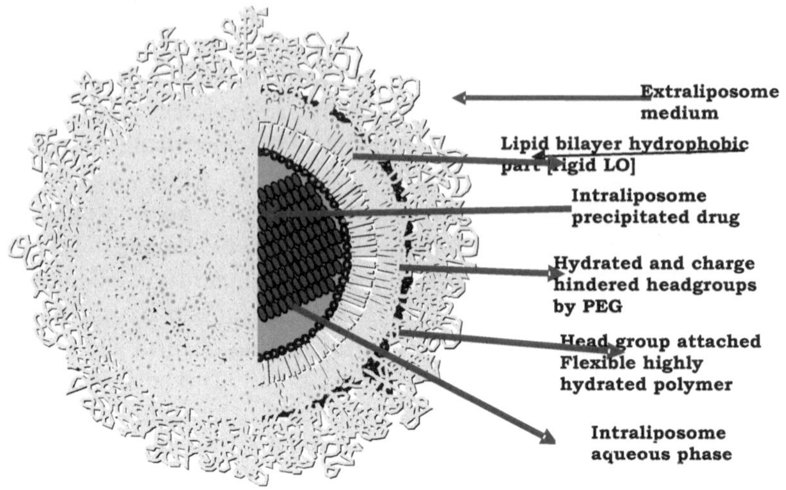

Figure 12.7 A cartoon of Doxil® = pegylated nano (<100 nm) unilamellar liposome. It is based on cryo-TEM, SAXS, WAXS, DLS, compressibility, and doxorubicin absorbance and fluorescence (Lasic et al., 1992, 1995; Haran et al., 1993; Tirosh et al., 1998). See also Color Insert.

A calculation based on the lipid molar concentration of the components and on liposome size reveals that 1 mL of the Doxil dispersion contains 2.3×10^{14} liposomes and each liposome contains ~10,000 molecules of doxorubicin, above 95% of which is in the crystalline phase.

12.4.8 Doxil-Related I.P.

It is important to note that Doxil® is based on two families of patents. One family covers the effect of adding the lipopolymer PEG-DSPE as a liposome lipid component on liposome circulation time (Woodle et al., 1991; US patent 5,013,556).

The second patent family is on the transmembrane-driven remote loading of amphipathic weak bases such as doxorubicin (Barenholz and Haran, 1993, 1994, US patents 5,192,549 and 5,316,771). Namely, there is no direct patent on Doxil!

It took seven and a half years from the submission of these two families of patent applications in 1988/1989 till Doxil approval in November 1995. As remote loading patents were extended till March 9, 2010, Doxil enjoyed 14 years of patent protection.

12.5 Doxil Performance in Humans

12.5.1 Pharmacokinetics and Passive Targeting to Tumors

The data presented in Figure 12.8 are the first proof of passive targeting due the EPR effect in humans (Gabizon et al., 1994a).

Doxorubicin when administered as Doxil show and high and selective tumor localization as was first demonstrated in the our "first in man Doxil" study, conducted by us in Jerusalem in 1991–1994 and published in *Cancer Research* in 1994 (Gabizon et al., 1994a).

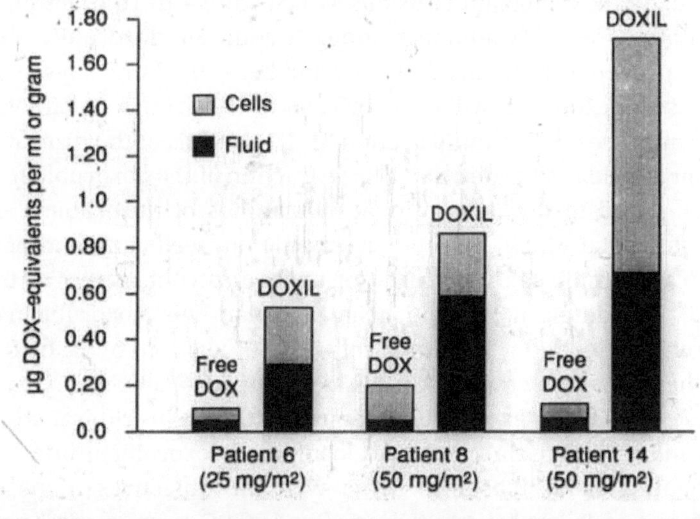

Figure 12.8 Doxorubicin levels in patients' tumor biopsies, comparing free doxorubicin and Doxil (from Gabizon et al., 1994a, 1995).

This pilot study, which includes 53 courses of Doxil (average three per patient spaced 3 to 4 weeks apart) was aimed to characterize and compare in cancer patients the pharmacokinetics and accumulation of doxorubicin in malignant effusions after administration of Doxil or of free drug (DOX). It clearly demonstrated much higher levels of doxorubicin both in cells and interstitial fluids of the tumor after Doxil administration than after DOX administration. Using the cationic ion exchanger Dowex-50 (Druckmann et al., 1989; Amselem et al., 1990), we found that more than 98% of the plasma doxorubicin after Doxil i.v. administration is liposome associated. Pharmacokinetics was determined for 25 and 50 mg/m^2. The plasma elimination time of Doxil followed a biexponential curve with half-lives of 2 and 45 h (median values), most of the dose being cleared from plasma under the longer half-life. A large difference in volume of distribution was also found (4 L for Doxil versus 254 L for free DOX. Similarly, doxorubicin derived from Doxil showed a much slower rate of clearance (compare 0.1 L/h for Doxil with 45 L/h for free DOX).

The types of Doxil-derived doxorubicin metabolites in patients' urine were identical to those of patients injected with free DOX; however, the overall urinary excretion in the Doxil group was significantly reduced. Most encouraging are the results on the levels of drug in the malignant effusions, which were 4 to 16 times higher than after free DOX administration. In addition, doxorubicin level there peaked after Doxil administration between 3 to 7 days, which means the exposure of the tumor cells to the drug is much longer than after free DOX administration. HPLC analysis of the drug at the tumor site demonstrated that a large fraction of the doxorubicin was metabolized to the conventional metabolites of doxorubicin. The fact that doxorubicin is metabolized only intracellularly and not in the plasma indicates internalization of the doxorubicin derived from Doxil. Two different mechanisms may explain this: doxorubicin can be released outside the tumor cell and be taken up by it, or Doxil can be taken up by the tumor cell, and then doxorubicin is released. These data are in excellent agreement with our preclinical studies and indicate that stable remote loading of doxorubicin into long-circulating nano-liposomes serve well the objectives of passive targeting of doxorubicin to tumors. Our 1994 *Cancer Research* paper is the first demonstration of the of EPR relevance in cancer patients to antitumor therapy by nano-drugs.

The localization of Doxil in humans' tumors was further supported by direct fluorescence microscopy of patient biopsies (Symon et al., 1999).

For extended information on the superiority of the pharmacokinetic (PK) performance of Doxil, see Gabizon et al. (2003). That review summarizes the PK profile in humans at doses between 10 and 80 mg/m^2. The PK has one or two distribution phases: an initial phase, with a half-life of 1–3 h, and a second phase responsible for most of the clearance, with a half-life of 30–90 h. The AUC after a dose of 50 mg/m^2 is approximately 300-fold greater than that with free drug. Clearance and volume of distribution are drastically reduced (at least 250-fold and 60-fold, respectively). These studies indicate the importance of utilizing the distinct pharmacokinetic parameters of pegylated liposomal doxorubicin in dose scheduling.

12.5.2 Doxil Tolerability

It was already demonstrated in our *Cancer Research* publication (Gabizon et al., 1994a) that, overall, Doxil is well tolerated and shows a distinct superiority over free DOX in most evaluated side effects. However, two side effects not typical of what is observed for conventional doxorubicin treatment were observed. The first of these shows up as flushing and shortness of breath; it is also referred to as acute infusion reaction or pseudo-allergy (Gabizon et al., 2008; Szebeni and Barenholz, 2012, this book) and is reduced by reducing rate of infusion. This side effect was recently reviewed by Szebeni and Barenholz (2012) (this book). The second effect that results is grade 2 or 3 of desquamating dermatitis and is referred to as Palmar Plantar Erythrodysthesia (PPE) or "foot and hand syndrome." The second effect increased with dose and was more pronounced for 3-week intervals than 4-week intervals between treatments (for more details, see Solomon and Gabizon, 2008). For more details on Doxil tolerability and side effects, see Doxil homepage (www.doxil.com) and drugs online (www.drugs.com/pro/doxil.html).

12.5.3 Doxil Therapeutic Indications

In this review, I will not discuss in detail Doxil clinical performance, which is covered in many scientific papers, reviews, and reports. As of today (April 4, 2011), Doxil has more than 171,000 Google citations, and most of them are related to clinical aspects.

A good starting point is a recent review by Solomon and Gabizon (2008) entitled "Clinical Pharmacology of Liposomal Anthracyclines: Focus on Pegylated Liposomal Doxorubicin". Current relevant websites are Wikipedia, Doxil homepage (www.doxil.com) and drugs online (www.drugs.com/pro/doxil.html). A summary of indications approved by the U.S. FDA and/or European Medicines Evaluation Agency (EMA) and approval year for Doxil is described as follows:

- AIDS-related Kaposi's sarcoma: Superior efficacy over former conventional therapy (1995).
- Recurrent ovarian cancer: Superior efficacy and improved safety profile over comparator drug (topotecan) (1998), as demonstrated first by Gordon et al. (2001) (Figure 12.9).
- Metastatic Breast Cancer: Equivalent efficacy and reduced cardiotoxicity compared with free doxorubicin (2003).
- Multiple myeloma: Equivalent efficacy and improved safety profile compared to free doxorubicin combo. Superior efficacy in combination with bortezomib over single agent bortezomib (2007).

In addition, regarding cardiac function, Doxil demonstrates major reduction of cardiotoxicity as compared to free doxorubicin in all settings (2000).

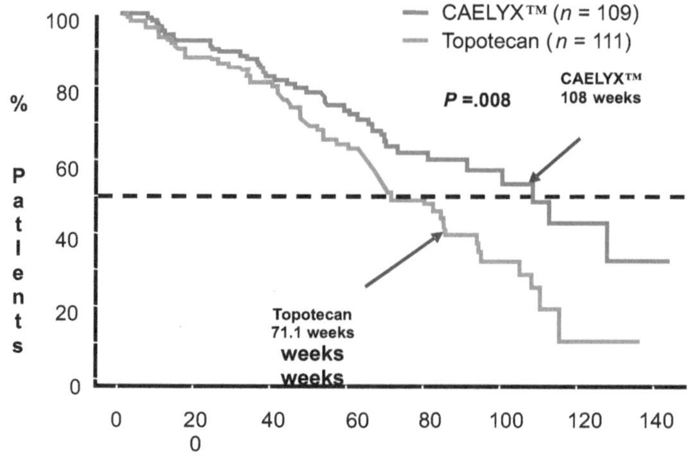

Figure 12.9 Caelyx^{TM} (= Doxil) is superior to topotecan in ovarian cancer (from Gordon et al., 2001). See also Color Insert.

12.6 Conclusions, Take-Home Lessons, and Future Directions

To sum-up, the anticancer nano-drug Doxil shows good clinical performance in a variety of neoplastic conditions due to its improved antitumor therapeutic efficacy and unique reduced safety profile, especially its impressive reduction in cardiac toxicity when compared with conventional doxorubicin. Of the >10 liposomal drugs approved (Zhang et al., 2001), Doxil has the most extensive clinical use.

Based on Doxil success, various novel drug formulations including modified Doxil, and other drugs or drug combinations with a similar approach to that of Doxil are now at different stages of development. These novel nano-drug formulations should have reduced (or no) side effect of acute infusion reactions or foot-hand syndrome. One approach to achieve the latter objective is to slightly reduce the half-life of the liposomal doxorubicin by replacing the sulfate counterion of the ammonium used for the remote loading with glucuronate. The use of glucuronate, which has a permeability coefficient similar to sulfate but does not induce intra-liposome drug precipitation, results in somewhat shorter circulation time of the doxorubicin, but without loss of therapeutic efficacy in tumor-bearing mice (Wasserman et al., 2007; Barenholz, 2007; Gabizon and Barenholz, 2005). This relatively small but distinct effect on the PK is expected to lower accumulation of doxorubicin in the skin, lowering hand and foot syndrome. Other ways to extend and improve nano-liposome-based anticancer therapy are to have better control of drug release (rev. in Barenholz, 2007) using external means, such as hyperthermia (Needham et al., 2000, 2001) or focused ultrasound (Schroeder et al., 2007, 2009a, 2009b); or to use a combination by remote loading of two drugs that act synergistically in one liposome (Zucker et al., 2010), or a combination of two different treatment modalities such as Doxil and interleukin 2 (IL-2) in liposome-based immunotherapy (Cabanes et al., 1999). The latter stems from the fact that doxorubicin when administered as Doxil is not toxic to the immune system and therefore IL-2 when delivered in liposomes is highly efficacious. The idea behind this chemo-immuno treatment combination is that the Doxil will take care of most of the tumor burden, while the immunotherapy elicited by the IL-2 will activate the intact immune system enabling it to kill the residual tumor cells (Cabanes et al., 1999). The use of liposomal IL-2 results in lower toxicity of the IL-2 and prolongation of IL-2 circulation time without loss of its potency (Kedar et al., 1994a, 1994b). A very promising approach is the one used recently by Jain and coworkers (Diop-Frimpong et al., 2011). Accordingly, losartan, which inhibits collagen I synthesis, was used to modify the interstitial tumor environment, leading to increase in Doxil (and other nano-particulates) accumulation in tumors, thereby increasing Doxil therapeutic efficacy.

The story of Doxil's development carries two important messages. The first one is that Doxil's successful development opens the way to major improvement in tumor therapy and especially it served as a gold standard in the new field referred to as nano-medicine. The second one is that development of such a complex drug system requires having a highly multidisciplinary team that can deal in an integrative way with the many kinds of expertise needed (Gabizon et al., 1995, 1999; Barenholz, 2003, 2007). Not less important is the recognition that the understanding and optimal utilization of physicochemical principles are crucial to the successful development of such a complex drug product.

12.7 Doxil: Historical Perspectives

Pre-Doxil era	(Liver passively targeted by liposomal doxorubicin)
1979	Gabizon and Barenholz start basic research on liposomal doxorubicin
1984	First clinical trials with liposomal doxorubicin (OLV-DOX and not Doxil)
1985	LTI licensed the OLV-DOX technology
1987	Clinical trial of OLV-DOX failed
1988	Barenholz developed and Yissum, R & D Company of the Hebrew University of Jerusalem, Israel, patented new concept of doxorubicin remote loading, the basis of Doxil (Barenholz and Haran, 1993, 1994); patents were licensed to LTI
1989	LTI patented the Stealth concept and registered Stealth®
1989	Gabizon and LTI start to develop sterically stabilized (Stealth) liposomes
1989	LTI, Gabizon, and Barenholz start Doxil® development
1991–1992	Doxil "First in man" clinical trial in Jerusalem
1994	Gabizon and Barenholz major publication on Doxil clinical trial (*Cancer Research*)
1995	(November 17) FDA-approved Doxil
1996	First Doxil sales in USA and Europe
2009 (March)	US patent expired

12.8 Personal Touch

The road to the development of Doxil® involved many people; most of them became my personal friends with whom I interacted for many years. This story started in 1984 when I met Dimitri Papahadjopoulos from the University of California, San Francisco (UCSF), a long-time friend and colleague "liposomologist." We had met at various conferences since 1974, when I was on an extended sabbatical (1973–1976) at the Department of Biochemistry of the University of Virginia (UVA) Medical School, at Charlottesville, VA. The reason for me to come to UVA for sabbatical was that this department, headed by Thomas Thompson, was one of the world centers (and considered a Mecca) of membrane and liposome biophysical research. Thomas Thompson and other scientists of UVA, especially Chien Chien Huang and Burt Litman, were leading membrane and liposome physical chemists. An important part of my Ph.D. research was carried out in 1969 at the Animal Research Council (ARC) Institute at Babraham near Cambridge, UK, under the supervision of Rex Dawson and Peter Quinn, from whom I learned about lipid monolayers at the air/water interface, and Alec Bangham, who introduced me to liposomes. I believed that lipid and membrane physical chemistry are crucial to membrane research, and that is why I decided to spend my first sabbatical at UVA. The UVA group was in tight competition with the UCSF group although the interests of the two groups were only partially overlapping, as the UVA focused on lipid biophysics and physical chemistry and the UCSF group focused more on biologically relevant topics such as fusion, interaction of liposomes with cells, etc. Every time Dimitri and I met, we talked extensively about science (mainly membrane and liposome research), as well as on culture, art, history, food, and wine. Dimitri kept telling me about Liposome Technology Inc. (LTI) a start-up located at Menlo Park, CA, which focuses its R&D in the field of liposome-based diagnostic and medical applications. Dimitri and his former student Frank Szoka were the scientific founders and mentors of this company. Nick Arvanitidis was convinced by Dimitri to be LTI CEO, and Frank Martin, another student of Dimitri's, was the first LTI employee. Nick brought with him Sally Davenport , Carl Grove, and Kathy, who had worked in Nick's previous R&D company, to deal with LTI administration. Dimitri asked me if I would be interested to spend a sabbatical at LTI. He told me that it is a great challenge but also a large reward regarding satisfaction. He already knew about our efforts in the field of drug delivery and that we were close to the "first in man" experiment, but he was more interested in my knowledge and experience in lipid and liposome biophysics and physical chemistry, as he well understood that this is the heart of the matter of developing liposomal products. I hesitated as, so far, most of my research was academic in nature. Dimitri proposed that I come to his laboratory at UCSF, give a seminar there, and he will organize my visit at LTI so I will be able to judge for myself if spending a sabbatical at LTI is of any interest to me. I also got a formal invitation from Nick, LTI CEO, to visit LTI and spend a day there. As things looked serious, I consulted with Hanna, my wife, who supported me and encouraged me to evaluate this interesting proposition. I knew this was not easy for her, as it meant that I may be away from home (in California) for long periods of time and she would have to take care, alone, of our four daughters, the dog, and our home, which is not easy. With her encouragement, I accepted Dimitri's and Nick's offers to visit. My visit at Dimitri's and at LTI was organized for December 1984. My seminar at Dimitri's lab was on glycosphingolipid biophysics, which was followed by discussion with Dimitri's lab people. The next day, Dimitri drove me to LTI in Menlo Park, which at that time was a startup company of about 40 people, where I spent the whole day talking with many company employees. After dinner with Nick and some good wine, Nick and I had a long conversion in which Nick was trying to convince me to spend my sabbatical at LTI. Nick is Greek, and as such he understood well the Mediterranean mentality and way of thinking, so we understood each other very well. Without going into detail and possibly with the aid of the good wine served continuously by Nick, late at night I agreed to seriously consider his proposal. Nick drove me to my San Francisco Hotel very late that night. The excitement, together with the 10-hour-long jetlag, made it very difficult for me to sleep.

Returning to Israel, I discussed Nick's proposal with Hanna, and with her support and encouragement I accepted it. I told Dimitri and Nick that I would not be able to come unless LTI would support our OLV-DOX program. It took a short time until the LTI board decided to accept my request. Frank Szoka, Dimitri, and Nick called me from the board meeting at 02:00 AM, Israel time, and woke me up, to tell me that LTI had accepted my request. But their condition was that I assure them of my continuous involvement in their relevant research and R&D programs. LTI support meant what was considered a large grant at that time, which would allow us to continue our OLV-DOX research, and especially the "first in man" clinical trial. So, it seemed we had a deal, the small details of which still needed to be finalized. At about that time, I was approached by another US company that proposed to license from us the OLV-DOX technology and product. Their proposal was tempting, as it involved what I considered then a large sum of money up front and reasonable royalties. However, this company requested that Alberto and I would be used only as consultants and not be involved in the research and development of the product. I did not like this idea, as we looked upon the product as a baby we have to nurture to maturity. I preferred LTI to the other company as I believed that our day-to-day involvement in the product development is crucial to the program's success. The future would show that I was right. So I convinced Moshe Vigdor, CEO of Yissum (the Research and Development Company of The Hebrew University of Jerusalem), to accept LTI's proposal. It did not take Nick long to come to Israel and finish the first license agreement, between LTI and Yissum, which was the basis of a master agreement that continued for 21 years. It started with LTI, with Nick as CEO, and went all the way to Johnson & Johnson. After Doxil's approval by the FDA, there was a change of management at LTI, and Craig Henderson, a top-level oncologist from UCSF (who had been involved in Doxil's clinical development), became LTI CEO. Then the company name was changed to Sequus. Craig and others sold Sequus to ALZA, Mountain View, CA (a major drug delivery company), with Doxil (due to its increasing sales) being one of the main reasons for the deal. It did not take a long time for ALZA to be bought by Johnson & Johnson, which until then was hardly involved in drug delivery systems. Again, Doxil was one of the main reasons for the deal. The rest is history!

During this fantastic very long voyage of 43 wonderful years of active research, I met many fascinating people, with whom I interacted and/or collaborated, and many of them remain lifelong friends. The 15 years I worked on liposomal doxorubicin, of which 50% was dedicated to Doxil development, was a unique experience I will never forget. It enabled me to be involved in a very complicated and complex process of drug development and to see its approval worldwide. The reward in terms of satisfaction is unmatched by any of my other achievements. I am trying hard to transfer my experience, part of which is summarized in this review, to many students and others worldwide.

Special Acknowledgments

This review is dedicated to my wife, Hanna. Without her encouragement, advice, patience, dedication, and support throughout our 52 years of life together, I would not have been able to accomplish my part of Doxil development.

I also want to thank my four daughters, Chagit, Ayelet, Tamar, and Avigail, who grew up during the years described in this review; their husbands, Uri, Perri, Ron, and Assaf; and last but not least, our 12 grandchildren, Yael, Yuval, Amit, Omri, Inbar, Mika, Rotem, Guy, Eyal, Gal, Dror, and Kfir, who give us so much joy. Our daughters and grandchildren were my escape during periods of despair.

Professionally, I would like to thank a few of the many people who deserve my gratitude: Alberto Gabizon, a 32-year partner in exciting research including Doxil development, and a friend (the many shared papers and patents with him are excellent evidence of our highly productive collaborative interaction) the late Demetrios (Dimitri) Papahadjopoulos, for his friendship and intellectual stimulus; and Nick Arvanitidis, from whom I learned about priorities in applied research and for the many heated disputes we had.

References

Abuchowski, A., McCoy, J.R., Palczuk, N.C., van Es, T., and Davis, F.F., Effect of covalent attachment of polyethylene glycol on immunogenicity and circulating life of bovine liver catalase, *J. Biol. Chem.* **252**(11), 3582–3586 (1977).

Allen, T.M., Liposomes with enhanced circulation time, U.S. Patent 4,837,028 (1989).

Allen, T.M., From fusion to magic bullets: the influence of Dimitri Papahdjopoulos, *J. Liposome Res.* **5**, 657–667 (1995).

Allen, T.M., and Chon, A, Large unilamellar liposomes with low uptake by reticuloendothelial system. *FEBS Lett.* **223**, 42–46 (1987).

Amselem, S., Cohen, R., Druckmann, S., Gabizon, A., Goren, D., Abra, R.M., Huang, A., New, R. and Barenholz, Y., Preparation and characterization of liposomal doxorubicin for human use. *J. Liposome Res.* **2**, 93–123 (1992).

Amselem, S., Cohen, R. and Barenholz, Y., 1993a. In vitro tests to predict in vivo performance of liposomal dosage forms. *Chem. Phys. Lipids* **64**, 219–237 (1993a).

Amselem, S., Gabizon, A. and Barenholz, Y., Evaluation of a new extrusion device for the production of stable oligolamellar liposomes in a liter scale. *J. Liposome Res.* **1**, 287–301 (1989–90).

Amselem, S., Gabizon, A., and Barenholz, Y., Optimization and upscaling of doxorubicin-containing liposomes for clinical use. *J. Pharm. Sci.* **79**, 1045–1052 (1990).

Amselem, S., Gabizon, A., and Barenholz, Y., A large-scale method for the preparation of sterile and nonpyrogenic liposomal formulations of defined size distributions for clinical use, in *Liposome Technology*, 2nd Edition, Vol. I, *Liposome Preparation and Related Techniques* (Gregoriadis, G., ed.), CRC Press, Boca Raton, FL, pp. 501–525 (1993b).

Andrews, P.A., Brenner, D.E., Chou, F.T., Kubo, H., Bachur, N.R., Facile and definitive determination of human Adriamycin and Daunorubicin metabolites by high-pressure liquid chromatography, *Drug Metab. Dispos.*, **8**, 152–156 (1980).

Avnir, Y., Ulmansky, R., Wasserman, V., Even-Chen, S., Broyer, M., Barenholz, Y., and Naparstek, Y., Amphipathic weak acid glucocorticoid prodrugs remote loaded into nano sterically stabilized liposomes: a novel approach to treat autoimmune arthritis. *Arthritis Rheum.*, **58**(1), 119–129 (2008).

Bandak, S., Ramu, A., Barenholz, Y., and Gabizon A., Reduced UV-induced degradation of doxorubicin encapsulated in polyethylene glycol-coated liposomes, *Pharm. Res.* **16**, 841–846 (1999).

Bangham, A.D., Liposomes: the Babraham connection, *Chem. Phys. Lipids* **64**, 275–285 (1993).

Barenholz, Y., Liposome production: historic aspects. In: *Liposome Dermatics* (Braun-Falco, O., Korting, H.C., and Maibach, H.I., eds.), Springer Verlag, Berlin, pp. 69–81 (1992).

Barenholz, Y., Design of liposome-based drug carriers: from basic research to application as approved drugs. In: *Medical Applications of Liposomes.* (Lasic, D.D., and Papahadjopoulos, D. eds.) Elsevier Science, Amsterdam, 541–565 (1998).

Barenholz, Y., Liposome application: problems and prospects. *Curr. Opin. Colloid Interface Sci.* **6**, 66–77 (2001).

Barenholz, Y., Relevancy of drug loading to liposomal formulation therapeutic efficacy, *J. Liposome Res*, **13**, 1–8 (2003).

Barenholz, Y. Amphipathic weak base loading into preformed liposomes having a transmembrane ammonium ion gradient: from the bench to approved Doxil. In: *Liposome Technology*, 3rd Edition, Gregoriadis, G., ed., Vol. II, Informa Healthcare, New York, pp. 1–26 (2007).

Barenholz, Y., and Amselem, S., Quality control assays in the development and clinical use of liposome-based formulations. In: *Liposome Technology*, 2nd Edition, Vol. I, *Liposome Preparation and Related Techniques*. (Gregoriadis, G., ed.), CRC Press, Boca Raton, FL, pp. 527–616 (1993b).

Barenholz, Y., Amselem, S., Goren, D., Cohen, R., Gelvan, D., Samuni, A., Golden, E.B., and Gabizon, A., Stability of liposomal-doxorubicin formulation: problems and prospects. *Med. Res. Rev.* **13**, 449–491 (1993a).

Barenholz, Y., and Crommelin, D.J.A., Liposomes as pharmaceutical dosage forms. In: *Encyclopedia of Pharmaceutical Technology*. (Swarbrick, J., and Boylan, J.C., eds.), Vol. 9, Marcel Dekker, New York, pp. 1–39 (1994).

Barenholz, Y., and Cohen, R, Rational design of amphiphile-based drug carriers and sterically stabilized carriers, *J. Liposome Res.*, **5**, 905–932 (1995).

Barenholz, Y., Druckmann, N.S., Cohen, R., Amselem, S., Sulkes, A., and Gabizon, A., Complete pharmacokinetic analysis of liposome-associated doxorubicin in cancer patients. In: *Recent Advances in Chemotherapy: Antimicrobial Section 1: Proceedings of the 16th Int'l Congress of Chemotherapy*, (Rubinstein, E., and Adam, D., eds), E. Lewin-Epstein Ltd. p. 303.1 (Jerusalem, 1989).

Barenholz, Y., and Gabizon, A., Liposome/doxorubicin composition and method, U.S. Patent 4,898,735 (February 6, 1990).

Barenholz, Y., and Gabizon, A., Liposome/anthraquinone drug composition and method, U.S. Patent 5,043,166 (August 27, 1991) (also see US Patent 4,797,285).

Barenholz, Y., and Haran, G., Method of amphipathic drug loading in liposomes by pH gradient, U.S. Patent 5,192,549 (March 9, 1993).

Barenholz, Y., and Haran, G., Liposomes: efficient loading and controlled release of amphipathic molecules, U.S. Patent 5,316,771 (May 31, 1994) (also Europe and Israel).

Barenholz, Y., Naparstek, Y., Avnir, Y., and Ulmansky, R., The use of liposomal glucocorticoids for treating inflammatory states, U.S. Patent 7,744,920, 2010, (June 29, 2010).

Bassermann, R., Changes of vascular pattern of tumors and surrounding tissue during different phases of metastatic growth, *Recent Results Cancer Res.*, **100**, 256–257 (1986).

Beijnen, J.H., Rosing, H., de Vries, P.A., and Underberg, W.J.M., Stability of anthracycline antitumor agents in infusion fluids, *J. Parenter. Sci. Technol.*, **39**, 220–222 (1985).

Belchetz, P. E., Crawley, J. C., Braidman, I. P., and Gregoriadis, G., Treatment of Gaucher's disease with liposome-entrapped glucocerebroside: beta-glucosidase. *Lancet* **8029**, 116–117 (1977).

Blum, R.H., Carter, S.K., Adriamycin: a new anticancer drug with significant clinical activity. *Ann. Intern. Med.*, 1974, 80, 249–259.

Blume, G., and Cevc, G., Liposomes for sustained drug release *in vivo*, *Biochim. Biophys. Acta* **1029**, 91–97 (1990).

Bolotin, E.M., Cohen, R., Bar, L.K., Emanuel, N., Ninio, S., Lasic, D.D. and Barenholz, Y., Ammonium sulfate gradients for efficient and stable remote loading of amphipathic weak bases into liposomes and ligandoliposomes, *J. Liposome Res.* **4**, 455–479 (1994).

Cabanes, A., Even-Chen, S., Zimberof, J., Barenholz, Y., Kedar, E., and Gabizon, A., Enhancement of antitumor activity of polyethylene glycol-coated liposomal doxorubicin with soluble and liposomal interleukin 2. *Clin. Cancer Res.* **5**, 687–693 (1999).

Clerc, S., and Barenholz, Y., A quantitative model for using acridine orange as a trans-membrane pH gradient probe, *Anal. Biochem.*, **259,** 104–111 (1998).

Diop-Frimpong, B., Chauhan, V.P., Krane, S., Boucher, Y., and Jain, R.K., Losartan inhibits collagen I synthesis and improves distribution and efficacy on nanotherapeutics in tumors. *PNAS*, on line (2011).

Druckmann, S., Gabizon, A., and Barenholz, Y., Separation of liposome-associated doxorubicin from non-liposome-associated doxorubicin in human plasma: implications for pharmacokinetic studies, *Biochim. Biophys. Acta* **980**, 381–384 (1989).

Emanuel, N., Kedar, E., Bolotin, E.M., Smorodinsky, N.I., and Barenholz, Y., Preparation and characterization of doxorubicin-loaded sterically stabilized immunoliposomes, *Pharm. Res.* **13**, 352–359 (1996a).

Emanuel, N., Kedar, E., Bolotin, E.M., Smorodinsky, N.I. and Barenholz, Y., Targeted delivery of doxorubicin via sterically stabilized immunoliposomes: pharmacokinetics and biodistribution in tumor-bearing mice, *Pharm. Res.* **13**, 861–868 (1996b).

Even-Or (Flasterstein), O., Samira, S., Rochlin, E., Balasingam, S., Mann, A.J., Lambkin-Williams, R., Spira, J., Goldwaser, I., Ellis, R., and Barenholz, Y., Immunogenecity, protective efficacy and mechanism of novel CCS adjuvanted influenza vaccine, *Vaccine*, 28, 6527–6541 (2010).

Forssen, E.A., and Tokes, Z.A. *In vitro* and *in vivo* studies with adriamycin liposomes, *Biochem. Biophys. Res. Commun.*, **91**, 1295–1301 (1979).

Forssen, E.A., and Tokes, Z.A., Use of anionic liposomes for the reduction of chronic doxorubicin induced cardiotoxicity, *Proc. Natl. Acad. Sci. USA*, **78**, 1873–1877 (1981).

Forssen, E.A., and Tokes, Z.A., Improved therapeutic benefits of doxorubicin by entrapment in anionic liposomes, *Cancer Res.*, **43**, 546–550 (1983).

Gabizon, A., Amselem, S., Goren, D., Cohen, R., Druckmann, S., Fromer, I. Chisin, R. Peretz, T., Sulkes, A., and Barenholz, Y., Preclinical and clinical experience with doxorubicin with a doxorubicin liposome preparation, *J. Liposome Res.* **1**, 491–502 (1991b).

Gabizon, A.A., and Barenholz, Y., Adriamycin-containing liposomes in cancer chemotherapy. In: *Liposomes as Drug Carriers* (Gregoriadis, G., ed.) Wiley, New York, pp. 365–379 (1988).

Gabizon, A., and Barenholz, Y., Liposomal anthracyclines — from basics to clinical approval of pegylated liposomal doxorubicin. In: *Liposomes: Rational Design* (Janoff, A.S., ed.), Marcel Dekker, New York, pp. 343–362 (1999).

Gabizon, A., and Barenholz, Y., A method for drug loading, WO 2005/046643 A2 (2005).

Gabizon, A.A., Barenholz, Y., and Bialer, M., Prolongation of the circulation time of doxorubicin encapsulated in liposomes containing a polyethylene glycol-derivatized phospholipid: pharmacokinetic studies in rodents and dogs, *Pharm. Res.*, **10,** 703–708 (1993).

Gabizon, A., Catane, R., Uziely, B., Kaufman, B., Safra, T., Cohen, R., Martin, F., Huang, A., and Barenholz, Y., Prolonged circulation time and enhanced accumulation in malignant exudates of doxorubicin encapsulated in polyethylene-glycol coated liposomes, *Cancer Res.*, **54**, 987–992 (1994).

Gabizon, A., Chisin, R. Amselem, S., Druckmann, S., Cohen, R., Goren, D., Fromer, I., Peretz, T., Sulkes, A., and Barenholz, Y., Pharmacokinetic and imaging studies in patients receiving a formulation of liposome-associated Adriamycin, *Br. J. Cancer*, **64**, 1125–1132 (1991a).

Gabizon, A., Dagan, A., Goren, D., Barenholz, Y., and Fuks, Z., Liposomes as *in vivo* carriers of Adriamycin: reduced cardiac uptake and preserved antitumor activity, *Cancer Res.* **42**, 4734–4739 (1982).

Gabizon, A., Goren, D., and Barenholz, Y., Investigation on the anti-tumor efficacy of liposome associated doxorubicin in murine tumor models, *Isr. J. Med. Sci.* **24**, 512–517 (1988).

Gabizon, A., Goren, D., Fuks, Z., Barenholz, Y., Dagan, A. and Meshorer, A., Enhancement of Adriamycin delivery to liver metastatic cells with increased tumoricidal effect using liposomes as drug carriers, *Cancer Res.* **43**, 4730–4735 (1983).

Gabizon, A., Goren, D., Fuks, Z., Meshorer, A., and Barenholz, Y., Superior therapeutic activity liposome-associated Adriamycin in a murine metastatic tumour model, *Br. J. Cancer* **51,** 681–689 (1985).

Gabizon, A., Goren, D., Ramu, A., and Barenholz, Y., Design, characterization and anti-tumor activity of Adriamycin-containing phospholipid vesicles. In: *Targeting of Drugs with Synthetic Systems* (Gregoriadis, G., Senior, J. and Poste, G., eds.), NATO ASI Series, Plenum, New York, pp. 229–238 (1986a).

Gabizon, A., Huang A., Martin, F., and Barenholz. Y., Doxorubicin encapsulation in polyethylene glycol-coated liposomes: initial clinical pharmacokinetic studies in solid tumors. In: *Stealth Liposomes* (Lasic, D.D., and Martin F., eds), CRC Press, Boca Raton, FL, Chapter 21, pp. 245–255 (1995).

Gabizon, A., Meshorer, A., and Barenholz, Y., Comparative long-term study of the toxicities of free and liposome-associated doxorubicin in mice after intravenous administration, *J. Natl. Cancer Inst.* 77, 459–469 (1986b).

Gabizon, A., and Papahadjoupoulos, D., Liposome formulations with prolonged circulation time in blood and enhanced uptake by tumors, *Proc. Natl. Acad. Sci. USA*, **85**, 6949–6953 (1988).

Gabizon, A., Peretz, T., Sulkes, A., Amselem, S., Ben-Yosef, R., Ben-Baruch, N., Catane, R., Biran, S., and Barenholz, Y., Systemic administration of doxorubicin-containing liposomes in cancer patients: phase I study, *Eur. J. Cancer Clin. Oncol.*, **25**, 1795–1803 (1989a).

Gabizon, A., Shmeeda, H., and Barenholz, Y., Pharmacokinetics of pegylated liposomal doxorubicin: review of animal and human studies, *Clin. Pharmacokinet.*, **42**, 419–436 (2003).

Gabizon, A.A., Sulkes, A., Peretz, T., Druckmann, S., Goren, D., Amselem, S., and Barenholz, Y., Liposome-associated doxorubicin: preclinical pharmacology and exploratory clinical phase. In: *Liposomes in the Therapy of Infectious Diseases and Cancer* (Fidler, I.J., and Lopez-Berestein, G., eds.) A.R.L., New York, pp. 391–402 (1989b).

Garbuzenko, O., Barenholz, Y., and Priev, A., Effect of grafted PEG on liposome size and on compressibility and packing of lipid bilayer, *Chem. Phys. Lipids*, **135**, 117–129 (2005).

Goormaghtigh, E., and Ruysschaert, J.M., Anthracycline glycoside membrane interaction, *Biochim. Biophys. Acta*, 779, 271–188 (1984).

Gordon, A.N., Fleagle, J.T., Guthrie, D., Parkin, D.E., Gore, M.E., and Lacave, A.J., Recurrent epithelial ovarian carcinoma: a randomized phase III study of pegylated liposomal doxorubicin versus topotecan, *J. Clin. Oncol.*, **19**(14), 3312–3322 (2001).

Gordon, A.N., Granai, C.O., Rose, P.G., Hainsworth, J., Lopez, A., Weissman, C., Rosales, R., Sharpington, T., Phase II study of liposomal doxorubicin in platinum- and paclitaxel-refractory epithelial ovarian cancer, *J. Clin. Oncol.*, **18**(17), 3093–3100 (2000).

Goren, D., Liposomes as doxorubicin carriers: a means to improve the therapeutic index of the drug, Ph.D. thesis submitted and approved by the Hebrew University of Jerusalem (1990).

Goren, D., Gabizon, A., and Barenholz, Y., The influence of physical characteristics of liposomes containing doxorubicin on their pharmacological behavior, *Biochim. Biophys. Acta*, **1029**, 285–294 (1990).

Gabizon, A., Isacson, R., Rosengarten, O., Tzemach, D., Shmeeda, H., and Sapir, R., An open-label study to evaluate dose and cycle dependence of the pharmacokinetics of pegylated liposomal doxorubicin, *Cancer Chemother. Pharmacol.*, **1**(4), 695–702 (2008).

Grant, G.J., Barenholz, Y., Bansinath, M., and Davidson, E.M. A novel liposomal Bupivacaine formulation to produce ultralong-acting analgesia, *Anesthesiology*, **101**, 133–137 (2004).

Grant, G.J., Barenholz, Y., Piskoun, B., Bansinath, M., Turndorf, H., and Bolotin, E., DRV liposomal bupivacaine: preparation, characterization and *in vivo* evaluation in mice, *Pharm. Res.*, **18**, 336–343 (2001).

Gregoriadis, G., and Senior, J., Liposomes *in vivo:* a relationship between stability and clearance? In: *Targeting of Drugs with Synthetic Systems* (Gregoriadis, G., Senior, J., Poste, G., eds), London, Plenum, pp. 183–192 (1986).

Gregoriadis, G., Swain, C.P., Wills, E.J., and Tavill, A.S., Drug-carrier potential of liposomes in cancer chemotherapy, *Lancet*, **1**, 1313–1316 (1974).

Gundersen, S., Kvinnsland, S., Klepp, O., Kvaloy, S., Lund, E., Host, H., Weekly Adriamycin versus VAC in advanced breast cancer. A randomized trial, *Eur. J. Cancer Clin. Oncol.*, 22, 1431–1434 (1986).

Haran, G., Cohen, R., Bar, L.K., and Barenholz, Y., Transmembrane ammonium sulfate gradients in liposomes produce efficient and stable entrapment of amphipathic weak bases. *Biochim. Biophys. Acta* **1151**, 201–215 (1993).

Hashizume, H., Baluk, P., Morikawa, S., McLean, J.W., Thurston, G., Roberge, S., Jain, R.K., and MacDonald, D.M., Openings between defective endothelial cells explain tumor vessel leakiness, *Am. J. Pathol.*, 156, 1363–1380 (2000).

Horowitz, A.T., Barenholz, Y., and Gabizon, A.A., *In vitro* cytotoxicity of liposome-encapsulated doxorubicin: dependence on liposome composition and drug release, *Biochim. Biophys. Acta*, **1109**, 203–209 (1992).

Hunt, C.A., and Papahadjopoulous, D.P., Method for producing liposomes in selected size range, US patent 4,529,561 (July 16, 1985).

Hwang, K.J., Liposome pharmacokinetics. In: *Liposomes: From Biophysics to Therapeutics* (Ostro, M.J., ed.), Marcel Dekker: New York, p. 109 (1987).

Joseph, A., Itskovitz Cooper, N., Samira, S., Flasterstein, O., Eliyahu, H., Simberg, D., Goldwaser, I., Barenholz, Y., and Kedar, E. A new intranasal influenza vaccine based on a novel polycationic lipid ceramide carbamoyl spermine (CCS). I. Immunogenicity and efficacy studies in mice, *Vaccine*, **24**, 3990–4006 (2006).

Kedar, E., Braun, E., Rutkowski, Y., Emanuel, N. and Barenholz, Y., Delivery of cytokines by liposomes. II. Interleukin-2 encapsulated in long-circulating sterically stabilized liposomes: immunomodulatory and anti-tumor activity in mice. *J. Immunother.* **16**, 115–124 (1994).

Kedar, E., Rutkowski, Y., Braun, E., Emanuel, N., and Barenholz, Y., Delivery of cytokines by liposomes. I. Preparation and characterization of interleukin-2 encapsulated in long-circulating sterically stabilized liposomes, *J. Immunother.*, **16**, 47–59 (1994).

Kenyon J, 2008. Chemotherapy and cardiac toxicity — the lesser of two evils, Doctors Lounge Website, available at http://www.doctorslounge.com/index.php/blogs/page/14030.

Klivanov, A.L., Maruyama, K., Torchilin, V.P., and Huang, L., Amphipathic polyethyleneglycols effectively prolong the circulation time of liposomes, *FEBS Lett.*, 268, 235–237 (1990).

Kumai, K., Takahashi, T., Tsubouchi, K., Shino, K., Ishbiki, K.K., and Abe, O., Selective hepatic arterial infusion of liposomes containing anti tumor agents. *Jpn. J. Cancer Chemother.*, **12**, 1946–1948 (1985).

Lasic, D.D., On the history of liposomes. In: *Handbook of Non-Medical Applications of Liposomes* (Lasic, D.D., and Barenholz Y., eds), Vol. 1, CRC Press, Boca Raton, FL, pp. 1–12 (1996).

Lasic, D.D., Valner, J.J., and Working, P.K, Sterically stabilized liposomes in cancer therapy and gene delivery, *Curr. Opin. Mol. Ther.*, **1**, 177–185 (1999).

Lasic, D.D., Ceh, B., Stuart, M.C.A., Guo, L., Frederik, P.M., and Barenholz, Y., Transmembrane gradient driven phase transitions within vesicles: lessons for drug delivery, *Biochim. Biophys. Acta*, **1239**, 145–156 (1995).

Lasic, D.D., Frederik, P.M., Stuart, M.C.A., Barenholz, Y., and McIntosh, T.J., Gelation of liposome interior. A novel method for drug encapsulation, *FEBS Lett.*, **312**, 255–258 (1992).

Lasic, D.D., and Martin, F. (eds), *Stealth Liposomes*, CRC Press, Boca Raton, FL (1995).

Lichtenberg, D., and Barenholz, Y., Liposomes: Preparation, characterization, and preservation. In: *Methods of Biochemical Analysis* (Glick, D., ed.) Wiley, NY, **33**, pp. 337–462 (1988).

Lopez-Berestein, G., Fainstein, V., Hopfer R, *et al.*, Liposomal amphotericin B for the treatment of systemic fungal infections in patients with cancer: a preliminary study. *J. Infect. Dis.*, **151**, 704–710 (1985).

Mace, K., Mayhew, E., Mihich, E., Ehrke, M.J., Alterations in murine host defense functions by Adriamycin or liposome-encapsulated Adriamycin. *Cancer Res.*, 48, 130–136 (1988).

Maeda, H., Bharate, G.Y., and Daruwalla, J., Polymeric drugs for efficient tumor-targeted drug delivery based on EPR-effect, *Eur. J. Pharm. Biopharm.*, **71**, 409–419, (2009).

Martin, F., Caignard, A., Olson, O., Jeanin, J.F., Leclerc, A., Tumoricidal effect of macrophages exposed to Adriamycin *in vivo* and *in vitro, Cancer Res.*, **42**, 3851–3855 (1982).

Matsumura, Y., and Maeda, H., A new concept for macromolecular therapeutics in cancer chemotherapy: mechanism of tumor tropic accumulation of proteins and antitumor agent SMANCS, *Cancer Res.* **46**, 6387–6392 (1986).

Mayhew, E., and Rustum, Y., The use of liposomes as carriers of therapeutic agents. In: *Molecular Basis of Cancer. Part B: Macromolecular Recognition, Chemotherapy and Immunology* (Rein, R., ed.), Alan R. Liss, New York, 301–310 (1985).

Mayhew, E., Rustum, Y., and Vail, W.J., Inhibition of liver metastases of M5076 tumor by liposome-entrapped Adriamycin, *Cancer Drug Deliv.,* **1**, 43–58 (1983).

Mayhew, E.G., Goldrosen, M.H., Vaage, J., and Rustum, Y.M., Effects of liposome-entrapped doxorubicin on liver metastases of mouse colon carcinomas 26 and 38, *J. Natl. Cancer Inst.*, **78**, 707–713 (1987).

McKelvey, E.M., Gottlieb, J.A., Wilson H.E. *et al.,* Hydroxyldaunomycin (Adriamycin) combination chemotherapy in malignant lymphoma, *Cancer,* **38**, 1484–1493 (1976).

Minotti, G., Menna, P., Salvatorelli, E., Cairo, G., Gianni L, Anthracyclines: molecular advances and pharmacologic developments in antitumor activity and cardiotoxicity,. *Pharmacol. Rev.* **56** (2), 185–229 (June 2004).

Needham, D., Anyarambhatia, G., Kong, G., and Dewhirst, M.W. A new temperature-sensitive liposome for use with mild hyperthermia: characterization and testing in human tumor xenograft model. *Cancer Res.*, 60, 1197–1201 (2000).

Needham, D., and Dewhirst, M.W., The development and testing of new temperature-sensitive drug delivery system for treatment of solid tumors. *Adv. Drug Deliv. Rev.*, **53**, 285–305 (2001).

Olson, F., Mayhew, E., Maslow D., Rustum, Y., and Szoka, F., Characterization, toxicity, and therapeutic efficacy of Adriamycin encapsulated in liposomes. *Eur. J. Cancer Clin. Oncol.*, 1982, 18, 167–176.

Perez-Soler, R., Lopex-Berestein, G., Kasi, L.P., *et al.*, Distribution of technetium-99m labeled multilamellar liposomes in patients with Hodgkin's disease, *J. Nucl. Med.*, **26**, 743–749 (1985).

Peng, X., Chen, B., Lim, C.C., Sawyer, D.B., The cardiotoxicology of anthracycline chemotherapeutics: translating molecular mechanism into preventative medicine, *Mol. Intervent.* **5** (3): 163–171 (June 2005).

Peleg-Shulman, T., Gibson, D., Cohen, R., Abra, R., and Barenholz, Y., Characterization of sterically stabilized cisplatin liposomes by nuclear magnetic resonance, *Biochim. Biophys. Acta*, **1510**, 278–291 (2001).

Poste, G., Liposome targeting *in vivo:* problems and opportunities, *Biol. Cells*, **47**, 19–38 (1983).

Poste, G., Bucana, C., Raz, A., Bugelski, P., Kirsh, R., and Fidler, I.J., Analysis of the fate of systemically administered liposomes and implications for their use in drug delivery, *Cancer Res.,* **42**, 1412–1422 (1982).

Rahman, A., Carmichael, D., Harris, M., and Roh, J.K., Comparative pharmacokinetics of free doxorubicin and doxorubicin entrapped in cardiolipin liposomes, *Cancer Res.*, **46**, 2295–2299 (1986a).

Rahman, A., Fumagalli, A., Barbieri, B., Schein, P.S., and Casazza, A.M., Anti-tumor and toxicity evaluation of free doxorubicin and doxorubicin entrapped in cardiolipin liposomes, *Cancer Chemother. Pharmacol.*, **16**, 22–27 (1986b).

Rahman, A., Kessler, A., More, N., et al., Liposomal protection of Adriamycin-induced cardiotoxicity in mice, *Cancer Res.*, **40**, 1532–1537 (1980).

Rahman, A., More, N., and Schein, P.S., Doxorubicin-induced chronic cardiotoxicity and its protection by liposomal administration, *Cancer Res.*, 42, 1817–1822 (1982).

Rahman, A., Roh, J.K., and Treat, J., Preclinical and clinical pharmacology of doxorubicin entrapped in cardiolipin liposomes. In: *Liposomes in the Therapy of Infectious Diseases and Cancer* (Lopez-Berestein, G., and Fidler, I.J., eds.), Alan R. Liss, New York, 367–389 (1989).

Rahman, A., White, G., More, N., Schein, P.S., Pharmacological, toxicological, and therapeutic evaluation in mice of doxorubicin entrapped in cardiolipin liposomes, *Cancer Res.*, **45**(2), 796–803 (February 1985).

Richardson, V.J., Ryman, B.E., Jewkes, R.F. *et al.*, Tissue distribution and tumor localization of technetium-99M labeled liposomes in cancer patients. *Br. J. Cancer*, **40**, 35–43 (1979).

Schroeder, A., Avnir Y., Weisman, S., Najajreh, Y., Gabizon, A., Talmon, Y., Kost, J., and Barenholz, Y., Controlling liposomal drug release with low frequency ultrasound: mechanism and feasibility, *Langmuir*, **23**(7): 4019–4025 (2007).

Schroeder, A., Honen, R., Turjeman, K., Gabizon, A., Kost, J., and Barenholz, Y., Ultrasound triggered release of cisplatin from liposomes in murine tumors, *J. Control. Release*, **137**, 63–68 (2009a).

Schroeder, A., Kost, J., and Barenholz, Y., Ultrasound, liposomes, and drug delivery: principles for using ultrasound to control the release of drugs from liposomes, *Chem. Phys. Lipids*, **162**, 1–16 (2009b).

Sculier, J.P., Coune, A., Brassine, C., *et al.*, Intravenous infusion of high doses of liposomes containing NSC 251635, a water-insoluble cytostatic agent. A pilot study with pharmacokinetic data, *J. Clin. Oncol.*, **4**, 789–797 (1986).

Sculier, J.P., Coune, A., Meunier, F., *et al.*, Pilot study of amphotericin B entrapped in sonicated liposomes in cancer patients with fungal infections, *Eur. J. Cancer Clin. Oncol.*, **24**, 527–538 (1988).

Skeel, R.T., *Handbook of Cancer Chemotherapy*, 5th Edition, Lippincott Williams & Wilkins, Philadelphia, pp. 100–101 (1999).

Storm, G., Roerdink, F.H., Steerenberg, P.A., de Jong, W.H., and Crommelin, D.J.A., Influence of lipid composition on the antitumor activity exerted by doxorubicin-containing liposomes in a rat solid tumor model. *Cancer Res.* **47**, 3366–3372 (1987).

Stein, W.D., *Transport and Diffusion Across Cell Membranes*, Academic Press, Orlando, FL, Chapter 2 (1986).

Solomon, R., and Gabizon, A.A., Clinical pharmacology of liposomal anthracyclines: focus on pegylated liposomal doxorubicin. *Clin. Lymphoma Myeloma*, **8**, 21–32 (2008).

Symon, Z., Peyser, A., Tzemach, D., Lyass, O., Sucher, E., Shezen, E., and Gabizon, A, Selective delivery of doxorubicin to patients with breast carcinoma metastases by Stealth liposomes, *Cancer*, **86**, 72–78 (1999).

Szebeni, J., and Barenholz, Y., Chapter 11, Complement Activation, Immunogenicity, and Immune Suppression as Potential Side Effects of Liposomes, This book (2011).

Szebeni, J., Alving, C.R., Rosivall, L., Bunger, R., Baranyi, L., Bedocs, P., Toth, M., and Barenholz, Y., Animal models of complement-mediated hypersensitivity reactions to liposomes and other lipid-based nanoparticles, *J. Liposome Res.* **17**, 1–11 (2007).

Takimoto, C.H., Calvo, E., Principles of oncologic pharmacotherapy. In: *Cancer Management: A Multidisciplinary Approach*, 11th edition (Pazdur, R., Wagman, L.D., Camphausen, K.A., and Hoskins, W.J., eds.), UBM Medica, Norwalk, CT (2008).

Tirosh, O., Barenholz, Y., Katzhendler, Y., and Priev, A., Hydration of polyethylene glycol-grafted liposomes, *Biophys. J.*, **74**, 1371–1379 (1998).

Tirosh, O., Kohen, R., Katzhendler, J., Gorodetsky, R. and Barenholz, Y., Novel synthetic phospholipid protects lipid bilayers against oxidative damage: role of hydration layer and bound water, *J. Chem. Soc., Perkin Trans.* **2**, 383–389 (1997).

Treat, J., Greenspan, A.R., Rahman, A., Liposome encapsulated doxorubicin —preliminary results of phase I and phase II trials. In: *Liposomes in the Therapy of Infectious Diseases and Cancer* (Lopez-Berestein, G., and Fidler, I.J., eds.), Alan R. Liss, New York, pp. 353–365 (1989).

Van Hoesel, Q.G., Steerenberg, P.A., Crommelin, D.J., et al., Reduced cardiotoxicity and nephrotoxicity with preservation of antitumor activity of doxorubicin entrapped in stable liposomes in the LOU/M Wsl rat, *Cancer Res.*, **44**, 3698–3705 (1984).

Veronese, F.M., and Harris, J.M., Introduction and overview of peptide and protein pegylation, *Adv. Drug Deliv. Rev.*, **54**(4), 453–456 (2002).

Veronese, F. M. , and Pasut, G., Pegylation, successful approach to drug delivery, *Drug Discov. Today*, **10**(21), 1451–1458 (2005).

Wasserman, V., Kizelsztein, P., Garbuzenko, O., Kohen, R., Ovadia, H., Tabakman, R., and Barenholz,Y., The antioxidant Tempamine: *in vitro* antitumor and neuroprotective effects and optimization of liposomal encapsulation and release, *Langmuir*, **23**(4), 1937–1947 (2007).

Weiss, R.B., The anthracyclines: will we ever find a better doxorubicin? *Semin. Oncol.* **19**(6), 670–686 (1992).

Woodle, M.C., Surface-modified liposomes: assessment and characterization for increased stability and prolonged blood circulation, *Chem. Phys. Lipids*, **64**, 249–262 (1993).

Woodle, M.C., and Lasic D.D., Sterically stabilized liposomes, *Biochim. Biophys. Acta*, **113**, 171–199 (1992).

Woodle, M.C., Martin, F.J., Yau-Yang, A., Redmann, C.T., Liposomes with enhanced circulation time, U.S. Patent 5,013,556 (May 07, 1991).

Woodle, M.C., Newman, M., Collins, L., Redmann, C., and Martin, F., Improved long circulating (Stealth®) liposomes using synthetic lipids. *Symp. Control. Release Bioact. Mater.*, **17**, 77 (1990).

Zhang, Y.P., Ceh, B., and Lasic, D.D., *Liposomes in Drug Delivery in Polymeric Biomaterials*, 2nd edition (Damitziu, S., ed.), Marcel Dekker New York, Chapter 29, pp. 783–821 (2001).

Zucker, D., and Barenholz, Y., Optimization of Vincristine-Topotecan combination — paving the way for improved chemotherapy regimens by nanoliposomes, *J. Control. Release*, **146**, 326–333 (2010).

Zucker, D., Marcus, D., Barenholz, Y., and Goldblum, A., Liposome drug's loading efficiency: a working model based on loading conditions and drug's physicochemical properties, *J. Control. Release*, **139**, 73–80 (2009).

Index

Color Insert

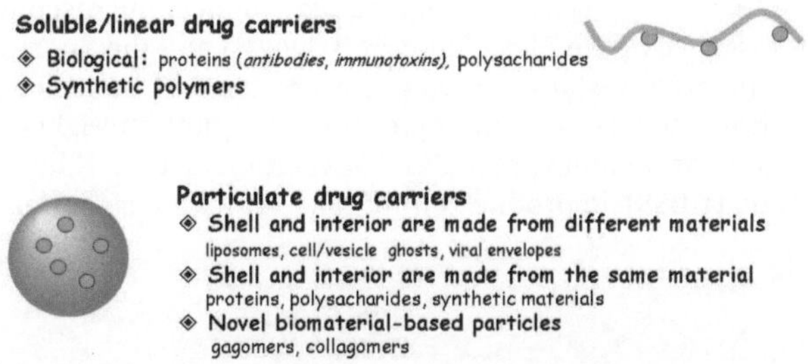

Figure 1.3 The two major categories of drug delivery systems.

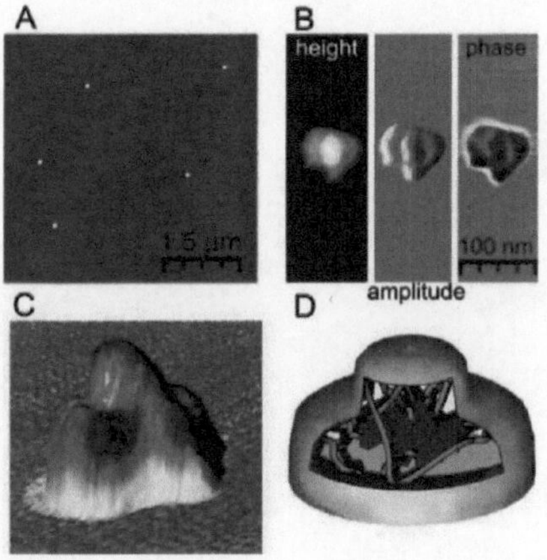

Figure 2.2 High-resolution AFM scan of individual SCNP: (A) Group of a few particles. (B) Height, amplitude, and phase images clearly indicating the complex geometry and raised core. (C) Three-dimensional height image with phase retrace overlay of this particle. (D) Cartoon depicting the possible particle morphology: 2-ureido-pyrimidinone (UPy)-urethane rich core (blue) immersed in a network of PMMA. Reproduced from ref. [35] with permission.

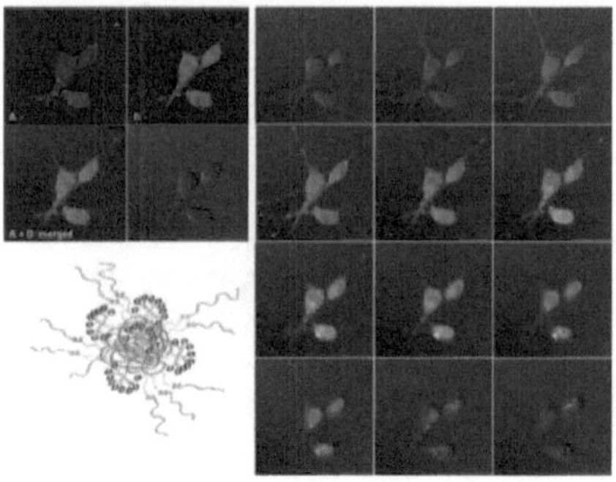

Figure 2.4 Cellular uptake experiments of nanoparticle transporter conjugate into NIH 3T3 cells investigated *via* confocal microscopy imaged for the fluorescence of the Alexa Fluor 568 dye (B) and the fluorescein (A), with complementing *z*-stack showing the presence of both fluorophores from the bottom (top, left) to the top of the cells (bottom, right). The cells were incubated for 30 min with a 37.2 μM solution of 15 in Hanks buffered saline solution (HBSS). Reproduced from ref. [31] with permission.

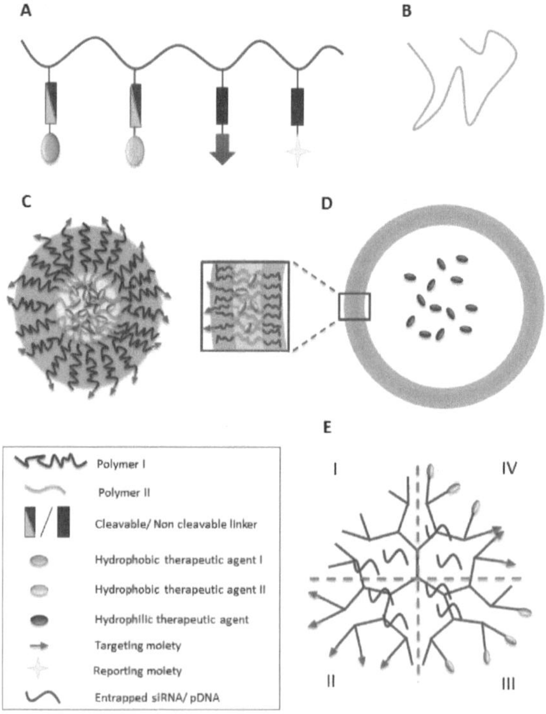

Figure 4.1 Structures of polymer therapeutics: (A) Modified Ringsdorf's model, (B) polymeric drug, (C) polymeric micelle, (D)polymersome, and (E) dendrimer.

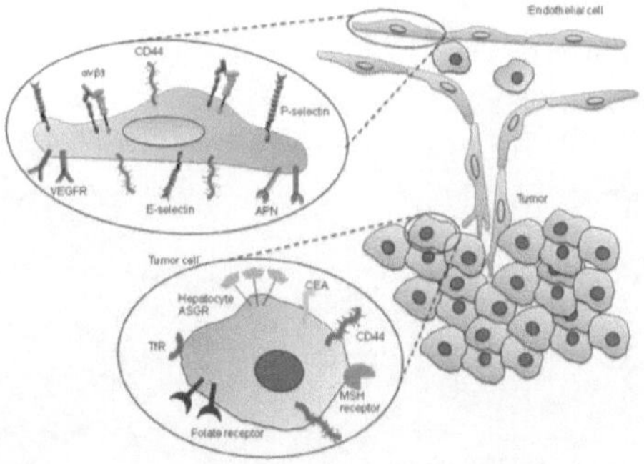

Figure 4.2 Molecular targets on tumor cells and on tumor endothelial cells.

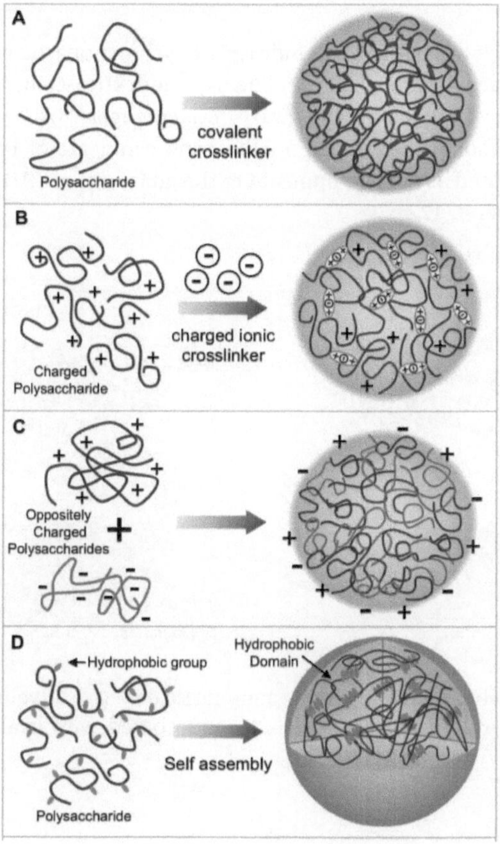

Figure 5.2 Common mechanism for polysaccharide based nanoparticle preparation. (A) Covalent cross-linking. (B) Ionic cross-linking. (C) Polyelectrolyte complexation (PEC). (D) Self-assembly of hydrophobically modified polysaccharides.

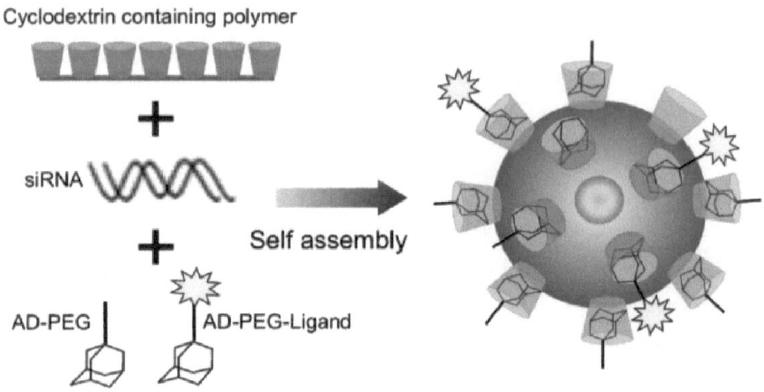

Figure 5.3 Self-assembly of cyclodextrin-based nanoparticle. The delivery components are a water-soluble, linear cyclodextrin-containing polymer (CDP), siRNA, an adamantane (AD)-PEG conjugate (AD-PEG), and the targeting component that is an adamantane conjugate of PEG that has a ligand conjugated at the end opposite to the adamantane (AD-PEG-Ligand). Modified from ref. 122.

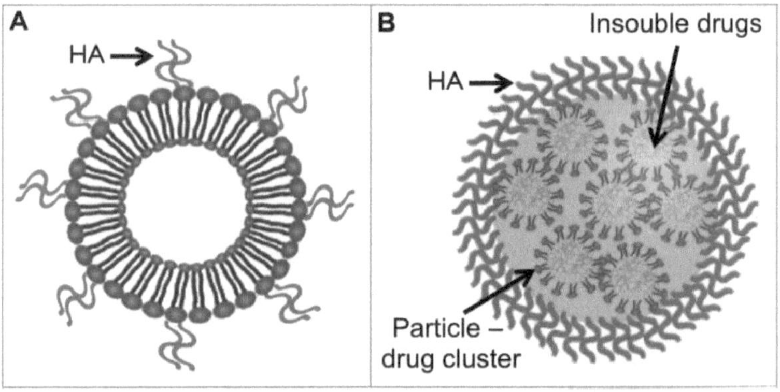

Figure 5.4 Hyaluronan-coated nanoparticles: (A) Hyaluronan-coated liposome (tHA-LIP). (B) Paclitaxel-clusters coated with hyaluronan (PTX-GAGs).

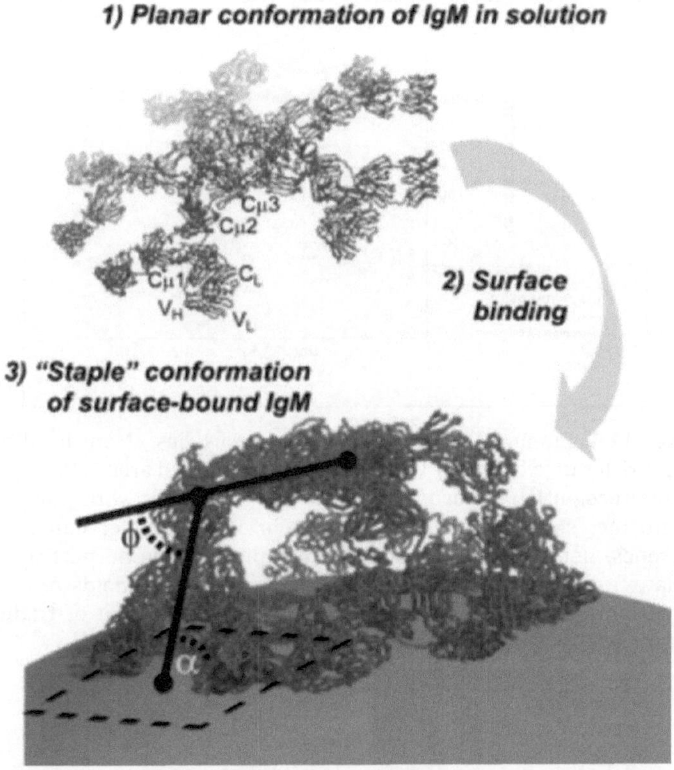

Figure 10.1 Three-step model for the binding of IgM to target surfaces. In solution IgM is a planar structure of five structural units each containing four constant (Cμ1-4) domains and one variable (V_H) domain in the heavy chain and one constant (C_L) and one variable (V_L) domain in the light chain. In 1) the planar structure described by Perkins et al. [4] is shown with indications of the approximate position of some of the structural domains. The dynamics of binding of IgM to target surfaces (2) is not well understood, but suggestions were [71] made that the process brings IgM into the "staple" conformation, which permits binding of the C1 complex and hence initiates complement activation. Perkins et al. suggested that the specific requirement would be that the angle ϕ takes a value of 60°. Pedersen et al. recently suggested that IgM binding to curved surfaces would regulate ϕ according to the curvature by assuming that the contact between epitopes and the variable domains in IgM is geometrically well defined with a characteristic angle α [70]. In (3), IgM is shown drawn to scale and bound to a sphere with a diameter of 66 nm (modified from [70]). The artwork was kindly made by Dr. T. Boesen, Aarhus University.

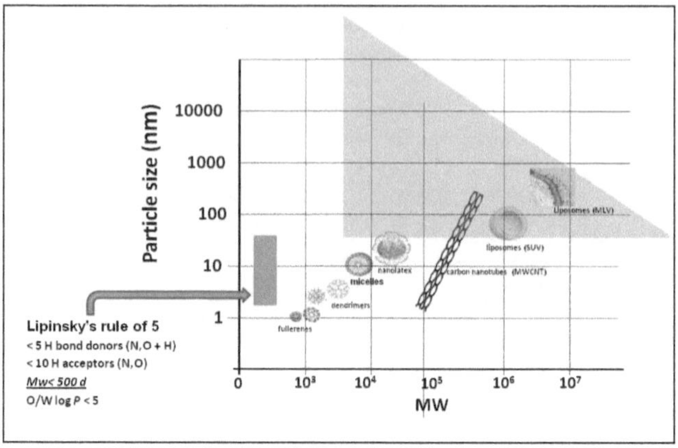

Figure 11.1 Immune recognition of nanoparticles. Map of different nanoparticles on a diameter vs. Mw chart; blue shaded area is the region of immune recognition. Liposomes and carbon nanotubes, with their length, fall into the "sight" of the immune system, while smaller nanoparticles (fullerenes, dendrimers, micelles and complex polymeric particles (e.g., nanolatex) are, in theory, below the size and Mw thresholds of immune recognition. The green "Lipinsky box" shows the position of traditional small-molecular weight drugs [62].

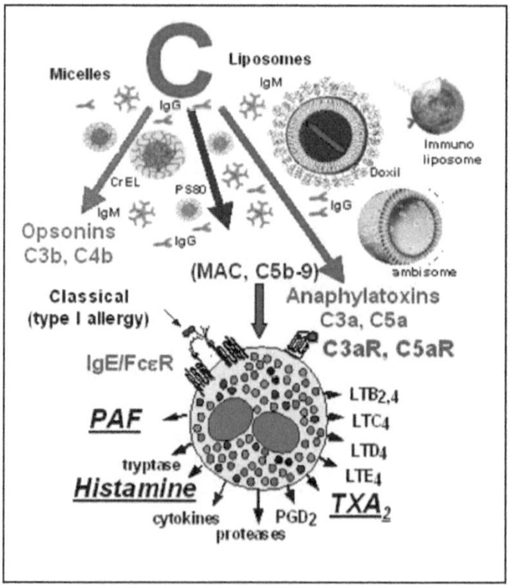

Figure 11.4 Mechanism of complement activation-related pseudoallergy (CARPA) caused by liposomes and micelles. Crel-Cremophor EL, PS80-polysorbate 80, R-receptor.

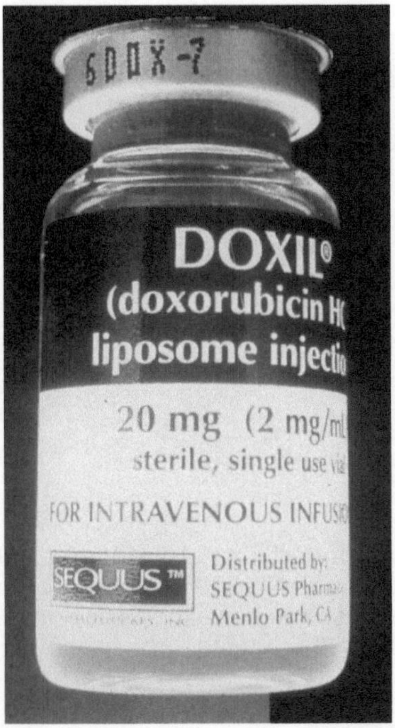

Figure 12.1 Doxil vial as sold by Sequus Pharmaceuticals (1996).

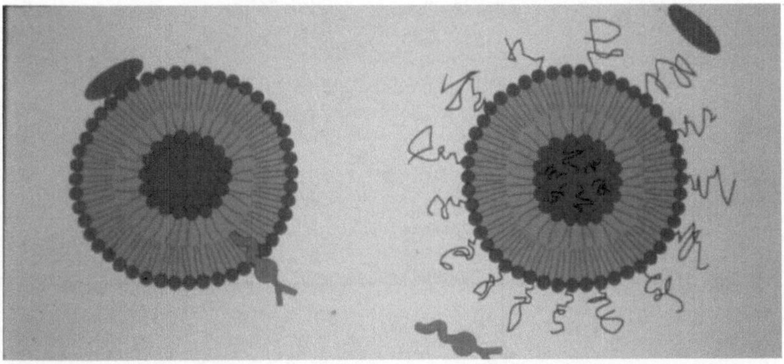

Figure 12.5 A cartoon showing a comparison between conventional and sterically stabilized (pegylated) liposomes (SSL, Stealth liposomes). (Courtesy of the late D. Lasic.) The cartoon shows lack of insertion of opsonins into the membrane of Stealth liposomes.

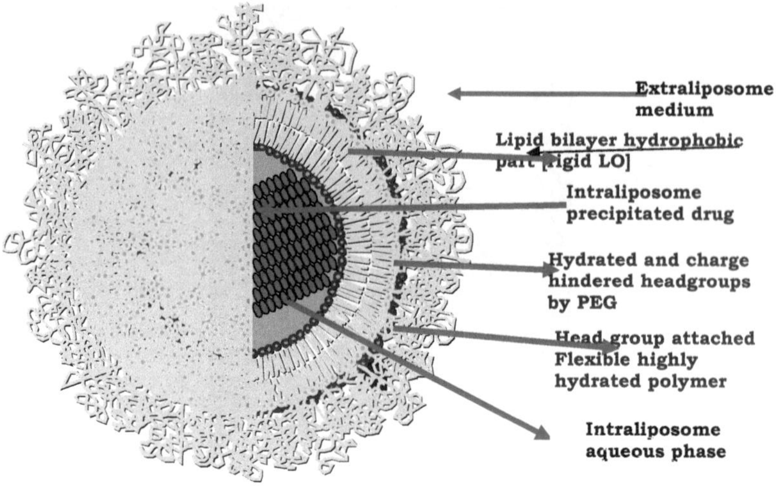

Figure 12.7 A cartoon of Doxil® = pegylated nano (<100 nm) unilamellar liposome. It is based on cryo-TEM, SAXS, WAXS, DLS, compressibility, and doxorubicin absorbance and fluorescence (Lasic et al., 1992, 1995; Haran et al., 1993; Tirosh et al., 1998).

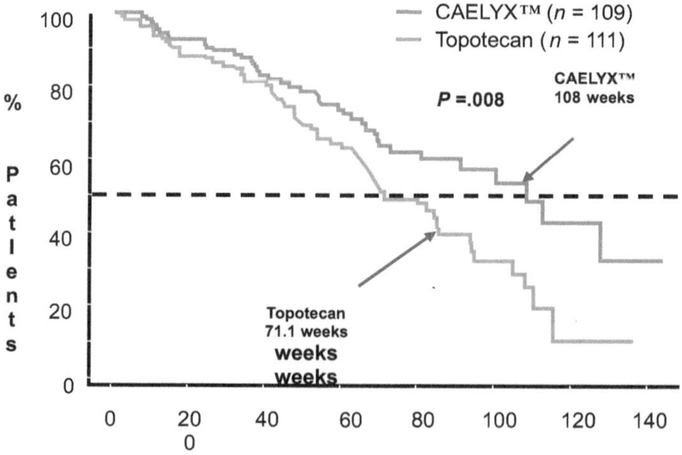

Figure 12.9 Caelyx^{TM} (= Doxil) is superior to topotecan in ovarian cancer (from Gordon et al., 2001).